W0235356

OXFORD HANDBOOK OF

Medical Education in Practice

Published and forthcoming Oxford Handbooks

OXFORD HANDBOOK OF
Medical Education in Practice

EDITED BY

Gabrielle M. Finn

Professor of Medical Education and Associate Vice President, University of Manchester

Megan E.L. Brown

Senior Research Associate in Medical Education, School of Medicine, Newcastle University

Matthew H.V. Byrne

University of Oxford, UK

Helen R. Church

Clinical Associate Professor in Medical Education, University of Nottingham, UK

Neel Sharma

GI Medicine Specialist with sub-specialty Interest in GI Oncology Cambridge University Hospitals University of Cambridge, UK

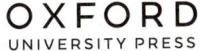

OXFORD
UNIVERSITY PRESS

OXFORD
UNIVERSITY PRESS

Great Clarendon Street, Oxford, OX2 6DP,
United Kingdom

Oxford University Press is a department of the University of Oxford.
It furthers the University's objective of excellence in research, scholarship,
and education by publishing worldwide. Oxford is a registered trade mark of
Oxford University Press in the UK and in certain other countries

© Oxford University Press 2025

The moral rights of the authors have been asserted

All rights reserved. No part of this publication may be reproduced, stored in
a retrieval system, or transmitted, in any form or by any means, without the
prior permission in writing of Oxford University Press, or as expressly permitted
by law, by licence or under terms agreed with the appropriate reprographics
rights organization. Enquiries concerning reproduction outside the scope of the
above should be sent to the Rights Department, Oxford University Press, at the
address above

You must not circulate this work in any other form
and you must impose this same condition on any acquirer

Published in the United States of America by Oxford University Press
198 Madison Avenue, New York, NY 10016, United States of America

British Library Cataloguing in Publication Data
Data available

Library of Congress Control Number: 2024939211

ISBN 978–0–19–284871–0

DOI: 10.1093/med/9780192848710.001.0001

Printed and bound in China by
C&C Offset Printing Co., Ltd.

Oxford University Press makes no representation, express or implied, that the
drug dosages in this book are correct. Readers must therefore always check
the product information and clinical procedures with the most up-to-date
published product information and data sheets provided by the manufacturers
and the most recent codes of conduct and safety regulations. The authors and
the publishers do not accept responsibility or legal liability for any errors in the
text or for the misuse or misapplication of material in this work. Except where
otherwise stated, drug dosages and recommendations are for the non-pregnant
adult who is not breast-feeding

The manufacturer's authorised representative in the EU for product safety is
Oxford University Press España S.A. of el Parque Empresarial San Fernando
de Henares, Avenida de Castilla, 2 - 28830 Madrid(www.oup.es/en).

Contents

Preface

The editors

The careers of health professionals are closely interlinked with education, where long initial periods of undergraduate education and postgraduate training lead to lifelong-learning to keep up with, and practice, evidence-based medicine. Given this educational journey, the learners you encounter while teaching can be highly variable. Educators may teach undergraduates, postgraduates, and experts; and these learners may be within your field, or they may be outside it.

Medicine is complex and its scope is vast. Healthcare professional students are required to learn about anatomy, physiology, and clinical conditions, as well as communication and practical skills. In postgraduate training and beyond, the skills and knowledge required for learners can be highly variable. Learners may need to have a wide breadth of knowledge or may be hyper-specialized. They may need to master technically challenging procedures or may never need to touch an instrument. Some learners may never see a patient, and others may need to communicate with entire populations.

The field of medical education itself is equally broad. Educators may deliver teaching one-on-one, to small groups, or to whole auditoriums. Teaching may be in classroom or clinical settings. It may be real or simulated, and formative or summative. Medical education also goes beyond what is taught. It is rooted within theory, and this can be used to inform our understanding of our own actions and the actions of others. The field of medical education is constantly evolving through medical education research, and because of this there are many different techniques that educators can use to maximize learning. Importantly, high-quality medical education has positive impacts on learners, educators, patients, and the communities that medicine serves.

The variety of learners, learning needs, and educational processes presents an exciting and unique opportunity for educators, and means that within medical education there are diverse opportunities for engagement for those with varied interests. In 2024, in the wake of significant change to medical education and patient needs, there is a pressing need for a contemporary, comprehensive, and accessible synthesis of what constitutes good practice within medical education.

We are delighted to present the Oxford Handbook of Medical Education in Practice, an essential guide for educators, students, and practitioners interested and involved in the training of healthcare professionals within both undergraduate and postgraduate settings. Drawing on the expertise of experienced scholars and educators internationally, and across stages of their educational and academic careers, this comprehensive volume offers advice within the key domains of medical education. These include: curriculum design, assessment, learning strategies, clinical teaching, educational theory, and the integration of technology. By synthesizing foundational research and practical wisdom, this Handbook provides a thorough understanding of the principles and practices that shape contemporary medical education.

This book aims to provide a practical, easy-to-read guide on medical education for doctors and healthcare professionals. Starting as an educator can be daunting and we hope it will help those who are beginning their journey within medical education, as well as those who are more experienced and seeking to develop their educational skillset.

Foreword

The publication of an Oxford Handbook is an important milestone in the establishment of Medical Education as a scholarly discipline. We have come a long way since entry to the profession was by apprenticeship, culminating in a licensing exam conducted in Latin. The preclinical education that preceded apprenticeships was notorious for students' fripperies. Kenneth Calman (1) describes students as 'a rowdy lot, callous and cynical. They behaved badly in classrooms, hissing and booing, and throwing things, even firing pistols'. Even in my own preclinical days, lectures could be rowdy affairs where students rained paper darts on unpopular lecturers. Fear of being sanctioned for unprofessional behaviour has, I suspect, mellowed students in recent times.

The relationship between the medical sciences, education, and practice has changed progressively. In late nineteenth-century America, there were 'sundown institutions,' which made it possible for 'the clerk, the street-car conductor, the janitor, and others … to obtain a medical degree' (2). All that changed after Flexner's landmark recommendation in 1910 that medical education should be a scholarly pursuit, grounded in science, from the moment of entry (2). It was safe for Flexner to assume that an education in science would improve clinical practice because clinicians themselves were eminent scientists. So medical education was inescapably oriented towards practice. The 'centre of gravity' of medical education has shifted progressively such that even clinician-educators in prestigious medical schools these days may not be scientists and scientists who teach medical students may not be clinicians. Medicine now mostly uses technologies developed with the help of sciences rather than being a science *per se*. Enter the emergent discipline of medical education, tasked with bridging a widening gulf within the scientifically informed, but pragmatically oriented practice of patient care.

The Editors of the Handbook—Gabrielle Finn, Megan Brown, Matthew Byrne, Helen Church, and Neil Sharma—have acknowledged the global reach of contemporary medical education by assembling an international team of authors. The scope of their expertise is commendably wide, ranging from existential philosophy to mixing Ispaghula husk and automotive anti-freeze to concoct simulated tissue. What I offer in this foreword is a hitchhiker's guide to the Handbook, which I hope may also provide a map of the terrain for those newly entering it. I identify seven themes in the Handbook: theory; curriculum; pedagogy; learning environments; tools and technologies; assessment (both of fitness to enter and progress to the next stage of medical education); and research and evaluation.

Theory comes first in my list of themes because, while the practices of medical education and patient care are to some extent consanguineous, there are important theoretical differences between them. These differences, I suggest, reflect the scholarship of medical practice being much more mature than the scholarship of medical education. Clinical practice is based on sciences, which have yielded mature technologies, whose effectiveness has been proven in clinical trials. You can design regimes of treatment without digging deep into clinical science. The learning sciences, in contrast, are young, to the extent that conflicting theoretical paradigms support competing educational approaches and there are few situations where we can make evidence-based choices between validated alternatives. Of course, advocates will try to persuade you that their approach is indisputably better than other ones but, until we know a lot more about how people become doctors, such advocates are not on solid ground. Good medical educators seek to understand how students learn and craft their approaches accordingly. Chapter 2 lays out theoretical considerations that can help them do so.

The authors of Chapter 12 define the term 'curriculum' as 'all the components that allow for teaching and learning to take place'. I think of it as an overall structure that shapes students' experiences. 'Pedagogy' is the name for the educational processes that curricula promote, educators conduct, and from which students learn. Even those whose job is to design, manage, and conduct educational processes use the word pedagogy surprisingly rarely, which makes me wonder how clearly they understand their task. My definition for the word pedagogy is 'what you do when you meet a learner, or a whole bunch of them'. Chapter 1 captures this nicely when it speaks of teachable moments: when an educator brings clinical and educational imperatives, perhaps briefly, into alignment with one another. Chapters 3 and 4 continue the theme. Chapter 3 gives practical advice and worked examples of the pedagogy of education in small groups, in and beyond the clinical contexts discussed in Chapter 1. Chapter 4 continues the theme, now regarding large groups. The exploration of factors that influence visual attention in Chapter 4 illustrates how, as I suggested earlier, theory can help us make practical educational choices. Large group teaching, Chapter 4 warns us, is a pedagogy to be used sparingly and skilfully. Chapter 5 locates simulation at an intersection between pedagogy and technology. It places simulation in the historical context of training pedagogies and offers a wealth of pedagogic advice that is applicable to training in general.

The term 'learning environment' is an important counterpart to the word 'teaching'. Whereas 'teaching' emphasizes 'the sage on the stage', who too often relishes transmitting their sagacity to passive learners, an emphasis on 'learning environments' represents a different pedagogic theory. The assumption, here, is that learners actively construct learning. They are helped to do so by what Billett calls the 'affordances' of the environment in which they learn. These affordances are of three types: organization of learners' experiences, a social climate that motivates students and boosts their confidence, and access to knowledge and skills that students can make their own. Don't be fooled by the lack of a chapter devoted to learning environments. Those three themes—good organization (curriculum), social support, and available knowledge and skills (pedagogy)—permeate the whole Handbook, particularly clearly exemplified by education in the most potentially hostile of all learning environments, clinical workplaces (Chapter 1).

Tools and technologies are considered in Chapters 9 (Technology-enhanced learning) and 11 (Educational portfolios), as well as Chapter 5 (simulation). Chapter 9's title places due emphasis on technology-enhanced LEARNING, which is important given the potential of technologies to seduce us into treating gizmos as the primary object of our attention. Chapter 9 provides coherence to the book by considering how technology intersects with curriculum, pedagogy, and assessment, and directs us towards the emerging role of communication technology, which showed its worth during the COVID-19 pandemic. Chapter 11 supplements Chapter 9, focusing on portfolios, not as 'filing cabinets', which they can too easily be, but on their role in *purposefully* collecting the products of learning.

Assessment is the topic of Chapters 6 and 7. Assessment is the exception to my rule that the scholarship of medical education is still quite young. The need to let the right people qualify as doctors and the right people enter medical education has fostered huge international research and development in medical assessment. The term 'Principles', as opposed to 'theory' was well chosen for Chapter 6, which leans heavily on the statistical discipline of psychometrics to define useful pragmatic rules that guide how to make reliable judgements. Chapter 7 goes yet further into educational practice, providing robust practical guidance to those tasked with managing assessments. If, though, we regard medical education as a scholarly pursuit, it is never too late to go back to fundamental questions. It might provoke an interesting debate if we were to ask the authors of this Handbook why the term 'pedagogy' (helping students learn) is so rarely used, while the term 'assessment' (measuring whether they have learned) is so often used! I suspect it's something to do with clinical educators' power.

If assessment is the province of certainty, research (a topic covered in Chapter 10) is the province of uncertainty. The authors provide an accessible overview of how to create new knowledge in a scholarly way, illustrating how theory can help us step back from our familiarity with education to identify important areas of uncertainty and provide answers. This chapter does novice medical educationalists a good turn by teasing out differences between research, evaluation, and scholarship. While this may seem rather abstract and removed from the day job, the contents of this chapter will come in very useful when it comes to preparing a case for promotion—which someone who seriously intends to rise through the academic ranks within medical education should start on day 1. The authors nicely bridge research theory and practice, introducing constructivist ways of thinking with which even well-established clinical researchers may be unfamiliar.

Chapter 12, a wide-ranging review of challenges in medical education, cross-cutting my seven themes, brings this commendable book to its conclusion. There are many walks of life where progress depends on younger people steering their 'elders and betters' in the right direction. In medical education, we depend on it heavily. The editors have done an important service by recruiting and tasking a cadre of writers, representing the spectrum of seniority, whose efforts will contribute importantly to progress. Take heed of what the authors suggest and enjoy the exhilaration of making medical education part of your career portfolio.

Tim Dornan
Emeritus Professor of Medical Education

References

1. Calman K. *Medical education. Past, present, and future.* Edinburgh: Elsevier, 2007.
2. Flexner A. *Medical education in the United States and Canada.* Carnegie Foundation for the Advancement of Teaching, 1910.

List of contributors

Yvette Annan
Imperial College Healthcare NHS
Trust, London, UK

Arabella Simpkin Begin
Fellow and Director of Studies in
Clinical Medicine at Lincoln College,
Oxford, UK

Jo Bishop
Associate Dean, Student Affairs
and Service Quality for the Health
Science and Medicine faculty, Bond
University, Australia

Megan E.L. Brown
Senior Research Associate in
Medical Education, School of
Medicine, Newcastle University, UK

Matthew H.V. Byrne
NIHR Academic Clinical Fellow
(Urology), Nuffield Department of
Surgical Sciences, Medical Sciences
Division, University of Oxford, UK

Charles Campion-Smith
Bournemouth University, UK

Myooran Canagaratnam
Consultant Psychiatrist in the
Lifespan ASC and Learning
Disabilities Service, Tavistock and
Portman NHS Foundation Trust,
London, UK

Julie Chen
Department of Family Medicine
and Primary Care/Bau Institute
of Medical and Health Sciences
Education, The University of Hong
Kong, Hong Kong, SAR, China

Helen R. Church
Clinical Assistant Professor, Faculty
of Medicine and Health Sciences,
University of Nottingham, UK

Iain Doherty
Senior Lecturer, Learning Futures,
Deakin Learning Futures, Australia

Chaoyan Dong
Assistant Director, Education
Office, Sengkang General Hospital,
Singapore

Luci Etheridge
Consultant paediatrician and
Honorary senior lecturer at St
George's Hospital and St George's,
University of London, UK

Gabrielle M. Finn
Professor of Medical Education and
Associate Vice President, University
of Manchester

Hossam Hamdy
Gulf Medical University,
Ajman, UAE

Marcus A. Henning
Associate Professor and
Postgraduate Academic Advisor at
the Centre for Medical and Health
Sciences Education, University of
Auckland, New Zealand

Karim Keshwani
University College London, UCL,
London, UK

Bob Klaber
Imperial College Healthcare NHS
Trust, London, UK

Marian C. Limacher
Professor Emerita, Former Senior
Associate Dean for Faculty Affairs
and Professional Development,
University of Florida College of
Medicine, Gainesville, FL

Matароria Lyndon
Senior Lecturer in Medical
Education, University of Auckland,
New Zealand

Kevin McLaughlin
University of Calgary,
Alberta, Canada

Eleana Ntatsaki
Consultant Rheumatologist at
Ipswich Hospital NHS Trust and
an Honorary Senior Lecturer at
University College London, UK

Rakesh Patel
Professor of Medical Education
and Head of MBBS, QMUL,
London, UK

Subha Ramani
Associate Professor of Medicine
at Harvard Medical School, and
Honorary Professor of Medical
Education at the University of
Manchester, UK

Gabriel Reedy
Programme Director for the
Master's in Clinical Education pro-
gramme, Kings College London, UK

David Sales
Freelance consultant in medical
assessment.
Former Chair of the Curriculum
Advisory Group, and RCGP
Assessment Fellow, UK

Bryony Sales
GP Partner and Trainer,
GP Associate Dean, Portsmouth
and Isle of Wight, UK

John Sandars
Professor of Medical Education,
Edge Hill University, Ormskirk,
Lancashire, UK

Affy Sepahzad
London North West Healthcare
NHS Trust, London, UK

Neel Sharma
GI Medicine Specialist with sub-
specialty Interest in GI Oncology
Cambridge University Hospitals
University of Cambridge, UK

Thomas Simpson
Research Fellow, Respiratory
Registrar, Kings College London, UK

Jessica Stokes-Parish
Assistant Professor, Bond
University, Australia

Chris Valerio UCL
University College London, UCL,
London, UK

Tim Vincent
Senior Learning Technologist,
Brighton and Sussex Medical
School, UK

Zareen Zaidi
Professor, General Internal
Medicine, Medical Education
George Washington School of
Medicine and Health Sciences,
Washington DC. Titles at the time
of authorship: Associate Professor,
Director of Longitudinal Portfolios,
Director Scholarship Department
of Medicine, Associate Chief Faculty
Development Division of General
Internal Medicine, Department
of Medicine, University of Florida
College of Medicine, Gainesville, FL

Elisa A. Zenni
Senior Associate Dean for
Educational Affairs, Designated
Institutional Official, Professor,
Department of Pediatrics,
University of Florida College of
Medicine—Jacksonville, FL

Ellen Zimmerman
Professor, Gastroenterology,
Hepatology and Nutrition,
Associate Dean for Faculty
Development, Vice Chair for
Academic Affairs, Department of
Medicine, University of Florida
College of Medicine, Gainesville, FL

Chapter 1

Teaching in the clinical setting

Bob Klaber, Hossam Hamdy, Affy Sepahzad, and Arabella Simpkin Begin

Introduction

The word 'doctor' is derived from the Latin *docere*, which means 'to teach'. The clinical setting provides a wealth of opportunities to prepare the next generation of doctors for their role as future healthcare providers, on whom high-value patient care undoubtedly depends. In particular, it offers an environment which invites participation, problem-solving, integration of basic and clinical knowledge, and active practice. Across clinical settings, there are a wealth of teachable moments, and the chance to model competent and knowledgeable patient care, together with qualities that are so critical in medicine: effective teamwork, curiosity, acceptance of uncertainty, engagement, integrity, and humility, to name a few. In the context of a rapidly changing healthcare environment, with expanding clinical responsibilities and shrinking time and support for educational endeavours, effective teaching in the clinical setting can feel ever more challenging. But we would argue that it is the very cornerstone of medical education.

∴ As Osler so wisely stated:

> '[Those] who stud[y] medicine without books sails an uncharted sea, but [Those] who stud[y] medicine without patients [do] not go to sea at all.'

The individual

Each individual in a learning interaction or encounter plays a distinct role.

Role of the teacher

The clinical teacher plays many roles simultaneously. In the clinical setting they are often managing patient care at the same time as overseeing learning opportunities for trainees. Effective educational and clinical supervision must have patient safety and quality of patient care as its primary purpose, but must also educate the trainee, promote high standards, identify trainee problems, support the trainee, and monitor their progress.

Role of the learner

Learning is an inborn ability that cannot be suppressed. No learner wakes up wanting to appear ignorant, incompetent, or disruptive in the clinical setting. However as humans, we are constantly attempting to influence others' perceptions of us by regulating and controlling information in social interactions. This can lead to deeply embedded actions, happening without conscious thought, to lower the risk of rejection or scorn and can manifest as a reluctance to ask questions, admit mistakes or weaknesses, or make suggestions. Unfortunately, this can seriously hinder the ability and opportunities for effective learning. Today's volatile, uncertain, complex, and ambiguous world requires continuous, and often self-directed, learning—there is, thankfully, no end to our medical education and we all remain, in some capacity, a learner forever.

Role of the patient

Patients are often at the heart of teaching in the clinical setting. Together with their families, friends, and loved ones, they can teach us about their lived experiences of diagnosis, treatment, living with long-term conditions, and advocacy. Patients provide invaluable perspectives for learners and their experiences can highlight the multiple elements and components of a patient's journey through the healthcare system. Involving patients in teaching often manifests as a symbiotic relationship, with both parties acting as resources for the other—when engaging patients in teaching is respectfully done, many patients enjoy being involved in educational experiences which contribute to student learning.

The clinical setting

The clinical environment consists of inpatient, outpatient, and ambulatory care settings (which includes General Practice and Community settings) each with their own distinct challenges and opportunities. It is in this environment that students learn what being a doctor means 'on the ground', or in practice. Optimal learning occurs when undertaking medical practice with appropriate supervision in an appropriate environment. Along with clinical knowledge, examination, and procedural skills, higher-order thinking skills, and the development of good team-working skills are critical for healthcare professionals. Healthcare occurs amidst constantly shifting configurations of people making up dynamic teams, in an environment that is rife with uncertainty. The art of communicating and coordinating effectively with people across boundaries of all kinds—expertise, status, and distance—is essential. This requires a psychologically safe workplace where learners are able to take the inherent interpersonal risks of candour, fully participating without fear. It also requires a workplace and environment that prioritizes value and respect, maximizing engagement and joy in practice, and celebrating medicine—the oldest learned profession in the world—a fascinating and dynamic profession with near limitless potential that is universal and eternal.

Teaching in the clinical setting

This chapter outlines theories that underpin learning and teaching, together with practical guidance on how to create a safe learning experience to maximize growth and opportunity across healthcare settings and clinical domains. It also includes thoughts for the future, considering the rapid acceleration of technology and its inevitable impact on teaching in the clinical setting.

▶ We hope to inspire commitment and enthusiasm that you can carry with you to learning encounters, whether in acute settings, on the wards, or in clinics, giving answers to the questions: What forms of teaching, guidance, or experience are most likely to help our trainees make the most of their individual talents and interests? How can we maximize each learning opportunity? How can we inspire life-long, self-directed learning? How can we maximize curiosity for learners and teachers alike? How can we best teach and engage in the clinical setting?

Attributes of an effective teacher

According to Bandura's social learning theory, individuals learn by observing others. The degree to which they incorporate observed behaviours into their own practice depends on both their self-efficacy for the behaviour to be learned and the environmental response to their attempts at the new behaviour.

Role model

A role model is defined in medical education literature as a person who is seen by another, or by a group, as demonstrating a standard of excellence to be imitated. Today, role modelling is thought to be an integral component of medical education and an important factor in shaping the values, attitudes, behaviour, and ethics of medical trainees. Many of the attributes associated with being an excellent role model are related to skills that can be acquired and to modifiable behaviour.

Attributes of a positive role model

Patient care qualities
- Excellent, experienced clinicians with expressed empathy for patients
- Positive interactions with patients, patients' families, and other healthcare workers
- Proficiency as a diagnostician

Teaching qualities
- Commitment to the growth of learners
- Humanistic style of teaching
- Creates safe environment
- Ability to explain difficult subjects
- Non-threatening style, approachable
- Repertoire of teaching methods

Personal qualities
- Enthusiasm
- Integrity
- Leadership ability
- Sense of humour
- Compassion
- Organized

Teaching effectiveness

'Effective' teaching is difficult to define and evaluate, prone to subjective rating ∴ context specificity is important, and teachers are more likely to be rated as effective when they are:
- Knowledgeable
- Value teaching
- Communicate effectively with learners
- Demonstrate concern for the well-being of learners
- Provide effective feedback
- Inspire learners

❶ It is important to acknowledge that ratings of effectiveness are prone to bias. Minoritised clinical teachers, e.g., Black women, are often subject to biases that can negatively impact their evaluations, irrespective of their actual teaching abilities. ▶ Ratings of teacher effectiveness may not always be a fair or accurate representation of skills and may reflect biases held by those evaluating them. Criteria used to evaluate teaching effectiveness may also be biased, favouring approaches to teaching that may not be beneficial for diverse learners, and undervaluing relational teaching styles, or culturally responsive approaches to teaching. Using multiple metrics and raters to assess teaching effectiveness, and making meaningful efforts to identify and address biases may be beneficial. Steps may include:

- Where evaluators are educators, training educators to recognize and reflect on their own biases, and engaging in conversations regarding addressing biases identified
- Employing a diverse panel of evaluators
- Reviewing and revising evaluation criteria to account for the diverse ways effective teaching can manifest

Levels of supervision

Supervision includes observation, continual feedback, and sharing of clinical judgement. The exact nature of supervision depends on both what the trainee is doing and how experienced they are:

- Modelling: observing the consultation
- Interaction: asking questions and debriefing
- Direct supervision: supervisor present
- Arm's length supervision: supervisor nearby and immediately available
- Local supervision: supervisor on the premises, available immediately via telephone, and able to come within a short period of time
- Distant supervision: supervisor on call and available for advice, able to come to assistance in an appropriate time

❶ Avoiding the pitfalls of clinical teaching

The following are common issues in clinical teaching which must be avoided to optimize learning:

- Lack of clear objectives and expectations
- Teaching pitched at the wrong level
- Focus on recall of facts rather than problem-solving
- Lack of active participation by learners
- Inadequate direct observation of learners and feedback
- Insufficient time for reflection and discussion
- Lack of congruence with the rest of the curriculum

Further reading

⊃ Bandura A. Social cognitive theory. In: Vasta R (Ed.), *Annals of child development. Vol. 6. Six theories of child development* (pp. 1–60). Greenwich, CN: JAI Press, 1989.
⊃ Boendermaker PM, Schuling J, Meyboom-de Jong BM, Zwierstra RP, Metz JC. What are the characteristics of the competent general practitioner trainer? *Fam Pract* 2000;17:547–553.
⊃ Wright SM, Kern DE, Kolodner K, Howard DM, Brancati FL. Attributes of excellent attending-physician role models. *N Engl J Med* 1998;339:1986–1993.

Maximize your teaching potential

Reflecting on your strengths and areas for development as a clinical teacher is critical.

Domains of knowledge

There are six domains of knowledge which an effective clinical teacher will apply. You can use these domains to reflect on your strengths and areas for development.

Knowledge of medicine

Integrating the patient's clinical problem with background knowledge of basic sciences, clinical sciences, and clinical experience.

Knowledge of patients

Familiarity with disease and illness, drawn from past experience.

Knowledge of the context

Awareness of patients in their social context and at their stage of treatment; the clinical context creates different opportunities for learning.

Knowledge of the learners

An understanding of the learner's level of training, together with an understanding of their curriculum requirements for that stage.

Knowledge of pedagogy and the general principles of teaching

An understanding of methods for teaching adult learners and the theoretical basis for teaching — the 'how' and 'why' of teaching.

Knowledge of case-based teaching scripts

The ability to present the patient as a representation of a certain clinical problem, using information specific to the case, and also contributing additional knowledge and experiences to expand learning about the condition.

Future domains

As the environment changes at exponential rates, with acceleration of technology, machine learning, and biomedical artificial intelligence, the domains of knowledge may expand .. perhaps 'knowledge', which suggests 'black-and-white', concrete information, will be transformed to include 'knowledge of uncertainty' and 'knowledge of analysis'. The physician's role may evolve from provider and purveyor of knowledge to supervisor of care and purveyor of humanism.

Further reading

Irby DM. What clinical teachers in medicine need to know. *Acad Med* 1994;69:333–342.
Irby DM. Excellence in clinical teaching: knowledge transformation and development required. *Med Educ* 2014;48:776–784.

Cognitive load theory

Cognitive load theory suggests the human brain can only process a certain amount of information at once. Individuals constantly take in information through their senses and hold this temporarily in working memory. As the capacity of working memory is finite, information must be processed and stored in long-term memory for later use. Here it is organized into schemas of increasing complexity, allowing individuals to retrieve schemas for use in working memory as single constructs. Cognitive load theory divides learning further into the intrinsic load of the information to be learned and the extrinsic load required to process it.

Intrinsic cognitive load

The complexity of the information itself. This is highest for novice learners and for complex tasks with interacting elements (e.g., managing a patient on mechanical ventilation).

Teachers can help by starting with simpler examples with fewer elements or by chunking many elements into more manageable parts. Learners can be provided partially worked examples, so they only need to supply a few missing parts.

Extrinsic cognitive load

Germane load: The cognitive work of organizing new information into schemas, i.e., the cognitive load beneficial to learning.

Extraneous load: The effort required to process new information due to the way in which it is presented.

This is the cognitive load most easily controlled by the teacher and should be reduced when intrinsic and germane load is high to free up space for processing complex information. In the clinical setting, extraneous load can be particularly high due to the complexity of auditory and visual stimuli on the ward or in the clinic. When teaching new, complex content, teachers should minimize these distractions (i.e., silencing unnecessary alarms, discouraging disruptions to rounds) whenever possible and teach learners how to recognize the impact of these distractions on their thought processes. Where content is familiar, teaching learners to work in an environment with high extraneous load (given this replicates actual practice) can be beneficial.

Era of big data

As there is an exponential growth in information available, there is a challenge to our ability to processing everything. There is a risk that the noise increases faster than the signal. The volume of data adds to cognitive load as we need to work harder to distill the most poignant signals.

Further reading

⮡ Gooding H, Mann K, Armstrong E. Twelve tips for applying the science of learning to health professions education. *Med Teach* 2017;39(1):26–31.
⮡ Leppink J, Duvivier R. Twelve tips for medical curriculum design from a cognitive load theory perspective. *Med Teach* 2016;38:669–674.

Teaching techniques

There is an industry of ever-evolving frameworks, models, and techniques for teaching. Included here are three that are popular and widely used. This is not intended as an exhaustive list, but rather a selection of practical models promoting excellence in teaching.

Stanford faculty development model for clinical teaching

Promoting a positive learning climate
Learning climate defined as tone or atmosphere of the teaching setting.

Control of session
Refers to the way the teaching interaction is focused and paced, influenced by the teacher's leadership style.

Communication of goals
Setting goals provides a structure for the teaching process, guides teachers in planning the teaching, and provides a basis for assessment.

Promoting understanding and retention
Understanding is the ability to correctly analyse, synthesize, and apply whereas retention is the process of remembering facts or concepts.

Evaluation
The process by which the teacher assesses the learner's knowledge, skills, and attitudes, based on educational goals previously established. Evaluation can be formative (to assess ongoing learner's progress towards educational goals) or summative (for final assessment to judge learner's achievement of goals).

Feedback
The process by which the teacher provides learners with information about their performance for potential improvement.

Promoting self-directed learning
Facilitating learning initiated by learner's needs, goals, and interests to ensure continued learning beyond the time of formal education.

▶ The one-minute preceptor

Named in view of the short time available for teaching in the clinical environment, the one-minute preceptor provides a simple framework for daily teaching during patient care that emphasizes higher-order learning such as clinical reasoning. These steps can be used to structure effective short clinical teaching encounters that last five minutes or less as well as to address problems that arise. The original model uses a five-step approach. Not every step needs to be used in every encounter, and the order of the steps is flexible.

Step 1. Getting a commitment
Initial buy-in from learner is critical, establishing investment in the case. The teacher encourages learners to articulate their opinions on the differential diagnosis and management rather than giving their own conclusions and plans. A safe learning environment must be created so learners feel safe enough to risk a commitment—even if it's wrong.

Step 2. Probing for supportive evidence

Evaluates a learner's knowledge and clinical reasoning, encouraging learners to 'think out loud', giving their rationale for the commitment they have made to diagnosis, treatment, or other aspects of the patient's problem. Validate commitments or reject them gently if flawed.

Step 3. Teaching general rules

Teachers can guide learners to understand how learning from one patient can be applied to other future situations.

Step 4. Reinforcing what was done well

Effective reinforcement should be specific, and behaviour based, not vague. Positive feedback also builds the trainee's self-esteem.

Step 5. Correcting mistakes

Negative or constructive feedback is often avoided by clinical teachers, but it is vital to ensure good patient care. Encouraging self-assessment is a good way for learners to realize mistakes themselves and if they have identified their errors, they can be given positive feedback on their self-reflective capabilities. If the teacher has to point out mistakes, this must be specific, timely, and entirely behaviour based.

Time-efficient teaching

Planning

Sharpen expectations; clarify roles and responsibilities; select appropriate patients for the teaching; allocate time for instruction and feedback; focus learners on important priorities and tasks.

Teaching

Common teaching methods used, depending on context and needs of learners: teaching from clinical cases; using questions to test learners' capacity for recall, and promote analysis, synthesis, and application; use advanced learners to participate in the teaching; using illness and teaching scripts; acting as role models at bedside or in clinic rooms.

Evaluating and reflecting

Observing learners directly is an important prerequisite for effective feedback. Positive and negative feedback should be included, and teachers need to promote self-assessment by learners.

Further reading

- Irby DM, Bowen JL. Time-efficient strategies for learning and performance. *Clin Teach* 2004;1:23–28.
- Neher J, Gordon KC, Meyer B, Stevens N. A five-step 'microskills' model of clinical teaching. *J Am Board Family Practitioners* 1992;5:419–424.

Creating a safe learning environment

As will be outlined in Chapter 2, Maslow's Hierarchy of needs explains how a learner's emotional state affects the physiological processes of learning. ● Although high-arousal, negative-emotion states such as fear can enhance memory for events, ▶ they can also impede problem-solving. There is robust evidence that feeling safe in a learning environment leads to more creative problem-solving and greater learning, particularly in team learning and in groups with hierarchical membership. Psychological safety allows learners to answer questions or ask for help without threats to their dignity or worthiness. Learners must feel valued and respected, with a sense of interpersonal trust allowing them to be comfortable being themselves. A psychologically safe environment does not mean accepting substandard performance from learners.

▶ Emotional and psychological safety

Teachers can help create a sense of emotional and psychological safety through verbal and non-verbal communication:

- Promote emphasis on learning and improvement
- Recognize and validate range of emotions experienced by learners
- Develop positive and supportive relationships with learners
- Make sure the learner knows how to contact you
- Hold learners accountable for achieving learning objectives, but without resorting to humiliation, hostility, or intimidation: 'It's okay to not know yet'
- Uncover learners' existing knowledge and skills in order to pose questions or problems to them that are challenging but do not surpass their current developmental stage
- Ensure sufficient time to allow for the strategic use of silence after posing questions, during which learners have the opportunity to consider the question, reflect on their knowledge, or think aloud
- Ensure distractions and outside influences are eliminated
- Encourage engagement from all team members and promote

Further reading

↪ Ashauer SA, Macan T. How can leaders foster team learning? Effects of leader-assigned mastery and performance goals and psychological safety. *J Psychol* 2013;147:541–561.

↪ Edmondson A. Psychological safety and learning behaviour in work teams. *Adm Sci Q* 1999;44(2):350–583.

Knowing your student

Learning should begin with the learner. It is thus important that educators are aware of different learning preferences that exist for learners.

Principles of adult learning theory

Adults:
- have a specific purpose in mind
- are voluntary participants in learning
- require meaning and relevance
- require active involvement in learning
- need clear goals and objectives
- need feedback
- need to be reflective

The Kolb learning styles

'Learning is a process whereby knowledge is created through the transformation of experience'

Learning results from the way people perceive and then process information, making it their knowledge. Kolb (1984) described four different learning styles:

Diverging (feeling and watching):
Tend to prefer to watch rather than do, gathering information, and using imagination to solve problems; perform well in situations that require idea generation.

Assimilating (watching and thinking):
Involves a concise, logical approach, with good clear explanation rather than a practical opportunity; interested in ideas and abstract concepts; enjoy having time to think things through.

Converging (doing and thinking):
Tend to use learning to find solutions to practical issues; like to experiment with new ideas, to simulate, and to work with practical applications.

Accommodating (doing and feeling):
This learning style is hands-on and relies on intuition rather than logic, enjoying taking a practical, experiential approach.

The experiential learning cycle
- Concrete experience: a new experience or situation is encountered or a re-interpretation of an existing experience
- Reflective observation of new experience: particular importance should be paid to any inconsistencies between experience and understanding
- Abstract conceptualization: reflection gives rise to a new idea, or a modification of an existing abstract concept
- Active experimentation: the learner applies their ideas to the world around them to see what happens

Ideally, a learner should be able to use each of the four different kinds of abilities to gain the most effective learning results for each situation. However, influenced by nature and nurture and different experiences and demands in the past and present, learners tend to develop preferences in one or more of the four learning styles.

Multilevel learner groups

In many clinical settings, a variety of trainees are present in a team. It can be challenging ∴ to engage the entire team while avoiding teaching that any particular trainee would perceive as too simple or too complex. There are strategies that can be employed to develop different learners' clinical skills and independence:

- Encourage all learners to contribute to teaching, filling knowledge gaps for those on the team. Interprofessional staff offer unique clinical perspectives
- Collectively review new guidelines, studies, and protocols
- Explicitly role-model humanism, professionalism, communication, and diagnostic bias by reflecting out loud and demonstrating vulnerability
- Ask questions to learners based on their anticipated knowledge base to build shared understanding
- Pair medical students with trainees to create coaching relationships
- Promote autonomy among all team members by delegating duties appropriate to each learner's level of training, encouraging team members to speak up with concerns

Further reading

➲ Curry L. Individual differences in cognitive style, learning style and instructional preference in medical education. In: Norman G. van der Vleuten, CPM, Newble D (Eds.), *International handbook of research in medical education* (pp. 263–276). Norwell, MA: Kluwer Academic Publishers, 2003.

➲ Knowles MS. *The adult learner: a neglected species*, 4th edn. Houston, TX: Gulf Publishing, 1990.

➲ Quigley PD, Potisek NM, Barone MA. How to 'ENGAGE' multilevel learner groups in the clinical setting. *Pediatrics* 2017;140(5):e20172861.

Feedback

Feedback is an essential part of education, defined as the 'transmission of evaluative or corrective information about an action'. Without it, learners cannot be sure of their progress, nor of developmental opportunities they may have missed. It is a crucial step in the acquisition of skills allowing strengths to be reinforced and errors corrected. When done well, feedback also serves to promote self-reflection and self-assessment. Providing timely, detailed, specific, constructive, non-judgemental feedback contributes to increased quality and utility of feedback. Despite continued calls for feedback, it is something that many struggle to deliver effectively. The key player, however, is not the giver of feedback, but rather the receiver of feedback. They are in control of how much of the feedback they absorb and whether they choose to change. The ability to accept feedback is a learned skill that anyone can develop.

For an in-depth discussion of feedback, and further practical tips, see Chapter 8.

Types of feedback
- Formal or informal
- Blunt or subtle
- Brief and immediate or long and scheduled
- Formative or summative

Kinds of feedback
- Appreciation—recognizes and values good practice and motivates the learner
- Coaching—offers advice or promotes self-reflection to help learners improve
- Evaluation—assesses and measures how well the learner completes a task

▶▶ Framing questions
- What was done well?
- What was not done so well?
- How can improvement be made for next time?

Approach to giving feedback in the clinical setting
- Be learner-led: ask the learner if, when, and how they would like to receive feedback; give options if they appear unclear; ensure discussions are interactive and keep returning to learner self-perception and agenda. Understand that unwanted feedback and feedback given at the wrong time, place, or style is not conducive to learning.
- Be flexible: be adaptable and responsive in real-time.
- Focus on achieving outcomes/improvements/change: ensure you support learners to continually seek improvement, however impressive their performance is; summarize how to achieve improvements.
- Structure is important, but avoid being predictable: there can be little gained if a feedback structure, such as the 'feedback sandwich' where positive feedback is positioned either side of an area for improvement, is used for the sake of it.

- Be specific, descriptive, balanced, and objective: avoid becoming personal.
- Relate to principles, concepts, and evidence: if the opportunity arises, relate specific feedback points to wider concepts and evidence as a useful way of contextualizing them.
- Separate evaluation from coaching and appreciation.
- Close the feedback conversation with a commitment, such as an action plan, with benchmarks and new strategies.

Barriers to giving feedback

One of the greatest barriers to effective feedback is lack of direct observation of the learner. Frequently feedback is non-specific and unhelpful to learners, in part as teachers can feel hesitant to provide detailed negative feedback as they feel uncomfortable, vulnerable, and risky contemplating highlighting problematic issues with a learner. Feedback usually comes from two places: observable data and interpretations of that data based on our own life experiences, assumptions, preferences, and priorities. Too often the feedback giver jumps unconsciously from data to interpretation, which is deeply coloured by our own understanding of what we're rating others on, our own sense of what looks good for a particular competency, our harshness or leniency as raters, and our own conscious and unconscious biases. Recognizing this tendency is essential whenever feedback is given.

The feedback receiver

The feedback receiver is key in determining the success of feedback. They decide whether your feedback will be heard, understood, digested, and finally acted upon to make improvements. Empowering learners to take a proactive part in any feedback is essential.

- Ask clarifying questions to truly understand what the feedback means and where it comes from; what data led to the interpretation?
- Separate the feedback from the relationship
- Understand own temperament and how we are wired
- Keep feedback in perspective
- Remember that traits and abilities are not fixed, but are amenable to change; avoid thinking 'this is just who I am'
- Recognize that emotions, triggered particularly by negative feedback, distort our thinking about the past, present, and future
- Reflect on your own 'feedback footprint' and how you typically respond
- Cultivate a growth mindset: see failures as a step in helping you make necessary progress; see challenges as opportunities

Barriers to understanding feedback

- Feedback is vague: too often feedback is generic and unhelpful
- Giver and receiver have different interpretations resulting in a mismatch between what is heard and what is meant
- It is unclear where feedback comes from or where it is going: specific feedback that has a past and a future is essential

Further reading

Klaber B. Effective feedback: an essential skill. *Postgrad Med J* 2012;88(1038):187–188.
Stone D, Heen S. *Thanks for the feedback: the science and art of receiving feedback well*. New York, NY: Penguin Books, 2014.

The patient

Contact with patients lies at the heart of clinical education. Changes in healthcare delivery, rising student numbers, and a drive for more equal partnership with patients has forced medical educators to consider new ways of involving patients and the patient experience for learners. Learning in context motivates through relevance and plays a major part in developing clinical reasoning by exposing learners to a range of presentations, including variations from so-called textbook cases. Contact with patients helps students form professional skills, develop their professional identity, and recognize the breadth of sociodemographic characteristics and cultural backgrounds that patients encompass.

Real patients

Real patients form the bedrock and hallmark for clinical teaching, fostering empathy, and forcing the student to look beyond the disease to see illness in a wider context.

❶ *Challenges*
- Unsuitable: problems may be too complex, especially in the early stages of medical education
- Unusable: increasing hospital turnover and an ageing population can mean that inpatients are too transient, sick, or frail
- Unpredictable: a problem if a degree of standardization is required
- Unwillingness to participate
- Lack of availability of translation services to overcome language barriers

Simulated or standardized patients

Simulated or standardized patients can enhance the value of real patients in the student's learning.

Simulated patients

Simulated patients can be real patients coached to modify their presentations, lay volunteers, faculty members, students, trained actors, high-fidelity mannequins, and more recently virtual patients. The emphasis for simulated patients is in portraying the signs and symptoms of real patients.

Standardized patients

A standardized patient is a broader term that includes simulated patients and actual patients who have been coached to present their own illnesses in a standardized, unvarying way. The emphasis is on consistency.

▶ *Advantages*
- Can be available at any time and in any setting, including non-clinical areas
- Presents the same problem for all students making it possible to provide students with equivalent patient experiences instead of the random experience of cases presenting in the clinical setting
- Avoids mistreatment of real patients when they are used for educational purposes. The standardized patient is prepared for students to perform inadequately and use them as a teaching tool
- Students can work without embarrassment about their novice status as they are learning to take histories and perform examinations

- Can practice with difficult and sensitive medical conditions that you would not allow the student to work with in real patient settings; and can practice advanced communication skills and learn how to handle emotionally charged situations in controlled settings. Opportunities for student support where situations involve emotional processing
- Can prepare students for actual clinical problems in a less threatening environment
- Allows interruption and restarting of the encounter to permit feedback and practice
- Can pause the encounter to discuss, with 'time outs', a variety of things that would perhaps not be discussed in front of a real patient
- The passage of time can be ignored so students can learn continuity of practice at one setting

Patient educators

It is possible to build a 'bank' of clinical volunteers with appropriate histories and stable clinical signs who will attend clinical teaching sessions when invited. These patients are not currently undergoing active treatment. In this model, the patient's contribution can more readily be focused on student learning needs. They can often give feedback to the learner about the accuracy and completeness of the workup and show how physical findings might be better elicited.

Factors to consider when working with all patients

- Get appropriate consent from real patients and patient volunteers
- Be prepared and meet with the patient before the clinical teaching session; coach patient on what is expected from them
- Be mindful that patient volunteers or real patients are not trained; they might have their own agendas and be vulnerable; they might also be looking to 'please' their healthcare providers who are the teachers. You must be mindful of the power you wield in these encounters
- Facilitate direct feedback from the patient to the learners
- Provide feedback to standardized or simulated patients to ensure ongoing quality
- Align patient experiences and conditions with goals of teaching session

Virtual patients

Virtual patients in online tools are now being used in clinical skills medical education, including platforms with virtual reality functions.

▶ High-quality platforms will involve patients with lived experience of the conditions or experiences represented in their design and development.

Further Reading

⊃ Hudson J and Ratnapalan S. Teaching clinical skills with patient resources. Canadian Family Physician. 2014;60:674-677
⊃ Spencer J. Patients in medical education. The Lancet. 2004;363:1480

Humanistic, patient-centred care

The practice of medicine combines the life sciences with humanism, defined as 'a doctrine, attitude, or way of life centred on human interests or values'. ► There is increasing recognition of the link between a humanistic doctor-patient relationship and key healthcare outcomes. Clinical teaching interactions can be structured in a manner that creates opportunities for teaching the human dimensions of patient care.

Educational strategies for teaching humanistic patient care

Establish a culture of humanism

- Encourage presentations that integrate relevant psychosocial as well as biomedical information and management strategies
- Move clinical round discussions to the bedside (where possible) and encourage presentations that recognize the presence of the patient, eliminate unnecessary jargon, and engage input from the patient
- Get to know learners as people and address their individual and human needs
- Promote a cooperative, respectful, and supportive environment where team members are encouraged to admit their mistakes and communicate their learning needs

Recognize and use influential events

- Giving bad news: recognize, elicit, clarify, and deal with feelings, concerns, and expectations
- Focus attention on the use of excellent communication skills or recognizing (and cautioning against) the use of dehumanizing language

Role model

- Demonstrate desirable skills or behaviours
- Comment on, and explain, what you have done

Actively engage the learner

- Involve learners in tasks that require humanistic skills, such as eliciting the ideas, concerns, and expectations of patients
- Ask questions and encourage learners to reflect on and discuss what they have done and what they have observed
- Engage learners in projects that are likely to include the human dimensions of care
- Utilize the arts and humanities (e.g. poetry) to promote reflection on the lived experiences of patients, and on learners' own experiences

Be practical and relevant

- Respect the limitations of time and resources
- Make a humanistic approach integral and relevant to patient care
- Focus on humanistic behaviours that are likely to improve outcomes

Further reading

➲ Branch WT, Kern D, Haidet P, Weissmann P, Gracey CF, Mitchell G, Inui T. Teaching the human dimensions of care in clinical settings. *JAMA* 2001;286:1067–1074.
➲ Finn GM, Brown ME, Laughey W. Holding a mirror up to nature: the role of medical humanities in postgraduate primary care training. *Educ Prim Care* 2021;32(2):73–77.

Role of the environment

The clinical environment consists of inpatient, outpatient, and ambulatory care settings, each rich in opportunities for learners to transfer theory to practice and learn the art of medicine. Both planned and unplanned experiences and opportunities must be considered. Learners need to feel welcomed and accepted, safe in an environment that will enhance their growth across all domains, with constructive feedback and coaching for development. ▶ A supportive environment is important for optimal learning.

Impact of the environment

Joy and flourishing in practice

The clinical environment has been shown to be a major determinant in provider well-being, with implications to self, learners, colleagues, and the delivery of patient care of the highest quality and safety. Creating a culture of wellness, by promoting self-care, personal and professional growth, and compassion for colleagues, patients, and self, and restoring joy to the healthcare environment and workforce are critical. When everyone is engaged in an equitable and diverse environment, they feel as though they can listen to what matters to patients, colleagues, and learners; comfortably ask questions, request help, or challenge what's happening; and use teamwork to successfully solve challenges. All of these contribute to a positive work experience and enable the entire team to experience joy in work, and flourish as people and practitioners.

● Science of resilience

The clinical environment can be stressful for learners and healthcare professionals alike. Recognizing this and empowering coping strategies is an important component of clinical teaching. **Personal** resilience to stress is a complex multidimensional construct, defined by the American Psychological Association as 'the process of adapting well in the face of adversity, trauma, tragedy, threats, or even significant sources of threat'. An enriched environment with consistency of support provides an atmosphere that fosters exposure to novelty and responding to challenges—stressors that are controlled and addressed can have a stress insulating effect, developing in learners an adaptive stress response which results in increased resilience for future events.

> 'It is not the strongest of the species that survive, nor the most intelligent, but the ones most resilient and responsive to change'
>
> Charles Darwin

Personal resilience-promoting factors in the clinical environment

- Effective role-modelling of resilience: openly discuss challenges and how they were addressed
- Cognitive flexibility: demonstrate the ability to cognitively reframe and extract meaning from adverse situations
- High-coping self-efficacy: discuss 'psychological toolkit' to promote self-care in the face of challenging environments
- Strong social support: encourage team bonding, and social support outside work
- Attention to physical health and support needs

Factors that motivate learners to increase satisfaction and performance in the clinical environment

- Autonomy: desire and opportunities to be self-directed, which increases engagement
- Mastery: the urge to get better and better at something that matters, and support to do so
- Purpose: desire to do something that has meaning and is important, and oppprtunities to find and exercise this purpose

❶ The discussion of personal resilience is one piece of the puzzle in relation to improving trainee well-being. ▶ Only making steps to promote personal resilience in harmful environments is futile and can imply that trainees are to blame if/when they cannot cope in the face of extreme environmental difficulties. Educators must also advocate for system-level changes to improve working conditions and environments, or **system** resilience. Recognizing the complexity of wellness and need for system-level change with trainees is important, as is discussing the actions you are taking to advocate for positive change.

Flourishing

Flourishing is a newer concept in medical education, which is gathering pace as a different, more holistic way to discuss wellness with trainees. Given tension surrounding the concept of personal resilience, it may be more fruitful to discuss flourishing with trainees, than to discuss resilience.

There is no consensus definition of flourishing within medical education, but Younie describes flourishing as involving 'authentic connection with our values, meaningful engagement in the world, the pursuit of excellence, and personal growth through challenges'. Where personal resilience is focused solely on individual coping during adversity, flourishing extends beyond survival to encompass a more holistic approach to well-being, accounting for trainees' emotional, intellectual, cultural, access, spiritual etc. needs.

Flourishing-promoting factors in the clinical environment

- Supportive leadership: leadership that values holistic approaches to well-being, that see beyond a focus soley on personal resilience
- Team cohesion: collaborative and supportive teams that encourage open communication, and acknowledge and reward the efforts of team members
- Work-life balance: policies and practices that enable reasonable and accessible scheduling, and flexible working
- Skill development and career progression: supported (including financially supported) opportunities for continuing education and career advancement
- Autonomy: ensuring clinicians have appropriate autonomy in relation to decision-making
- Values-consistent practice: a work environment that aligns with clinicians' ethical beliefs and values, including mission-based values
- Creating spaces for meaningful reflection: creating physical and psychological safe spaces for meaningful reflection (reflection that is not assessed, and may include creative approaches to reflection)

- Inclusivity: an inclusive and diverse environment that values all individuals, that takes meaningful and tangible action to improve working conditions

Challenges of the clinical environment

Teaching in the clinical environment comes with its own set of ❶ challenges:

- Time constraints
- Work demands—teachers maintain other clinical, research, or administrative responsibilities while being called upon to teach
- Often unpredictable and difficult to prepare for
- Engaging multiple levels of learners (students, resident doctors, etc.)
- Patient related challenges: short hospital stays; patients too sick; patients unwilling to participate in teaching encounter
- Lack of incentives and rewards for teaching
- Physical clinical environment not comfortable for teaching
- Culture or chaos of the clinical environment can act as impediment

Further Reading

- Hargreaves DH. *On-the-job training for physicians: a practical guide.* London: Royal Society of Medicine, 1997: xv, 151.
- Pink D. *Drive: the surprising truth about what motivates us.* New York, NY: Riverhead Books, 2009.
- Ramani S, Leinster S. AMEE Guide no. 34: teaching in the clinical environment. *Med Teach* 2008;30:347–364.
- Southwick SM, Charney DS. The science of resilience: implications for the prevention and treatment of depression. *Science* 2012;338:79–82
- Spencer J. Learning and teaching in the clinical environment. *Br Med J* 2003; 326:591–594.
- Younie L. When I say flourishing in medical education. *Br J Holistic Med* 2020;17(2):44–46.

Acute setting

The acute setting provides inherent challenges to effective education and training as distractions and interruptions pose potential obstacles that do not exist in more static educational environments. These interruptions, however, can provide unique opportunities for teachers to model non-technical skills and enhance instruction.

Shadowing

Shadowing a resident doctor on the unit where they will subsequently be working has become a required part of the final year programme for medical students in the UK (termed, 'the assistantship'). Opportunities exist to share in carrying out ward tasks, formulating management plans, and observing good practice. ▶ Active involvement in tasks should be facilitated where possible to enhance learning. Opportunities to reflect and debrief on experiences while shadowing are also important both for trainee well-being, and for highlighting learning needs, and can be done informally.

Case-based

Real-time case-based teaching provides the opportunity for clinical teachers to demonstrate the thought processes that are involved in clinical reasoning. Adult learning theory suggests that learning is best accomplished by repeated, deliberate exposure to real cases, with the participation of a teacher to augment the value of the educational experience. Real cases often reflect the false leads, the polymorphisms of actual clinical material, and the misleading test results encountered in everyday practice. This fosters the teaching and learning of the diagnostic process, the complex trade-offs between the benefits and risks of diagnostic tests and treatments, and cognitive errors in clinical reasoning. It emphasizes the uncertainty that is rife in the clinical environment.

Supervised learning

Supervised learning events are designed to highlight achievements and areas of excellence, provide immediate feedback, suggest areas for further development, and demonstrate engagement in the educational process. Trainees may be required to complete a minimum number of supervised learning events spread evenly throughout their placements, with different trainers and covering diverse acute and long-term clinical problems. Some training programmes have now removed minimum numbers, in favour of a competency-based approach, but the need to demonstrate breadth of clinical experience through supervised learning events remains.

Further reading

◉ Kassirer JP. Teaching clinical reasoning: case-based and coached. *Acad Med* 2010;85(7):1118–1124.

Bedside teaching

Bedside teaching has always been one of the main pillars for clinical learning, epitomizing the classic view of medical training. Before beginning, it is important that the team is introduced to the patient with an explanation that the encounter is primarily intended for teaching and that certain theoretical discussions may not apply to their illness.

Small group bedside teaching

Preparation
- Patients: Invite to participate without coercion and with opportunity to decline. Consideration must be given to patients needs and possibility that other healthcare staff or visitors may need to see them.
- Students: Between two and five students is optimal number. Students should comply with appropriate professional appearance and behaviour. Some may feel intimidated by an unfamiliar environment and fearful of criticism of inadequacies and may position themselves towards the back to avoid participation, while more confident students dominate conversation. An observant tutor will be aware of this behaviour, redressing the balance to ensuring all participate.
- Tutors: Consultant staff, resident doctors, nurses, or student peers.

Orientation and introduction
Orientate learners and introduce everyone, including the patient.

Interaction and observation
Role-model a doctor-patient interaction. Watch how the students are proceeding. ❗ Avoid demonstrating inappropriate 'shortcuts'.

Models of bedside teaching
- Demonstrator model: the clinical tutor demonstrates aspect of the case history and physical examination to the students.
- Tutor model: the clinical tutor stands to the side and critiques each student in turn as they enquire into aspects of the history and carry out aspects of the physical examination.
- Observer model: the clinical tutor stands back from the student-patient interaction and observes, providing feedback at the end.
- Report-back model: students take a history and examination without supervision and report back to the tutor in a separate room.

Instruction and summary
Provide instruction and tell the students what they have been taught.

Debriefing and feedback
Answer questions, provide clarifications, and engage in feedback.

Reflection
Evaluate what went well and what was less successful.

Further reading

➲ Ramani S. Twelve tips to improve bedside teaching. *Med Teach* 2003;25:112–115.

Ward teaching

Teams often represent a diverse group of people (multi-departmental and multi-professional) with varying levels of clinical experience creating a wide range of learner expectations.

It is essential ∴ on the first day of a student's placement or rotation to establish clear expectations for knowledge, technical skills, presentation style, and feedback. A clear description of the responsibilities for each team member (clinical and educational) encourages team bonding, prevents frustration, and optimizes teaching.

Ward-based teaching

Ward-based teaching forms one of the central pillars of clinical medicine, yet students often struggle to maximize the vast array of opportunities presented to them. With a multitude of healthcare professionals and patients who are often willing to aid medical students and trainees, a placement on a ward, regardless of specialty, is a chance for students to immerse themselves and engage in a fruitful experience. ∴ it is not only an important place to aid clinical knowledge and awareness, but also an opportunity to appreciate the organizational processes that take place to enable the smooth-running of the hospital.

Opportunities:
- Practice examinations
- Improve history-taking skills
- Refine clinical competencies
- Develop teamwork and professional attributes

Questions to ask before each teaching encounter:
- What do you hope to accomplish?
- What is your point of view?
- How will your learners be engaged?
- How will you meet the needs of each learner?
- How will rounds be organized?
- How will you make the time?

Challenges of ward-based teaching
- Can be difficult to set and meet teaching goals, as unanticipated events occur frequently, and the round may be too busy
- Ward team often composed of varying levels of learners
- Patients too sick or unwilling to participate in teaching encounter
- Patient stays are too short to follow natural history of disease, or to follow patient journey through and across care settings
- Teachers could compromise trainee-patient relationship if they dominate the encounter
- Trainees and teachers may feel insecure about admitting errors in front of the patient and the rest of the medical team
- Tendency by many clinical teachers to lecture rather than practice interactive teaching
- Engaging all learners simultaneously can be difficult
- Teachers need to pay close attention to learner fatigue, boredom, and workload

Business ward round

This is a challenging activity for both clinicians and students. Little time is available for formal teaching, observing student performance, or providing feedback.

Teaching ward round

This specially created ward round is aimed at taking students to a small number of selected patients to provide opportunities for them to see physical signs and hear aspects of the case history.

Patient allocation models

Students attached to a ward for a period to time can be allocated a certain number of patients, each of whom they initially admit and then follow throughout their time in the hospital. They are made responsible for presenting them on ward rounds, and opportunities exist for them to practice examination and communication skills. Patients can be followed to investigations and to surgery, and even visited at home on discharge so the student can assess the impact of illness and sociodemographic aspects of healthcare. This is easier to achieve in models of clinical education which are more longitudinal in design, where students have longer periods of time based with your clinical team and can experience the continuity of responsibility and care this brings (e.g. within placements known as 'Longitudinal Integrated Clerkships').

▶ Upside-down ward round

In this model the supervising doctor takes on the role traditionally given to the most junior member of the team (e.g., the note-taker) and everyone else in the team reverses their roles. This allows the most junior members of the team to practice their communication and clinical skills in a setting that is supportive and safe. Importantly this model provides an excellent opportunity for junior members of the team to practice and build leadership skills and inherently builds a culture of psychological safety where any member of the team can do any task.

Further reading

⮑ Bharamgoudar R, Sonsale A. Twelve tips for medical students to make the best use of ward-based learning. *Med Teach* 2017;39(11):1119–1122.

⮑ Ende J. What if Osler were one of us? Inpatient teaching today. *J Gen Intern Med* 1997;12(Suppl 2):S41–48.

Handover

Handing over responsibility for patients has always been part of medical practice. While definitions tend to focus on the transfer of responsibility to ensure effective continuity of care and patient safety, handover also epitomizes a time when teams meet, have the opportunity to communicate, support each other, and learn. There is huge potential educational value for handover, which often occurs several times a day in the clinical setting.

Handover as an educational activity

Planned

Unlike many areas of clinical practice, handover is a predictable part of the day which makes it more amenable to planning for learning than, for example, practical medical emergencies.

Encompasses action, reflection, extrapolation, and planning

Handover should include summarizing cases, reporting clinical assessments, investigations, completed and planned actions, and formulating plans for the shift ahead. There may also be opportunities to explore theoretical extrapolations (what if I had managed the patient this way instead of that?). It mirrors models, such as Kolb's learning cycle.

Longitudinal

Patients are often presented in the morning and again in the afternoon with discussion on the progression of the situation. This gives real potential for developmental learning. ►The challenge is to maximize these opportunities and develop strategies for when key learners (such as those who worked overnight) are not at the next handover.

Useful

Trainees need to feel the learning in handover has benefited them and their learning needs. This is a key principle of adult learning theory.

Meaningful

In making learning meaningful there needs to be alignment between the aims of what the individual or department is trying to teach, what the trainee feels they need, what actually happens, and how it is assessed—so-called ► constructive alignment. If trainees find that either their discussions are curtailed or that raising such issues is seen as demonstrating a lack of clinical confidence, they will become disillusioned. If they put thought and effort into a handover that is then rushed or cancelled, they will become resentful.

Communication

Represents an ideal opportunity for trainees to be taught the operational and communication skills of handing over: prioritizing of information, summarizing, presenting and questioning skills.

Further reading

➲ Klaber RE, Macdougall CF. Maximising learning opportunities in handover. *Arch Dis Child Educ Pract Ed* 2009;94:118–122.

Ambulatory care setting

Ambulatory care refers to any place where patients are seen without being admitted as inpatients. It provides many unique educational opportunities for learners, including more complete observation of chronic diseases, closer relationships between teachers and learners, and a more appropriate forum for teaching preventative medicine, medical interviewing, and psychosocial aspects of disease.

Training in ambulatory care centres includes a variety of training sites depending on the health system of the country, but includes treatments limited to hospitals and outpatient clinics, general practitioners' clinics, and primary healthcare centres, etc.

Home visits

A unique example of an ambulatory care setting is the patient's own home. Care of the patient in their own home used to be reserved for those who were unable to attend a clinic. ▶ Since the COVID-19 pandemic, and the advances in communication technology, many patients now access healthcare from home (and in other settings, such as work, school, or when travelling) through telephone, video conference, and sending photographs through SMS or email (e.g. of skin conditions).

Ambulatory care teaching settings

- Routine outpatient clinics
- Community/General Practice clinics (which include routine and urgent appointments)
- Multi-professional clinics where staff from a variety of disciplines see patients together
- Teaching clinics
- Accident and emergency departments
- Clinical investigation units, e.g. endoscopy suite
- Radiology and imaging suites
- Nurse-led clinics, e.g. for pre-assessment of surgical admissions
- Day surgery unit
- Dialysis unit
- Patient's home (home visit)

▶ Benefits of teaching in ambulatory care settings

- Outpatient facilities can offer large numbers of patients with common medical conditions who are not acutely unwell
- More space is usually available
- Often able to select patients appropriate for the students' stage of learning
- Increased student numbers can be accommodated
- Health education can be emphasized

❶ Challenges of teaching in ambulatory care settings

Ambulatory care settings are often busy and chaotic with very short teacher-learner interactions, with service requirements often outweighing teaching requirements.

- Busy clinical setting

- Teaching time often short, no time for elaborate teaching
- No control over distribution and organization of time
- Attending to several patients at the same time with multiple learners
- Brief teacher-trainee interactions
- Patient care demands usually take priority and must be addressed
- Multiple patient problems must be addressed simultaneously, so teachers cannot focus on one problem to teach
- Learning and service take place concurrently
- Organic and psychosocial problems are intertwined
- Diagnostic questions often settled by follow up of empiric treatment
- Teacher should be a guide and facilitator than information provider

Leaner-centred outpatient model (SNAPPS)

Wolpaw et al. (2003) described a model for learner-centred outpatient teaching where learners are equal (if not the leaders) of the teaching interaction.

Summarize briefly the history and physical exam findings
The learner obtains a history, performs an appropriate examination of a patient, and presents a concise summary to the teacher.

Narrow the differential diagnosis
For a new patient encounter, the learner presents two or three reasonable diagnostic possibilities. For follow-up or sick visits, the differential may focus on why the patient's disease is active, what therapeutic interventions might be considered, or relevant preventive health strategies. The formulation of the differential list will be driven by the learner's baseline knowledge.

Analyse the differential diagnosis
The learner should compare and contrast diagnostic possibilities and discriminatory findings. This discussion allows the learner to verbalize his or her thinking process and clinical reasoning and can stimulate an interactive discussion with the teacher.

Probe teacher by asking questions about uncertainties, difficulties, or alternative approaches
The learner initiates an educational discussion by probing the teacher with questions rather than waiting for the teacher to initiate the probing of the learner. The learner is taught to utilize the teacher as a knowledge resource that can readily be accessed.

Plan management for patients' medical issues
The learner initiates a discussion of patient management with the teacher and must attempt either a brief management plan or suggest specific interventions.

Select a case-related issue for self-directed learning
The learner may identify a learning issue at the end of the patient presentation or after seeing the patient with the teacher. The learner should check with the teacher to focus the reading and frame relevant questions.

Further reading

⬥ McGee SR, Irby DM. Teaching in the outpatient clinic. Practical tips. *J Gen Int Med* 1997;12(Suppl 2):S34–40.
⬥ Wolpaw TM, Wolpaw DR, Papp KK. SNAPPS: a learner-centred model for outpatient education. *Acad Med* 2003;78:893–898.

The clinic

Outpatient clinics offer trainees one of the most varied clinical experiences within the hospital setting where trainees can learn both technical aspects of practice and professional attributes. Learning in outpatient clinics is patient focused, as a scheduled clinic is usually made up of new or review patients or a mixture of both. There is usually a large number of patients attending with common clinical problems, but additional space for teaching may be limited.

Opportunities exist for students to: see patients independently; observe decision-making and the selection of appropriate investigations; be supervised in communication and examination skills; attempt simple practical procedures.

▶ Independent learning can be encouraged if sufficient rooms are available for students to see patients at their own pace and effective, one-on-one tuition is possible.

❶ Heavy service commitment can place time constraints on clinicians who are under pressure to see high volume of patients.

Clinical teaching model

Supervisors need to be aware of the importance of being a good role model, as trainees can pick up many hidden messages about clinical practice from their trainer. McGee and Irby describe practical tips for efficient teaching in the outpatient settings.

▶ *Prepare for the visit*

Define the learner's specific role in the clinic, outlining: the number of patients the learner should see; the time to spend with each patient; the parts of the physical examination to perform; the content and form of written note and case presentation; how to review the medical record efficiently; and when and how to consult the teacher.

Teaching during the visit

Ask questions

Show interest in the learner's thoughts and encourage the learner's clinical reasoning. Questions are a quick way to diagnose strengths and shortcomings to target teaching. Effective questions usually begin with a request for analysis of the case: 'What do you think is going on?' 'What would you like to do?' followed by request for supporting evidence: 'Why do you think that?'.

Select one specific teaching point

One useful technique is to consider the central question: 'What one teaching point do I want the learner to leave this patient's encounter with?'

Modelling

▶ When there are time constraints, modelling can help keep patients flowing through a busy clinic efficiently. The teacher simply thinks out loud, shares clinical hunches and insights, points out controversial issues, or provides a rationale for what to accomplish during the visit. It is important to specifically tell the learner what behaviour or technique to observe during modelling.

Provide feedback

Teaching after the visit

Answer questions that arise from specific patient problems, clarify what learners did not understand, refer to literature, and create reading assignments.

Clinic letter writing

Clinic letter writing is an important communication tool in the hospital out-patient setting, serving as a record of the consultation for the hospital, confirming the information gathered and the agreed outcome with the patient, and communicating progress to other healthcare professionals, such as the general practitioner, involved in the patient's care. Clinic provides an opportunity for this skill to be role-modelled, practiced, and refined. It is an essential skill for efficient, safe practice and develops the learner's clinical knowledge, management planning, and written communication.

Communicating advice

Increasingly, communicating advice occurs across modes of contact, including designated pathways between primary, secondary, and tertiary care units set-up through email to offer helplines for patient care. These can be used as valuable supervised learning events, where the trainee can draft responses to the provider and then go through the drafts with a supervisor who is able to give feedback, directly and immediately, regarding content, communication, resource suggestions, and phrasing. This not only serves to provide good service, but also promotes good learning: the perfect synergy between patient-centred care and student-centred education.

Further reading

➲ Williamson J. Teaching and learning in outpatient clinics. *Clin Teach* 2012;9:304–307.

Post-clinic learning and debrief

Bloom's taxonomy is presented here as a structured debrief approach which encourages learners to reflect on their experiences through demonstrating different levels of their understanding.

Questions to clarify concepts

Knowledge
- What is the nature of this?
- What exactly does this mean?

Comprehension
- Can you give me an example?
- What do we already know about this?
- How does this relate to what we have been talking about?

Questions to probe for rationale, reasons, or evidence

Application
- Can you give me an example of that?
- How do you know this?

Analysis
- Why is that happening?
- What do you think causes that?
- What evidence is there to support what you are saying?
- How does ___ affect ___?
- Then what would happen?

Questions to explore implications and consequences

Evaluation
- Why is that important?
- How does that fit with what we learned before?
- What are the implications of that?

Synthesize
- Based on the history and physical, can you put this together for me?
- What do we need to know to take care of Mrs Smith today?

Further reading

➲ Bloom BS, Englehart MD, Furst EJ, Hill WH, Krathwohl DR. *The taxonomy of educational objectives, handbook I: the cognitive domain*. New York: David McKay Co., Inc., 1956.

Opportunistic learning events

Clinical practice is rife with unpredictability. ▶ For many students the development of the ability to accept uncertainty and deal with it effectively is one of the most difficult adaptational tasks they face. Training for competence in routine situations is insufficient, trainees need to be equipped to contend with the myriad, unpredictable, non-routine situations they will confront in clinical practice. When unexpected events occur, they can provide an ideal opportunity to teach and model these skills—both in the moment, and in debriefing after the event.

Impromptu sessions

Impromptu sessions are flexible educational activities in response to an issue identified. They should be focused, cover one to two teaching points, and relate to the issue at hand. If possible, further reading suggestions should be provided.

Learning to embrace uncertainty

Clinical uncertainty is inherent to medicine. Doctors continually make decisions based on imperfect data and limited knowledge, which leads to diagnostic uncertainty, coupled with the uncertainty that arises from unpredictable patient responses to treatment and from healthcare outcomes that are far from binary. Unfortunately, we have an educational system that prioritizes and rewards certainty, and a culture in healthcare that too often equates uncertainty with ignorance or failure. The clinical environment provides an ideal setting to openly acknowledge and discuss uncertainty. Learning to recognize and becoming familiar with uncertainty is now highlighted as a core competency for students.

Tips to help learners embrace uncertainty

- Ask questions that focus on 'how' and 'why', not 'what' and 'when'— stimulating discussion that embraces the greyscale aspects of human health and illness, aspects that cannot be neatly categorized.
- Encourage learners' curiosity to explore and capacity to sit comfortably with uncertainty.
- Acknowledge that certainty is not always the end goal.
- Be explicit about the level of uncertainty.
- Speak about 'hypotheses' not 'diagnoses', changing expectations of certainty.
- Role model embracing the inherent uncertainty of clinical medicine.

'Medicine is a science of uncertainty and an art of probability'—Osler

Further reading

➲ Simpkin AL, Schwartzstein RM. Tolerating uncertainty—the next medical revolution? *NEJM* 2016;375(18):1713–1715.

➲ Veen M, Brown M. The serious healer: developing an ethic of ambiguity within health professions education, pp. 39–53. In: Brown M, Veen M, Finn GM (Eds), *Applied philosophy for health professions education: a journey towards mutual understanding*. Singapore: Springer, 2022.

Technology

Many learners have grown up in an age of technological convenience, with exposure to technology and electronic devices from the first day of life. Patient-centred use of technology should be an intentional part of core curricula to prepare physicians to use technology in meaningful ways.

Artificial intelligence

The arrival of artificial intelligence, deep learning, and forms of automation such as robotics are already transforming healthcare and education. The likelihood of further advances warrants thought in our clinical teaching as to what human health professionals will be doing in an age of thinking machines. ▶The importance of metacognition, situational awareness, and other higher human cognitive functions should be enhanced and focused on in teaching to facilitate safe and productive computer-human interactions.

Role of social media

The age of the internet has seen an explosion in online platforms to support and augment medical education. Instant messaging applications, online forums and networks, podcasts, and blogs are frequently used to share clinical teaching points, disseminate evidence-based medicine, and circulate materials to trainees. Increasingly medical schools and training programmes are using social media, although widescale adoption is still in early stages. By following physicians, journals, and institutions of interest, medical professionals can use social media as an efficient mechanism to receive relevant, high-yield content. There are, of course, challenges of data privacy, security concerns, time demands, misinformation concerns, and technology issues in implementing social media-based curricula. The usage of social media in continuing medical education is likely to become increasingly worthwhile as technology-savvy physicians enter the profession.

Eye-tracking as a training method

Oculomotor and eye gaze training as a teaching method was introduced in 2011 by Wilson et al. This enables expert-like gaze strategies highlighting critical areas of interest to be taught to novice learners and can lead to rapid improvement in task performance, particularly for procedural skills. In addition, gaze behaviour differences found between experts and novices can help guide development of training programs.

Further reading

⮕ Chan TM, Dzara K, Dimeo SP, Bhalerao A, Maggio LA. Social media in knowledge translation and education for physicians and trainees: a scoping review. *Perspect Med Educ* 2020;9:20–30.

⮕ Wilson MR, Vine SJ, Bright E, Masters RSW, Defriend D, McGrath JS. Gaze training enhances laparoscopic technical skill acquisition and multi-tasking performance: a randomised, controlled study. *Surg Endosc* 2011;25:3731–3739.

Theory in medical education

*Megan E.L. Brown, Matthew H.V. Byrne,
Helen R. Church, and Gabrielle M. Finn*

Introduction: Why is theory important?

'Experience without theory is blind, but theory without experience is mere intellectual play'

Immanuel Kant, Kritik der reinen Vernunft, 2nd Edition, Hoover translation, 1787

The philosopher Immanuel Kant is frequently quoted in support of the necessary balance between theory and practice. Though theory is seen by many as inaccessible and dense, only necessary within the ivory towers of academia, it is a way of making sense of the world that is extremely useful for both academics and practitioners alike.

For clinical teachers, theory helps cast light on why some approaches to teaching work, and others don't. Theory can give us something to aim towards, it can be an ideal that we design our teaching sessions and materials in pursuit of. Theory also provides us with a common language—a way of communicating with one another about why we have chosen to make certain educational choices, or why we do things in a certain way. ▶ Theory can also be practical. We can use theory to design, describe, and evaluate teaching and learning, and this helps increase the impact of research—your work is more likely to be wide-reaching, and international. Theories also help us to develop a body of knowledge, through which we can become increasingly evidence based.

The orientation of learning theory is towards practice. It should help us to understand how and why learning occurs, what the influence of various approaches to teaching and education are, and how to improve our practice to facilitate learning. Theory can help us to learn from the past, and to make predictions about the future. It helps us focus on how the choices we make might influence learners.

Educational theory (or theory which helps us to make sense of teaching and learning) speaks a different language to clinical medicine. Ways of thinking and viewing the world differ within medical education. Medical education is interdisciplinary in that it draws on theory and perspectives from a diverse range of fields (including sociology, psychology, philosophy, and the arts and humanities). Each of these disciplines have their own established traditions—their own respectable ways of viewing knowledge creation, reality, and the connections between teaching and learning. It can be overwhelming for a novice, or an early-career educator, to know where to start when it comes to educational theory, especially theory that seems to be written in an alien style, using an entirely different vocabulary.

The purpose of this chapter is to give you a grounding in the language of educational theory and offer an overview of common theoretical traditions used to conceptualize learning within health professions education. In doing so, we hope to help you create mental building-blocks, on which you can base theory use in later chapters of this book.

What is theory?

Theory is challenging to define, and ● scholars don't agree on its definition. How theory is viewed and used depends on the backgrounds and beliefs of the scholars that use the theory. However, within medical education, foundational work within the past decade has brought together variations in vocabulary and background and led to the creation of a now widely used definition.

Varpio et al.[1] define theory within medical education as concerning the connections between constructs and propositions (Box 2.1).

Simply put, theories explain the relationships between concepts. Concepts are ideas that describe particular events, objects, conditions, situations, people, or behaviour. Concepts can be defined through common experiences, by a discipline through research, or can be borrowed from other disciplines. In education, examples can include emotion, culture, community, etc.

Propositions, which are also mentioned in Varpio et al.'s definition, are statements which may be true or false, but not both. Propositions are sentences which declare a fact. ► Theories, in other words, should make claims of fact about concepts, and the ways in which they connect.

Two common concepts within medical education are the event of transition (e.g. between ward environments when a junior doctor moves jobs, or between medical school and practice as a new doctor), and the condition of well-being. A theory of how transition influences doctor well-being would have to explain the relationship between (make propositions about) these two concepts.

Karl Popper famously argued that theories should be falsifiable,[2] i.e. they propose something that can be tested. ► Varpio et al. also draw attention to the need for empirical support for learning theory within medical education—'the more data supporting the theory, the stronger it becomes'.[1] Continuing efforts within medical education research test theory in a variety of contexts, offering new insights on its use and limitations within our field. It is important to note that by 'testing' and 'data' in relation to theory, we do not mean that theory can be tested in a lab, or even a randomized controlled trial, settings in which we might be most familiar with these terms. The data we use to 'test' theories can be quantitative but is most usually *qualitative*—it consists of in-depth interview transcripts, field notes, diaries, videos, and images.

Box 2.1 A definition of theory in medical education

'A theory is a set of propositions that are logically related, expressing the relation(s) among several different constructs and propositions.'

Varpio L, Paradis E, Uijtdehaage S, Young M. The distinctions between theory, theoretical framework, and conceptual framework. *Acad Med* 2020;95(7):989.

Explanatory power

As explanations of how things work, theories can be classified according to 'explanatory power':

- Theory may be 'grand', i.e. when it attempts to explain a large social landscape. Grand theory provides an overall framework for structuring one's ideas about teaching and learning, or one's research;
- 'Mid-range', i.e. when theory seeks to connect high-level social theory to more specific aspects of human interaction. ▶ Middle-range theory can be useful when suggesting interventions within education or health and social care. Middle-range theories are used with particular frequency within medical education;
- 'Micro' when theory concerns individual-level phenomena or limited aspects of social organization. Micro-level theoretical framing is mostly provided by concepts. Micro-level theory will most likely concern an individual concept, like 'well-being', without exploring the connections between that concept and any other concept. However, micro-level theory should still make propositions about that concept that add to the understanding of how the concept is experienced or manifests. There may be limited reference to social organization or social structures.

Grand, mid-range, and micro-level theory exist on a continuum, where the increasingly grand a theory is, the more it can make abstract claims about teaching and learning that might fundamentally shift the way we think. However, these abstract claims are difficult to act on. The more micro-level a theory, the more it can make specific recommendations for changes in practice, but the less widely applicable the theory and these recommendations are. For an illustration of this continuum, see Figure 2.1.

See Box 2.2 for an example of a grand theory, a middle-range theory, and a micro-theory (and a brief description of each).

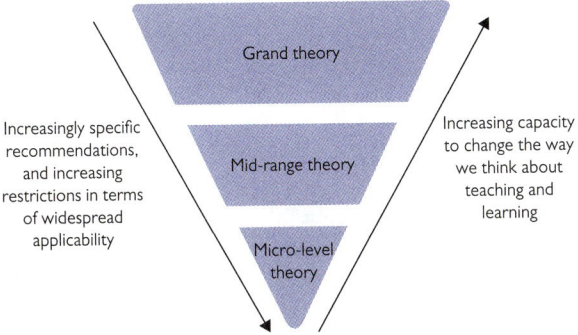

Increasingly specific recommendations, and increasing restrictions in terms of widespread applicability

Grand theory

Mid-range theory

Micro-level theory

Increasing capacity to change the way we think about teaching and learning

Fig. 2.1 The continuum of grand, mid-range, and micro-level theory. No permissions necessary.

Box 2.2 Examples of explanatory levels of theory

Grand theory—an abstract explanation of the uniformities of social be-haviour, organization, and change comprising definitions, concepts, variables, statements, and theoretical concepts, e.g. Theory of Human Caring—caring is a fundamental human need which involves connecting on a deep level to promote well-being and healing.

Middle-range theory—concepts (well-being, healing, etc.) plus variables (sex, class, race, role) and statements of fact or propositions (made up of concepts and variables): e.g. Healthcare professionals can promote patient well-being by providing holistic care attentive to patients' physical, emotional, social, and spiritual needs.

Micro-level theory—an exploration of singular concepts (e.g. healing), with reference to limited aspects of social organization: e.g. 'Healing in the con-text of pressure sores means improving patient comfort as well as promoting tissue care'.

(Adapted from Grbich, 2012[3])

Theory in research

Within evaluation of teaching and learning, and within medical education research, ▶ theory helps us anchor our findings in what is already known about a phenomenon or experience. Theory offers a common language, using which we can communicate the impact or importance of our approach to teaching and learning, or the findings of our research. Theory can be a starting point for medical education research—you can set out to 'test' or explore the relevance of a theory within a particular context—or be an aid to data analysis and interpretation, applied as a lens through which you view your findings, and discuss their importance.

Theory or paradigm?

It is important to note that the terms 'theory' and 'paradigm' differ.

Paradigms are sets of assumptions, values, beliefs, and practices that, together, form one way of viewing the world. They are typically shared by members of a community and inform how we view and discuss reality, and knowledge, and so how we believe we come to know about experiences and our environment. Within medical education, they are most frequently discussed within research, and so Chapter 10 explores the term paradigm, and the different paradigms common within medical education, further.

Theories differ in that they can be tested, and can be used to make predictions about teaching, learning, and various phenomena. They help us to explain the connections between what we observe, rather than tell us how we might go about observing those connections in the first place.

What are paradigms?

Paradigms inform how we view and use theories within medical education. Certain theories may have come about within the tradition (the ways of viewing reality and knowledge) of a particular paradigm. Though paradigms and theories differ, they are connected (Figure 2.2). We can add paradigms to our continuum of grand, mid-range, and micro-level theory as a foundational lens, through which we view and use theory.

Given this connection, ▶ it's important that we reflect on our own ways of viewing reality and knowledge before we use, and while using, theory. To align oneself with an established paradigm (school of thought on the nature of reality and knowledge) within medical education, one must consider their axiology, ontology, and epistemology.

- **Axiology**: what you value. Reflecting on axiology helps you to consider what you think ought to be within education and research. These ideas and values inform your practice as an educator, and any research you undertake.
- **Ontology**: assumptions you make regarding the nature of reality. We all make these assumptions, even if we don't consciously reflect on them. There are two broad ontological positions—realism and relativism.
  - Ontological realists believe that there is one reality—it exists irrespective of individuals' awareness and knowledge. This reality is driven by causal mechanisms that research attempts to unearth.
  - Ontological relativists believe that reality is subjective and that multiple realities exist. Any perception of reality—of right and

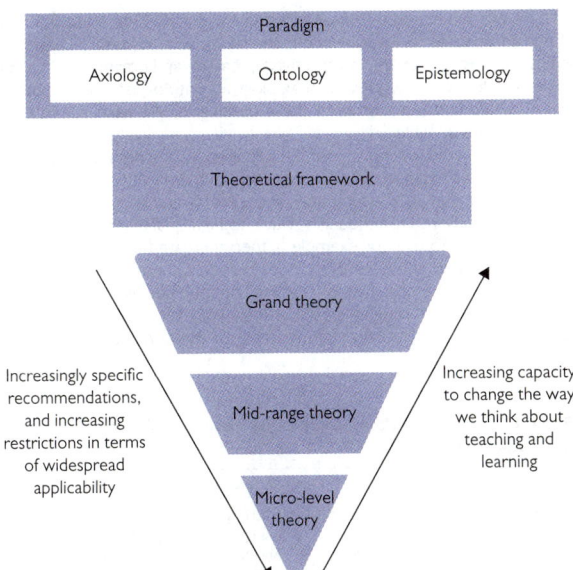

Fig. 2.2 The relationship between paradigms and theories. For more on theoretical frameworks, see Chapter 10 on Research, Evaluation, and Scholarship. No permissions necessary.

wrong, of causal mechanisms—are products bound intrinsically to their historical, social, and cultural contexts.

- **Epistemology**: assumptions you make regarding the nature of knowledge. Ask yourself: what is knowledge, and how is knowledge acquired? Three epistemological positions exist—objectivism, subjectivism, and constructionism.
  - Objectivism is the view that knowledge exists independent of human consciousness. Knowledge is absolute and, as such, causes, effects, and explanations are discoverable through careful research.
  - Subjectivism is the view that knowledge of human behaviour depends wholly on reconstructing the understanding that those performing the behaviour have. Meaning within subjectivism is individualistic—to understand human behaviour ∴ you must appreciate the meaning individuals uniquely assign to their actions and the world around them.
  - Constructionism is the view that social contexts are fundamental to the formation and acquisition of knowledge. Individuals and groups participate in the creation of knowledge. This knowledge is socially situated, contextually bound, and ever evolving as social interactions continue to occur.

There are five commonly used paradigms within medical education that inform approaches to teaching and research we wish to detail. These are: positivism, post-positivism, interpretivism, realism, and pragmatism. So that you can reflect on how your own axiological, ontological, and epistemological positions might align with these paradigms, we have summarized these positions in Table 2.1.

Having reflected on how your beliefs align with common paradigms within medical education, you are ready to use theory in a consistent way. ▶ Making sure that your assumptions about reality and knowledge are consistent in the way you use theory is critical to high-quality research.

If you choose to use, for example, a theory created by an interpretivist author (such as communities of practice theory, a theory which describes how newcomers become part of learning communities over time), but approach this theory through a positivist lens, your research findings would be confusing. It's not possible or desirable to measure participation in a

Table 2.1 Orientation of common paradigms within medical education. Adapted from Brown and Dueñas[4]

Paradigm	Axiology	Ontology	Epistemology
Positivism	All inquiry should be value-free, positivists should reflect on their values to make themselves as neutral as possible	There is a single, objective reality, observable through science	Neutral knowledge can be obtained through reliable and valid measurement tools
Post-positivism	All inquiry should be as value-free as possible, post-positivism should reflect on their values to minimize inevitable bias	There is a single, objective reality, only ever known imperfectly	Obtaining knowledge is subject to human error and interpretation—∴ only probable truths can be established
Interpretivism	Research is value-bound, a researcher is part of what is being researched or explored. All exploration is guided and influenced by researcher position and values	There are multiple, subjective realities, each of which is socially constructed by and between individuals or groups	Knowledge is subjective and formed at the individual or group level. There is not one knowledge, rather multiple ways of knowing or 'knowledges' that are socioculturally bound

Table 2.1 (Contd.)

Paradigm	Axiology	Ontology	Epistemology
Realism	All inquiry should pursue theories which are true. Realist exploration focuses on values—values are driven by mechanisms (which connect context, and outcomes), and can act as mechanisms	There is a real world, independent of our interpretations of it (though there are multiple, legitimate interpretations). The real world is driven by mechanisms, which may or may not be	Knowledge is socially and individually constructed, there is no such thing as a final truth or knowledge, as reality constrains our interpretations of it
Pragmatism	Values outcomes, all inquiry should attempt to solve practical problems of interest/ importance using the most practical and efficient approach	Pragmatism is not committed to a fixed ontology. The nature of reality is created and changes as individuals interact with the world. Reality is orientated towards solving practical problems	Pragmatism is not committed to a fixed epistemology. Knowledge is created and changes as individuals interact with the world. Knowledge creation should be directed towards solving practical problems

community of practice (a positivist approach), as this isn't the purpose of interpretivist theory, which aims, instead, to cast light on the rich experiences of individuals and groups within social contexts. At best, research or evaluation which uses theory within a different paradigm is confusing, at worst it is misleading and may lead authors to make inappropriate educational recommendations.

Theory in teaching and learning

How educators structure a teaching session, or create a learning environment depends, to some extent, on their view of learners and learning. Educational theory helps us to describe our views in these domains.

There are many theories on the topic of teaching and learning that attempt to explain how learning works, and why in various contexts. It is not the intention of this chapter to offer an overview of all of these theories, you will see that descriptions of key theories and explanations regarding their relevance to various topics (e.g. Miller's pyramid, which proposes a framework for assessing clinical competence thereby explaining the connections between competence and assessment) are interspersed throughout the chapters of this book. What you will likely note is that the theories explored throughout are either mid-range, or micro-level. Miller's pyramid, for example, is a mid-range theory.

Here, we offer an overview of the five most common *grand* theories within medical education that inform teaching and learning strategy. These grand theories have been developed through thoughtful appraisal of teaching and learning over many years. They direct thinking in our field, and the mid-range and micro-level theories we use are encompassed by these abstract perspectives on the goals and structure of medical education. It is ∴ critical that we appreciate the differences between these perspectives, and how they shape the theory we might be more familiar with.

Five common grand theories of learning

The five common grand theories of learning we have chosen to discuss are: behaviourism; cognitivism; constructivism; humanism; and socioculturalism.

Behaviourism

Behaviourism is learning through reinforcement. It is a grand theory of learning based on the idea that all behaviours are acquired through conditioning, and that conditioning occurs through interaction with one's environment. You might be most familiar with the term 'conditioning' from Pavlov's famous dog experiment (Figure 2.3) which, in 1890, marked the beginning of behaviourism as we know it.[5] Classical conditioning refers to the learning that occurs when a neutral stimulus comes to be associated with a stimulus that produces a certain behaviour. Pavlov saw that dogs began salivating while looking at the helpers who usually brought their food and began experimenting with associating other facets of the dog's environment with feeding (e.g. the sound of a bell), so that eventually the dogs would salivate at the sound of a bell. Pavlov's thinking on conditioning became the basis of current behaviourist learning theories, which emphasize how one's environment facilitates learning.

▶ Educational behaviourists discuss positive and negative reinforcement as ways of shaping student behaviour. This is a type of conditioning known as *operant* conditioning. Positive reinforcement is the use of rewards or praise to encourage good behaviour, while negative reinforcement is the use of punishment to decrease poor behaviour. Behaviourist educators are trainers, and this is an approach commonly used within skills-based instruction, e.g. cannula insertion. Repetition and practice (e.g. of cannulation)

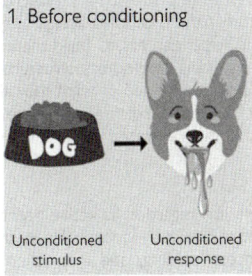

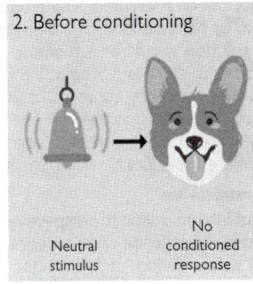

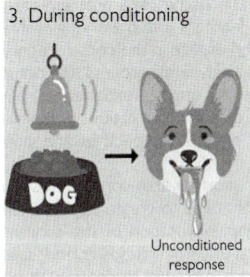

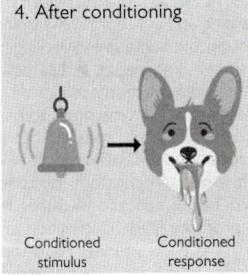

Fig. 2.3 Conditioning explained using Pavlov's famous dog experiment. No permissions necessary.

with feedback (which includes reinforcement) as students practise are critical to learning.

Behaviourists believe that only observable behaviour should be studied (such as Pavlov's dog's salivation), as thoughts and emotions are subjective and, so, of little use.

Cognitivism

Cognitivism is learning through knowing. It is a grand learning theory that describes how knowledge is received, structured, stored, and recalled by the mind. ∴ Learning, for cognitivists, is an internal, mental process, where learners actively make sense of information. Learner personality, motivation, and ability all influence learning.

The most common approach to cognitivist instruction is the traditional lecture. The assumption within a cognitivist approach is that learning can be done within large groups, because how information is organized and presented is what is important, rather than interaction. ▶ It is an educator's job to provide tools that help learners process information cognitively. Material (e.g. lecture slides) should be logical and clear to follow.

Information presented in different formats helps (e.g. providing a transcript and/or handout alongside delivering a lecture) and promotes accessibility. Instruction should be structured so that it helps learners to build mental models to store and process information (e.g. using mnemonics, structured ways of delivering content). Learners should be reminded of what they already know, so that they will connect new learning to existing knowledge.

Advice on how to manage cognitive load (a theory rooted in cognitivism) is offered specifically within Chapter 12.

Constructivism

Within constructivist perspectives, learners are regarded as active agents in the construction of knowledge. Knowledge is built by individual learners on a foundation of their prior experiences, learning, and interactions. Constructivism refutes the cognitivist notion that knowledge is something that can be delivered and received—rather, it is something that has to be actively constructed by learners.

As a result, constructivism underpins approaches like problem-based learning and collaborative learning, where learners (often working in small groups, but sometimes working individually) engage in the construction of their own knowledge. ▶ Learning is seen as a dynamic process that occurs as individuals actively reflect on their past and ongoing experiences, perspectives, and interactions, to make sense of new information. Given this, understanding and meaning can shift over time as perspectives and interactions continue to change and evolve.

It is not an educator's job to lecture or inform within constructivist approaches to education—rather, ▶ educators need to create opportunities to promote learner reflection and the deep exploration of the concepts they are encountering. Educators encourage learner curiosity and questioning, and learner self-directedness, which provides students with opportunities to construct their own understanding of the concepts they are studying. Where learners construct their own understanding, constructivism maintains that this knowledge is more likely to be retained long term.

Humanism

Humanism is learning through realising potential. As its name might suggest, humanism is a grand learning theory which focusses on teaching the whole 'human' (in education, the whole student). Humanism extends beyond a focus on behaviour (behaviourism), and on the mind (cognitivism), to focus on students' emotions, motivations, agency (the choices they make), and moral values. The central idea of humanism is that, through a broader focus, ▶ humanist educators help their learners achieve their full potential. Humanism places students and their experiences at the forefront of learning.

Humanism is an approach to education which requires teachers to become facilitators of learning. It might strike you as odd that direct teaching does not feature in humanist approaches—all learning should be as a result of the skilful questioning and mentoring that facilitation involves.

Humanism emerged in response to behaviourism, critiquing the approach for adopting a simplistic view of human behaviour, and neglecting human emotions. For humanists, punishing someone when they do something wrong (to disincentivise maladaptive behaviours) is not particularly helpful. Instead, ▶ carefully exploring why they have behaved that way—why things

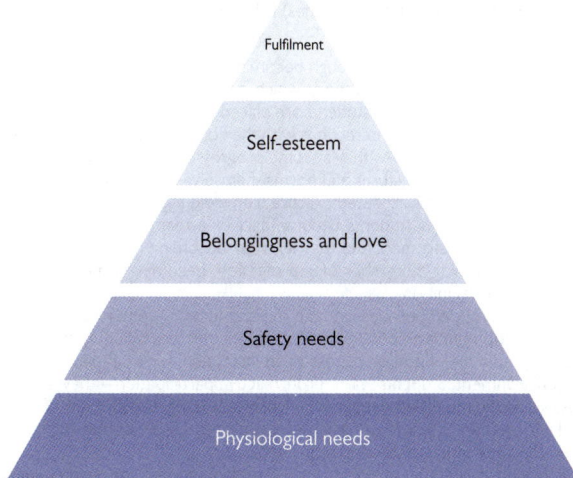

Fig. 2.4 Maslow's 1954 Hierarchy of Needs.[6] No permissions necessary.

have gone wrong—and addressing those problems or underlying factors is more appropriate and seen to have longer term positive influences on behaviour.

Maslow was an influential humanist within education. Many of us will be familiar with his Hierarchy of Needs (Figure 2.4), a widely used model which shows the fundamental conditions people need to experience fulfilment within their lives. Many modern representations of this model present human needs in a pyramid shape (though it is important to note that Maslow did not originally present these needs in this specific shape). Belonging and love are understood to be basic needs within the pyramid (basic needs are the bottom three levels, while growth needs are the top two levels), highlighting the importance of positive relationships, including within educational spaces, to success and fulfilment.

Humanist educators must consider how to foster inclusion within education. There are many ways to attend to inclusion and belonging. Some suggestions might include:
- Promoting small group work and activities which promote relationship-building
- Facilitating discussion amongst peers rather than prioritising didactic information giving
- Setting ground rules to promote group ownership
- Ensuring diversity in materials and resources used to promote belonging for those from minoritized backgrounds
- Celebrating learner success

- Teaching students about growth mindsets which emphasize that success comes from effort, and (sometimes) failure

Socioculturalism

Socioculturalism is learning through becoming. Socioculturalism is a newer, but popular, grand learning theory which suggests that ▶ students learn through experience. When students are placed in work environments, they observe others and their interactions with the norms, values, and structures of a social environment. As they become progressively more involved, they participate in these structures and norms themselves, learning how to navigate them and what is accepted practice from role models and community ways of working. As students become part of a team, their professional identities are transformed, and they learn by becoming (becoming a team member, becoming a member of a profession, becoming a member of a particular community).

Sociocultural perspectives on teaching and learning remind us that student development is embedded in the contexts within which they study and learn—within the education culture of an institution, for example, or a clinical environment. Students learn through active participation—they are not passive recipients of knowledge who learn only by the acquisition of facts and information.[7] They must have meaningful and authentic roles aligned to their future practice to develop as professionals.

Sociocultural perspectives encourage educators to step back and evaluate their educational environments. Educators can design opportunities for newcomers to be made welcome to their new environment—induction events, for example, that provide basic knowledge on how to navigate a ward or clinic, usual practice, and sources of support. Educators can be an access point for integration within a community, encouraging participation, assigning students appropriate and meaningful tasks, and continually re-evaluating (and upscaling, as necessary) the responsibility assigned to students. Including students in social events and taking the care to ensure they feel valued (introducing them to all members of the team, ensuring everyone knows their name and what they can do, providing them with access to changing facilities and bag storage etc.) are small actions that can make a big difference in regard to feeling like an involved and included member of the team.

Grand learning theories summarized

We have summarized these theories, for ease of reference, in Table 2.2, below.

Table 2.2 Five orientations to learning (adapted from Merriam and Caffarella, 1991, p. 138)[8]

	Behaviourism	Cognitivism	Constructivism	Humanism	Socioculturalism
Famous learning theorists Note: some of these learning theorists span traditions, e.g. some aspects of Piaget, Bruner, and Bandura's work could be considered cognitivist	Thorndike, Pavlov, Watson, Guthrie, Hull, Tolman, Skinner	Koffka, Kohler, Lewin, Ausubel, Gagne	Piaget (e.g. schemas), Bruner (e.g. scaffolding, discovery based learning), Bandura (e.g. social cognitive theory), Dewey	Maslow, Rogers	Bandura, Lave and Wenger, Engeström, Vygotsky
View of the learning process	Change in behaviour	Internal mental process (including insight, information processing, memory, perception)	An active and individualized process of knowledge construction in which learners construct understanding based on prior experiences and interactions	A personal act to fulfil potential	Interaction / observation in social contexts. Movement from the periphery to the centre of a community of practice
Locus of learning	Stimuli in external environment	Internal cognitive structuring	Between learners and past experiences	Affective and cognitive needs	Learning is in relationship between people and environment
Purpose in education	Produce behavioural change in desired direction	Develop capacity and skills to learn better	Promote active learning and develop deep understanding	Become self-actualized and autonomous	Full participation in communities of practice

(Continued)

Table 2.2 (*Contd.*)

	Behaviourism	Cognitivism	Constructivism	Humanism	Socioculturalism
Educators' role	Arranges environment to elicit desired response	Structures content of learning activity	Provide opportunities for exploration, reflection, and inquiry	Facilitates development of the whole person	Works to establish communities of practice in which conversation and participation can occur
Manifestations in medical education	Behavioural objectives, competency-based education, skill development, and training	Cognitive development, intelligence, learning how to learn	Problem-based learning, collaborative learning, simulation-based learning	Discussions of 'adult learning', self-directed learning, well-being initiatives	Socialization, social participation, induction planning/activities

Which theory is best?

There isn't a simple answer to the question of which theory is 'best'. The answer depends entirely on context—what you are trying to achieve, who your learners are, your setting, and your experience. ▶ The theory that is most effective in helping your learner master the specific task you'd like them to master is the 'best' theory.

Behaviourism, for example, is appropriate for skills-based learning (such as teaching someone how to insert a central line). Cognitive strategies are useful for assimilating information (e.g. teaching students how to diagnose depression through discussing history-taking in a lecture). Constructivist approaches are well-suited to encouraging problem solving and the development of lifelong learning skills (e.g. teaching using problem-based learning, or facilitating learning through exploratory questioning). Humanism is best suited to facilitating learning (e.g. mentoring, or developing a learner's perspective through skilful questioning). Sociocultural orientations promote the development of professional behaviours through authentic participation in clinical care or role play.

In sum, one should consider the use of theory comprehensively and critically. Attention should be paid to the interplay between the theory, the context, the interactions, and the associated implications.

Further reading

🎞 Learning theories map. HoTEL project. http://hotel-project.eu/content/learning-theories-map-richard-millwood

➲ Dornan T, Mann KV, Scherpbier AJ, Spencer JA. *Medical education: theory and practice*. London: Elsevier, 2011.

➲ Kaufman DM. Teaching and learning in medical education: how theory can inform practice. In: Swanwick T (Ed.), *Understanding medical education: evidence, theory, and practice* (pp. 37–69). New York: Wiley, 2018.

References

1. Varpio L, Paradis E, Uijtdehaage S, Young M. The distinctions between theory, theoretical framework, and conceptual framework. *Acad Med* 2020;95(7):989–994.
2. Popper KR. Science as falsification. In: Popper KR (Ed.), *Conjectures and refutations* (pp 33–39). London: Routledge, 1963.
3. Grbich C. Qualitative data analysis: an introduction. New York: Sage Publishing, 2012.
4. Kaufman ME, Dueñas AN. A medical science educator's guide to selecting a research paradigm: building a basis for better research. *Med Sci Educ* 2020;30(1):545–553.
5. Curzon LB. *Teaching in further education: an outline of principles and practice*. London: A&C Black, 2003.
6. McLeod S. Maslow's hierarchy of needs. *Simply Psychology* 2007;1:1–18.
7. Sfard A. On two metaphors for learning and the dangers of choosing just one. *Educ Res* 1998;27(2):4–13.
8. Merriam SB, Caffarella RS, Baumgartner LM. *Learning in adulthood: a comprehensive guide*. San Francisco, CA: Jossey-Bass, 1991.

Chapter 3

Small group teaching and learning

Myooran Canagaratnam, Charles Campion-Smith, and Subha Ramani

Introduction: Why learn in small groups?

Small groups are a valuable setting in which doctors can learn the range of skills required for professional practice. The strength of learning in a small group, compared with a large group, lies in the increased opportunities for interaction, both between teachers and learners, and between the learners themselves.

▶'Small group teaching' is not determined by any specific size of the group, but rather through fulfilling certain characteristics, which include: active learner engagement and participation, group interaction, group work on a specific task, and reflecting back on both group work and the group process.[1,2]

Small group teaching and learning theory

Small group learning supports the key principles of adult learning, described by Knowles.[3]

Specifically, teaching learners within a small group allows educators to more effectively:

- Identify and build on learners' prior knowledge and experience
- Establish learner-driven goals
- Tailor teaching so that it is relevant to learners' professional practice
- Assess what has been learnt at the end of each session
- Support learners to:
  - Devise their own learning strategies
- Solve problems independently
  - Seek out relevant resources to aid their further learning

Small groups also provide a context in which learners can be supported to engage in reflective practice.[4]

Role of small group teachers and facilitators

Small group teachers/facilitators have two major roles: ensuring that the group completes specific tasks effectively and efficiently, and that the group functions in a collaborative and effective manner.[2]

Examples of task maintenance activities include:
- Opening the discussion
- Planning group work
- Providing information as appropriate
- Inviting varied opinions
- Diagnosing difficulties in group work
- Summarizing
- Skilful use of questions to assess individual learners
- Explaining when concepts are not clear to learners

Examples of group maintenance activities include:
- Establishing ground rules and expectations
- Listening to all group members
- Ensuring participation from all group members
- Relieving tension and conflict
- Ensuring clarity in discussions
- Commenting on group process
- Building trust and rapport between group members
- Being available
- Providing feedback

▶ The small group facilitator can use the following questioning strategies to stimulate meaningful, deep learning[1,2]:
- Using open-ended questions to prompt critical thinking
- Ensuring questions are clear
- Adopting an encouraging tone
- Posing questions that require comprehension, analysis, and synthesis
- Using suitable follow-up probes and prompts
- Ensuring questions are pitched to the level of learners

Stages in group formation

▶ Tuckman has identified different stages in the functioning of small groups.[5] It must be emphasized that this is one of many models but is a good illustration that groups do not form and work as a team from the start. The stages include:

- **Forming**: At the start of a block/rotation/session, group members engage in informal conversations to get to know each other. This is essential before group work begins, teachers can facilitate introductions and icebreakers to ease this phase.
- **Norming**: Group members start establishing ground rules (see Box 3.1) formally or informally for group work, assign roles, express, or clarify learning goals and strategies for task completion. Teachers can facilitate by clarifying the task, educating the team on appropriate resources, and settling uncertainties in the group.
- **Storming:** After initial introductions, but before the work starts, group members start to work out each other's roles within the group, one or more members may compete to emerge as the group leader, based on their skills and interests. Conflicts could ensue at this stage before group members start recognizing each other's knowledge and skills and reach a consensus on who might be the most effective leader and ensure completion of their work.
- **Performing:** The group starts working together, assigning each other specific tasks and developing strategies on how to collaborate to achieve their goals effectively. Satisfaction is enhanced when goals are accomplished, and group tasks are completed.
- **Disbanding:** Small groups complete their work or project and then it is time to terminate the collaboration. Teachers can assist in this phase by reviewing successful accomplishments and providing feedback to individual members.

Box 3.1 Facilitator's checklist of ground rules/group agreements for small group learning

▶▶*Ground rules checklist*

(These are better suggested by participants prompted by 'If this group is to work well for you what ground rules will be helpful?' If time is short the facilitator may offer these for the group's endorsement).

- Agree confidentiality– be specific –no attribution of participants' views and no identification any patients mentioned but sharing of wider learning acceptable)
- Listen actively and attentively
- Show respect for your fellow group members and their opinions within communication
- Critique ideas not the person
- Own your statements and avoid generalizations—'I think' not 'Everybody knows'
- Avoid stereotyping such as 'nurses always' 'doctors never'
- Challenge and disagreement are acceptable, and discussion creative
- Ask for clarification if you are unclear
- Avoid jargon and acronyms—particularly important if patients/users or non-clinical staff are included
- Respectful use of time
- Avoid interruptions—mobile phone and bleeps/pagers to be switched off if possible—or at least in silent mode

Small group learning formats

There are a number of different formats in which small group learning can take place. Mckimm and Morris[6] have described these. Box 3.2 summarizes some of these.

Box 3.2 Small group formats

Small group formats

Tutorials: These are sessions with a small group of learners focused on a particular problem or topic, facilitated by a tutor. Commonly they may focus on solving a particular clinical problem or clinical material (e.g. videos, photographs, or X-rays) can be used to trigger more general discussion and debate. Video conferencing technology enables 'e-tutorials', as an alternative to traditional face-to-face meetings. Problem-based learning is a specific small group learning method which uses the tutorial format.

Seminars: Involve slightly larger groups of students of between 8 and 20. A student, group of students, or tutor may present a paper or report to introduce a subject, followed by a group discussion. Journal clubs follow this format. It is important that a paper is selected carefully. It must be of relevance to the participants, and all must have read it prior to the seminar.

Workshops: Meetings which involve interaction and exchange of information between participants. Often there may be an aim to generate an output such as a paper. Workshops may involve a number of different activities including role-plays, case studies and patient encounters to set the scene and stimulate discussion and debate.

Action learning sets: Action learning sets are often used to support the personal and professional development and learning of trained staff who are engaged in work activities of a similar nature. They usually comprise about six to eight people who bring work-related 'issues' to the group. The group then helps the individual to reflect, find solutions, and discuss options. ▶ Ground rules around time and participation are key. There may be a facilitator, but often the group facilitates itself.

Problem-based learning

Problem-based learning (PBL) is a specific small group learning method, which was first used at McMaster University in 1968.[7] PBL generally involves a clinical problem or scenario (e.g. a patient presenting to their GP with a lump in their neck) which is presented to the small group. The focus is on active learning—through group discussion the learners identify the areas that they need to explore to satisfactorily resolve gaps in their knowledge and understanding.

The manner in which PBL is conducted varies. Wood[8] describes a particular approach in which a PBL tutorial group of 8 to 10 students meet for a number of sessions facilitated by a tutor. For each PBL scenario, the group elects a chair and a scribe. The group then progress through seven steps, in accordance with the Maastricht model (see Box 3.3). ► Through this process, learners not only acquire knowledge and its application to practise, but they also develop skills in teamwork and communication skills, chairing a group, critically evaluating the literature, self-directed learning, and using resources and presentation skills

Role of faculty in PBL

Successful PBL depends, in part, on well written case scenarios. Dolmans[9] advises that cases should adapt to students' prior knowledge and be relevant to their future practice, encourage integration of knowledge of basic sciences, stimulate interest, discussion, and self-directed learning, and should match faculty objectives.

► The role of PBL tutor is more that of a facilitator, whose main role is to ensure the group functions well, and who should use their expertise subtly and sparingly.[10] Wood[8] states that the tasks of the PBL tutor may include helping the chair manage group dynamics, and move through the task, as well as helping the group define learning objectives consistent with the curriculum. The tutor may need to ask non-directive questions and restate ideas to help learners develop their thinking, provide additional material at an appropriate time, and provide support in identifying a suitable format for learners to present the results of independent study.

Box 3.3 PBL tutorial processes (see: Wood[8])

PBL tutorial processes

1. Identification and clarification of key terms, concepts etc.
2. The problem is defined
3. 'Brainstorming' session, in which group uses prior knowledge to generate possible explanations of the problem and identify areas of incomplete knowledge
4. Steps 2 and 3 are reviewed. Explanations are organized and arranged into tentative solutions
5. Group formulates and agrees shared learning objectives;
6. Students work independently or in subgroups, gathering information related to each learning objective
7. The group re-convenes a few days later to discuss the results of independent study. Evaluation of learning and assessment by tutor

Assessment in PBL

Assessment in PBL should follow general principles of assessment in using a range of methods and be aligned to curriculum outcomes.[7] More specifically, Wood[8] advises asking the group to reflect on its PBL performance including its adherence to the process, communication skills, respect for others, and individual contributions.

Assessment of the PBL group as a whole may be considered, with a group mark added to each learner's individual mark, in order to encourage achievement of the generic goals of PBL[8].

Small group facilitation techniques

There are various techniques employed by small group facilitators to promote learner discussion, participation, and interaction (see Box 3.4)

Box 3.4 Small group techniques (see: Jacques[11])

Small group facilitation techniques

Group rounds: each member of the group has a brief time (e.g. one minute) to say something in turn. The order in which people speak can be determined in various ways: e.g. by seating position ('going round the room'), by the contributors nominating the next person to speak, or it can be at random. This technique is often used as an icebreaker at the beginning of a session.

Brainstorming, or idea generation: the whole group is asked to generate thoughts or ideas. The focus is on quantity rather than quality of ideas, with no criticism. Each contribution may be written up on a flipchart. Evaluation of the ideas comes later.

Buzz groups: small groups of students (commonly pairs) discuss a subject between themselves for a very brief period. This can be useful in encouraging learners to speak in an unthreatening context, particularly sharing difficulties, or areas, which they don't understand that they would be unwilling to share with the whole group.

Snowball groups: an extension of buzz groups. Learners initially discuss a topic in pairs and then join another pair to discuss in a group of four, and then another four to form a group of eight. ▶ You should give increasingly complex tasks to the group as it gets larger to prevent learners becoming bored with discussing the same topic.

Cross over groups: Subgroups of students are initially each asked to discuss a different aspect. New subgroups are then formed, containing a member of each original subgroup to maximize sharing of information. Using a colour or number coding system for members of the original group helps this process.

Fishbowls: a group of learners sit in an inner circle discussing a topic, observed by an outer circle of learners. The outer group may be directed to observe for particular themes and patterns in the discussion, or to evaluate the arguments. The roles can then be reversed.

Role-plays: are a useful technique for developing communication skills and for enabling understanding of the different feelings and perspectives of individuals in an interaction (e.g. a clinical encounter). Commonly a role-play might involve three participants—a doctor, a patient, and an observer. ▶ See later in this chapter for an example of a role-play used during a small group workshop for primary care doctors and nurses focusing on challenging conversations.

Planning a small group learning session

Small group learning sessions can either be one-off standalone sessions or part of a series of sessions forming a course. Where small group sessions are 'one-off' sessions, there are particular challenges for the facilitator leader due to time constraints. Careful preparation is paramount. Spencer[12] describes four fundamental questions teachers should ask themselves when planning a teaching session:

1. Who am I teaching?

The number of learners and their study level or stage in training.

2. What am I teaching?

The topic or subject, the type of expected learning (knowledge, skills, behaviours).

3. How will I teach it?

Teaching and learning methods/formats, length of time available, location of teaching session, access to patients, internet resources, clinical skills models, etc.

4. How will I know if the students understand?

Informal and formal assessments, questioning techniques, feedback from learners.

In terms of content, Mckimm and Morris[6] describe how clinical learning can be based around specific topics or themes (e.g. diabetes), specific clinical cases, clinical problems, or situations (e.g. A middle-aged man presenting with chest pain), or tasks and skills (e.g. neurological examination).

Some of the different small group learning formats and facilitator techniques have already been described. Participants should have an idea of the process and the content of the session and clarity about expectations (e.g. attendance and participation) before attending the session.

Sessions should be clearly structured. Some guidelines around the introduction, main body, and ending of a session are given in Box 3.5.

Box 3.5 Structuring a small group session
Guidelines for structuring a small group session

Introduction
Establish a positive learning environment.

Introduction of the facilitator and any co-facilitators is mandatory and brief introductions of the participants is recommended.

An icebreaker task can be helpful.

Outline the learning objectives for the session and allocated timing.

If anyone has to leave before the end of the session it is good to know but they do not have to provide you with a reason why in front of the group.

Depending on the subject, participants could be asked to answer the question: 'If this session is really successful, what will you aim to take away?'

Some brief group agreements/ground rules are usually necessary—if time is short the leader must be prepared to offer some rather than waiting for participants to do so.

Being explicit about confidentiality and anonymity is important if people are to share specific experiences. This is to ensure maintenance of a safe learning environment. This is particularly relevant for interprofessional sessions or those in which patients or service-users are involved.

Main body
The main body of the session is where content is covered.

Try to vary the learning methods within even a brief session. Aim to ensure more active discussion. Limit the use of PowerPoint and enhance engagement with videos, audio and discussion as appropriate.

Explore opportunities to use the knowledge and experience the participants bring. At the same time, the facilitator will also need to manage the time, and ensure that the group is focused on the topic. A 'parking lot' where additional important topics are 'parked' for later discussion can be helpful.

A number of techniques may be used to stimulate discussion; these may prove useful for the more reserved learner who may find it easier to provide insights to a smaller group rather than to a larger audience.

Provision of regular allocated breaks or pauses gives a chance to check both mundane issues such as comfort, audibility, and visibility as well as pace, process, and progress towards learners' objectives.

Ending
Evaluation is essential, particularly if there are plans to repeat the workshop in the future. Paper evaluation forms distributed at the end of the session are more likely to be completed; online surveys used a few days later may allow for a greater degree of reflection following the learning event but completion rates may be lower.

Contacting participants some time after the session can capture whether there have been any changes in their clinical practice and benefit to patients as a result of the session.

Ensure adequate session closure. Take a few minutes for a concluding session with a brief review of the learning objectives and how they have been met. Thank your co-facilitators, venue, and administrative staff and participants. If you have used the 'parking lot' strategy, ensure you revisit it before finishing. Acknowledge anything not covered due to time and signpost additional learning resources.

Case example: A small group workshop for primary care doctors and nurses

The 'Challenging Conversations' workshop was developed as part of joint working between the National Council for Palliative Care and Macmillan Cancer Support and is used with permission. It was set up to support primary care doctors in their conversations with patients who were approaching the end of their lives. The stated aims were:

- to revise basic communication strategies
- to consider the application of these strategies with those approaching the end of their lives
- to practice these conversations in a safe learning environment

Preparation

- Review facilities available—physical space in which to conduct the teaching and availability of co-facilitators. Also, decide a maximum number of participants for the session. Determine what administrative/ secretarial support is available to prepare scenarios, administer attendance register and give certificates of attendance, indicate changeover times in role-play session and distribute scenarios. Strong administrative back-up from someone who is clear about the process is very helpful and contributes greatly to the success of a workshop.
- Recruitment: By letters/flyers/email to all target audience (e.g. by Integrated Care Board mail-list). Additionally direct approach to key directors of learning such as GP trainers and vocational training course organizers and continuing medical education tutors may be helpful.
- Initial publicity should make the aims and nature of the workshop clear and that it is a participatory session using role-playing scenarios to practise strategies in a safe environment.
- Letter of confirmation and welcome to successful applicants. Reminder of nature of workshop and expectation of active participation.
- Practical information: directions, parking arrangements, what food and refreshments will be available etc.
- Programme outline, with timings. Make the start time for the actual learning activities clear.
- Emphasize that it is expected that participants will attend for the whole session.
- Enquire about any special requirements or accessibility needs—mobility, hearing, or vision, dietary.
- Give pre-course preparation for participants. Ask that they listen to Atul Gawande's Reith Lecture on Medical Hubris to set the scene for the learning. Give a BBC iPlayer link.
- Ensure co-facilitators are clear about their role and are prepared for this. They may need information in writing or an opportunity to discuss their role in person or by phone/online meeting if unfamiliar with the format of this workshop.
- Prepare at least five clinical scenarios (or choose from a library of these available from Macmillan). Standard scenarios may need adaptation

to make them relevant to the environment the participants work in—
primary care, outpatient clinics etc.
- Determine which trio will do which three consultations.
- E.g. Trio 1. will do Scenarios A B & C, trio 2. BCD, trio 3. CDE, trio
  4. CDA etc.
- If possible, allocate people to the trios in advance so people work with
  those they know less well.
- Check with the venue about IT, seating arrangements break times, and
  catering.

Delivery

Welcome: Introduce yourself and co-facilitators and consider all participants if group not to large (5 minutes)

Outline programme, aims, breaks, and timing. 'Phones off if possible—or
at least silent'. Questions (5 minutes)

Introduction and background—few PowerPoint slides:
- Show patterns of 'hoped for' and 'actual place' of death in UK.
- Give the evidence that most patients do want to talk about what the
  future holds.
- Inform them that primary care professionals are often the people with
  whom patients want to talk.

Questions or comments (15 minutes)

Use PowerPoint and question and answer/discussion to revise good and
bad listening and communication behaviours.

Whole group or subgroups depending on numbers
(15 minutes)

Show video example of role-played consultation. Explain that this
was acted out by a generalist doctor and an actor playing the patient. ▶
Acknowledge the artificiality. Ask participants to focus on the communication not the clinical case and to note and write down behaviours and
strategies used (20 minutes)

Questions, comments, and feedback—whole group or subgroups (20 minutes)

Quick review of the workshop so far. Ask for comments or questions
about the temperature of the room, visibility of slides etc., and audibility of
presentations etc. *(5 minutes)*

Break (20 minutes)

Box 3.6 Role-play of scenario-based consultations
Role-play of scenario-based consultations

Introduction and explanation of process and timing (10 minutes)

Participants are allocated roles of professional, patient, and observer. Each participant will take each role in turn using a different scenario.

If there are sufficient facilitators (GP educators or trainers), ask one to monitor process with each trio. If not, the participant taking the observer role should be asked to manage timekeeping and remind the participants taking the professional and patient role about adherence to the 'rules'.

Explain that in each scenario the participant taking the professional role has one briefing sheet, the 'patient' another and the observer both—see example. Give each group the option of using an alternative scenario if any of the participants feel uncomfortable with the initial allocation because of personal or professional issues.

Explain that each participant will take the professional, patient, and observer roles in turn for three different scenarios. Arrange seating in groups of three to minimize disturbance from neighbouring trio. Using several breakout rooms is ideal but in larger rooms the trios can be widely space and screens can be used to lessen crosstalk.

Role-play practice (3 × 25 minutes)

The facilitator (or observer) allows role-played consultation to run for up to 10 minutes. The facilitator is encouraged to stop the consultation if it is running into real difficulties or has come to a natural end. The consultation is then reviewed using 'Oxford Rules'[13] for role-played consultation review:
1. The 'professional' says what they think went well
2. The 'patient' and observer are asked to add the positive points they noted (N.B. The observer will need to be mindful to ensure the positives are noted first).
3. The 'professional' is then asked to comment on areas of difficulty. Their view should be accepted and valued but the 'patient' and observer can be asked how they viewed the points raised
4. The 'patient' and observer are then asked to comment what could have been better—but no criticism should be made without a suggestion of how this phase might have been done better.

If the consultation has been stopped early because it was running into difficulties the patient and observer can be asked to suggest alternative actions and 'professional' can then be given the opportunity to re-run part of it

Emphasize that effective feedback to the consulter should be as specific as possible. Give examples of comments patient or observer might use to illustrate this such as:

'Your welcome and body language put the patient at ease ... ' 'Your reflective question when she said ... was very effective.'

'When I said ... I should have liked you to ask me to say more'.

Indicate time to change over to next scenario by ringing a bell or similar and giving out next set of scenario sheets. Help from an administrator can be helpful.

Review of consultations

Ask participants to share ways of dealing challenging questions that they have found successful. Be ready to offer your own strategies.

Conclusion of meeting

Signpost further training and resources. Encourage completion of initial evaluation (paper or online) and ask for suggestions for future workshops. If there is to be deferred evaluation to assess the impact on participants' practice explain the importance of this and encourage its completion. Thank the co-facilitators and participants. Invite final comments. *(5 minutes)*.

Running a course for a small group

Facilitating a course comprising a series of meetings allows the facilitator to build a relationship with the participants and for participants to build relationships between themselves. Understanding the group development process described earlier in this chapter is important. Participants also have the opportunity to apply learning to their workplace, and then reflect on the success and challenges of this with their fellow course members.

At the end of each session, ask the participants to complete a feedback form (see Chapter 8) to identify the areas about which they remain unclear or other topics the session has raised that they would like covered in future sessions.

▶ It is important for facilitators to have flexibility in the plan of the course to allow the organizers to respond to these identified needs for more information or further opportunities to practise skills. Learners can also provide useful feedback regarding style and learning methods.

Setting up a course

Decide the intended group for whom this course is intended. How many group members will there be? ▶ We suggest that 10–12 is the ideal.[14]

Identify the learning aims and objectives—what is it that the participants will know or be better able to do at the course conclusion? What will be the effect on their competence and confidence?

Consider what learning processes will be used. In such a course there is the opportunity to use several—including provision of information, practicing of skills, workplace-based tasks, paired or group reflection.

Decide timing for the course. Whole and half-days each have their advantages. If participants come from a larger area, whole day courses may be better. But if members are more local, they may find it easier to attend half day sessions—though there is the risk of practice work encroaching on the learning time. How many sessions will there be? Is it possible to avoid holiday times that may make attendance more difficult? ❶ In general, Mondays and Fridays are less accessible to those working in primary care.

Determine the venue. Consider practical considerations—what food and refreshments will be provided. Avoid days or times when travel will be particularly difficult. Ensure parking space is readily available and/or there is good public transport access, especially if the course is to be held in an urban area. Ensure there will be the facilities you require such as breakout rooms and information technology provision. Compile information regarding venue accessibility for disabled attendees, or attendees with accessibility needs.

Decide how much work the participants will be expected to do between the sessions.

Be clear whether this course will have closed membership, meaning that no-one will be able to join the course once it has started and that there is an expectation of consistent attendance.

Decide about the cost of attendance to the individual or employer. Is any assistance available for travel or other expenses?

Be clear about the selection of participants. Will this be on a 'first comers' basis, will participants be asked to state why they wish to attend or do you want to achieve a purposeful mix of participants representing a variety of work backgrounds? Will the course be uni-professional or interprofessional?

What administrative support will you require and who will provide this? Will you need an administrator to attend the sessions?

Will any kind of accreditation of learning be given?

How will you reach the intended participants?

How will you convey the essence of the content and process of the course to both participants and their employers or managers?

Ensure you are clear of the expectations of the participants and their organization.

What is the application process and deadline? When will the selection be made and successful/unsuccessful applicants informed?

Pre-course preparation by participants: This should help them arrive already engaged with the topic and having considered what their learning needs are.

Written or email confirmation of successful application.

Reiteration of expectations of full attendance and workplace support. Consider a formal written agreement for this signed by the individual and their employer or manager.

Consider some scene-setting by means of pre-course reading or online material. Pre-course work should be easy to access.

Decide whether a pre-course questionnaire or quiz will help you identify participants' current knowledge and clarify their learning needs

Confirm practical arrangements, start, and finish times and course administrator contact details. (See Box 3.7 Facilitator's checklist)

The initial meeting

It is vital that this is well managed as it will establish your relationship with the participants and their relationship with each other.

A warm welcome—individually on arrival if possible.

Introductory session emphasizing the collaborative nature of the course and the flexibility of the curriculum in line with learners' needs. Encourage

---

Box 3.7 Facilitator checklist

Facilitator checklist

Spare flip chart pens

Sticky notes

Any handouts or other written materials

Name badges: Do you want to prepare these or have people write their own? First or last names? Titles?

Attendance certificates

Note paper

Blu Tac

Presentations on USB sticks/accessible cloud-based storage system

Any DVD you intend to use if applicable, and if DVD facilities are available

Laptop, projector and speakers

Connecting leads

Any IT passwords needed

Phone numbers of the venue staff and fellow facilitators

participants to ask for clarification and also to say if the environment (heating or ventilation) or timing of breaks need adjustment.

Be specific about the timing of the day—including a guaranteed finish time.

Individual introduction. Facilitator and each participant should give a few details of their workplace, their experience, and its relevance to the topic and perhaps something about their personal circumstances and other interests (in our experience, people seem to prefer this to 'icebreaker' activities – although there are an option at this stage)

Introduce any administrative staff present and explain their role.

Outline the intended course in terms of objectives, content, and process. Acknowledge the experience and expertise that the participants bring.

▶ Make sure that there is time for whole group work to build ground rules or agreements for the course how they will work together. These are better coming from the participants themselves but the facilitators need a checklist so any rules not included can be offered to the group. If patients or carers are to be included in some sessions, this will need specific consideration (see guidelines checklist—Box 3.7.)

Plan an activity in pairs or trios to determine participants' hopes and expectations of the course. The following can be a useful prompt: 'If this course was really successful, what would be different for you at the conclusion?' What areas of the outline do they perceive as being of particular importance? Is anything missing?

If a pre-course questionnaire or quiz is used, ask how easy participants found this. Did it make them aware of learning needs and raise questions that they hope the course will answer? It may not be appropriate to give answers at this stage; an option is to say that by the end of the course the participants will have learnt so that they can answer these questions themselves.

It is good to have some topic specific input at this stage, so participants feel they have learnt something as well as establishing the agenda and process of the course.

Agree some relevant but not too demanding work to be done in the practice or workplace prior to the next session. Explain that subsequent sessions will start with a reflective exercise as participants share successes and challenges with this.

Allow time for immediate evaluation emphasizing the importance of this in determining future sessions.

Session closure. Thanks all for their active participation. Give your details if you wish to encourage contact between sessions.

Encourage participants to discuss the topic and the course between the sessions. Ask whether participants wish to share email addresses or set up some format for communication between them between sessions. Make it clear that anyone can opt out of this if they wish.

Subsequent meetings

These should follow a similar format but start with a response to the feedback forms picking up any points from the previous meeting that need clarification and planning how topics highlighted for inclusion in the course will be dealt with. There will then be group discussion of the experience of the in-practice work agreed at the previous session. What were the successes and challenges?

It is probably better to delay the introduction of practical skills practice or role-play until the later sessions when the group will have developed cohesion, mutual respect, and confidence. A clear and prescriptive structure for any role-play exercises is vital to maintain a safe and non-threatening learning environment.

Final meeting

This is an opportunity to review and celebrate the shared and individual learning and perhaps present this to an external audience of workplace colleagues, local commissioners, and sponsors.

A short comment from someone familiar with the context of the work but external to the course itself can be a powerful way of emphasizing relevance and value. Certificates of completion can be presented at this stage.

If a pre-course questionnaire was used, it can be useful to review this—so participants can see how their knowledge and understanding has changed. Reviewing the goals described in the initial sessions and repeating any self-assessment of knowledge and confidence used at the outset can make participants aware of their learning and development. Resources to meet further learning needs or interest stimulated by the course can be signposted at this stage.

It is good to offer the option of a follow up meeting several months later and also to inform the participants of any deferred evaluation and emphasize the importance of this to the development of the course for future participants. Discussion of how individuals will keep in touch and consideration of one-to-one buddying may be appropriate.

Small group learning in the clinical setting

The clinical environment provides rich opportunities for learning through real life experience of clinical problems and interactions with patients. Learners are also able to observe clinician-educators themselves demonstrating clinical skills, and role-modelling professional behaviours.

However, the clinical setting also poses challenges for the small group teacher. ❶ One of the biggest challenges is meeting the educational needs of learners, while maintaining a focus on clinical care. Clinical environments are frequently busy and stressful places, and educators need to establish a learning environment that is safe and that is conducive to learning. Educators should encourage learners to take responsibility, autonomy, and gain 'hands on' experience but need to match clinical activity to level of ability, provide the appropriate level of supervision, and intervene and take charge as appropriate to ensure safe effective care. This requires the educator to be highly aware of the composition of the group in terms of their level of knowledge, prior experience, and competence.

Often the small group may be a working team providing clinical care (e.g. in an in-patient setting). ∴ in such scenarios, the educator has the added responsibility of leading the clinical team, which includes managing group dynamics.

Small group teaching can take place in a number of different clinical settings including:
- Ward rounds
- Outpatient clinics
- Primary care consultations
- Operating theatres
- Home visits
- Clinical team meetings

Teaching and learning in the clinical setting may necessarily be more opportunistic than in other settings. However, as the following case examples illustrate how sessions preparation before the session and debriefing at the end are crucial to the process.

Case example: Small group teaching on the ward round

In the in-patient setting, the group is a working team providing patient care. The team works together for a certain duration—as short as a week or as long as a month. The teacher should ensure that group dynamics are established early on—as the goal of providing excellent care can be derailed by group conflicts. The following strategies could be useful to consultants who lead an in-patient team.[15]

Preparation

Ahead of the rotation, obtain basic information on the team members, their level of training and any specific needs of the team in order to maximize learning and ensure each team member is adequately supported. A brief pre-rotation email to team members followed by a day one meeting would set the stage for effective group work.

Negotiate group agreements, set ground rules, and establish learning contracts.

Though the teacher is the most senior team member with ultimate responsibility for patient care, resident doctors need to be mentored to be team leaders and teachers themselves.

Group work

Ideally the resident doctor or resident would lead daily rounds—observed and guided by consultant teachers.

The consultant should step away from the limelight, add clinical and teaching points as needed and establish an environment where a variety of opinions are welcomed and valued.

Decisions should be made on the length of case presentations, what details are essential, and in what order. ❶ Frequently, clinical trainees struggle with succinct case presentations—clarifying expectations is important.

Ward teams are interprofessional teams: explicit modelling of interprofessional communications and professionalism is critical.

❶ Typically, ward rounds are busy, and quick decisions about patient management can take priority over formal learning. Encourage all team members to write down their questions for later discussions in the event that the round moves on quickly.

Debriefing

Clarify any confusion on patient care plans to prevent team members from learning erroneous concepts of clinical medicine.

Since case presentations are usually complex, assignments to individual group members will set the stage for more in-depth discussions.

The structure of rounds should ensure that work occurs efficiently, patient care needs are met, and there are opportunities for teaching and learning on-the-fly.

Asking for one take-home message from each group member stimulates clinical reasoning and learning. The teacher can quickly assess what the group learned and steer them away from errors.

Emphasize the importance of teamwork.

Periodic discussions should ascertain that learning goals are achieved and all team members develop professionally. At these discussions, goals should be recalibrated, and ground rules revisited.

Case example: Small group teaching in the outpatient clinic

The outpatient setting is very different to the in-patient setting where one or more trainees work with supervising faculty in seeing and/or caring for individual patients. Though this setting is dominated by one-on-one communications and rapid-fire teaching, the teacher and a small group of learners may come together before or after the clinic for a dedicated teaching session.[16]

A team comprising one teacher and several learners do not usually care for a panel of patients, as is typical in in-patient settings. Instead, each learner works with a teacher as well as an interprofessional team consisting of clinic staff, nurses, and allied healthcare professionals for example.

Preparation

The following preparatory strategies can maximize efficiency in patient care, ensure efficient teaching and the smooth flow of patients:

A meeting at the start of the outpatient rotation should include all potential teachers and learners who will be working together.

During the team meeting, ▶ set ground rules and establish learning contracts. Each of the group members should state their goals for the rotation and discuss the roles of individual team members.

Before starting the outpatient session, establish expectations in terms of how much time to spend with each patient, prioritizing which medical needs are to be addressed at that visit, how to present cases etc. In addition, encourage learners to generate specific clinical questions to be answered immediately as well as questions that need to be looked up later.

Communicate how teaching will occur: on-the-fly and/or formal presentations, who will lead the teaching, and whether it will be one-on-one or in a small group.

Clarify what degree of autonomy is appropriate at different stages of training and how respectful interactions will occur in the presence of patients.

During the visit

Generally, there is no common clinical task performed by the group, but the group could come together to debrief patient cases and present relevant topics to each other. Teacher strategies for effective outpatient teaching could include:

Introduction of teacher role to patients especially if the learner is a postgraduate trainee or resident doctor

Skilled use of questions to invite learner input, stimulate clinical reasoning, assess knowledge and skills, and learn strengths and areas for improvement

Make quick teaching points as relevant to immediate patient management

▶ Gentle correction if the learner is moving in the wrong direction

Role-model physician–patient communication, interprofessional communication, clinical reasoning by thinking out loud, physical examination, and professionalism

Show respect for the learners and in the case of more senior learners, pay attention to their autonomy and relationships with patients

Debriefing

Stimulate self-reflection
Provide feedback
Assign topics for further reading and discussion
Obtain take-home points

Case example: Small group teaching at the bedside

The patient's bedside is often a venue for on-the-fly teaching during business rounds. In addition, the bedside is also used for dedicated clinical skills teaching where the team comes together purely for education without involvement in direct patient care.[17]

Preparation

Exploring the knowledge and clinical skill levels of all the learners

Deciding what particular system is to be taught at the bedside and what specific aspects are to be emphasized. Teachers may need to enhance their own skills and knowledge with some focused reading before the session.

Planning learning activities so that all learners are engaged and involved in the teaching and learning, even if only one or two learners may be directly interacting with or examining the patient.

Selecting patients for the bedside teaching exercise who are consistent with the learning goals and who consent to participate. It is best to obtain consent from patients, and explain the teaching activity to them prior to bringing a group of learners to the bedside.

Orient learners to the objectives of the exercise and the activities planned.

▶ Assign roles to each of the team members—this can prevent the chaos that sometimes invades a bedside teaching exercise and will also minimize the boredom felt by learners who may otherwise not feel fully engaged.

Learners need to be informed of the teacher's expectations and be educated about appropriate bedside manner. Team ground rules need to be established.

Any sensitive discussions need to be postponed and the entire team needs to be aware of this.

Orientation of the patient: patients need to know the objectives of the exercise, the role of the team that will be participating in these rounds—that is, whether they are the same team responsible for their clinical care or are just there as learners.

Group work

Introduce yourself and the team to the patient; emphasize the teaching nature of the encounter. Decide and communicate about the specific purpose of the session whether it is demonstration and role-modelling of a physician–patient interaction, observing learners communicate with or examining patients, or observing the teaching by a designated group member.

Role-model and emphasize professionalism and bedside manner at all times. Stepping out of the limelight and keenly observing is a necessary part of learner-centred bedside teaching. Respecting the experiences and knowledge of junior to senior members of the group is essential—this will encourage the group to be open to a variety of opinions. ▶ Admitting one's own lack of knowledge might set the tone for trainees to admit their limitations and engender a willingness to ask questions.

Challenge the learners without humiliating. Give gentle correction when necessary. Capture teachable moments: the bedside is the perfect venue for unrehearsed and unexpected triangular interactions between teacher, trainees, and the patient. Examples of such interactions might include demonstration of superb humanistic skills by a trainee, missed clues in the history or physical examination, or exhibition of communication skills requiring improvement by a trainee. Ensure patients have the opportunity to provide feedback on the encounter.

Before leaving the bedside, teachers need to summarize what was taught and learned during that encounter. Patients also need a summary of the discussion, explaining what applies and what does not apply to their illness and its management. Patient education and counselling can be done at this stage, albeit concisely.

Debriefing

This is the opportunity to discuss sensitive aspects of the patient's history or differential diagnosis. Learners will have an opportunity to ask questions, resolve confusion, and relax and decompress after an intense encounter.

Brief debriefing should focus on the strengths and deficiencies of the completed teaching encounter. This will serve to improve the quality of future teaching rounds, boost team morale, give a chance for trainees to express their frustrations and their deficits in knowledge or skills, and to change or modify teaching goals for the team.

For the teacher, taking the time to reflect on one's own strengths and areas for improvement at the bedside and formulate goals and objectives for future teaching encounters will be most helpful.

Challenges in small group learning

While the strength of small group learning lies in the opportunities for inter-action and in-depth discussion, this can also be the source of a number of challenges. ❶ Managing time and staying on topic can be a particular issue in this context when group discussion is free flowing. ❶ Engaging all par-ticipants can also be tricky especially when a group is of mixed ability and differing prior knowledge and experience. ❶ Issues may also arise around boundaries, for example when group members disclose personal or other-wise sensitive information.

The preceding pages have highlighted the importance of the role of the small group teachers and facilitators in careful preparation, communicating expectations to learners, and setting ground rules and facilitating discussion to promote optimal learning. This may go some way to mitigating these challenges though cannot eliminate their occurrence entirely.

A common challenge is dealing with difficult group members or with interpersonal issues within the group. McCrorie[18] describes a number of different types of challenging learners including those that are dominant, ag-gressive, or argumentative, offensive, overly jocular, disengaged, shy, overly dependent, or constantly late.

▶ There is no single best approach for dealing with interpersonal issues in the group, but understanding what may underlie the difficulty can help guide intervention. Edmunds and Brown[2] suggest asking four diagnostic questions to help choose which strategy to use:

1. Is there a problem beneath the problem?
2. Is the problem for the individual or the group?
3. What is the priority—group morale or the task?
4. What strategy or tactics can you use? Beforehand, On the spot, Privately, Privately afterwards, Reminders

McCrorie[18] advises that where possible the group should be encouraged to sort out its own problems. The tutor's role is then to raise the group's awareness of the issue, e.g. by asking the group to take a time-out to reflect generally on the way the group is working together. Sometimes the group leader does need to intervene, either addressing issues in the presence of the group or as a 1:1 outside of the group. The following case studies illus-trate how different approaches may be used depending on the situation.

Case studies: adapting to learners' needs

The disengaged student

A medical student, Sheila, frequently missed or arrived late for small group teaching sessions during a placement in psychiatry. When she did attend, she appeared distracted, uninterested, and disengaged, frequently checking her phone.

The tutor raised these issues with the student in a 1:1 meeting. She disclosed that she had had her own mental health issues in the past, and that the placement in psychiatry had evoked in her difficult feelings associated with this episode in her life. Exploration of the issue allowed the tutor to understand the student's lack of engagement as a response to these feelings and arrange appropriate emotional support. As a result, the student was able to engage more fully with learning and successfully complete the placement.

The dominant student

During small group teaching, one student, Ian, would often dominate discussions. When the tutor asked questions to the group, he would invariably answer at length, rather than allowing space for other members of the group to contribute. He would also dominate group discussions, sometimes interrupting the tutor and other students. He was an intelligent, knowledgeable, and articulate student; however, the other group members began to adopt more passive roles.

The facilitator considered the options of formally addressing the issue in the group, or individually with the student. However, in the first instance she felt a lighter touch intervention would be more appropriate. She reflected on her style of facilitation and began using techniques to encourage contributions of the whole group. This included buzz groups, and smaller group discussion around topics with feedback to the larger group. During whole group discussion, she would encourage contributions from the whole group, by intervening politely but firmly when Ian responded, with statements such as 'That's a very interesting point, Ian, what do other people think about that?' With these relatively gentle interventions, other students in the group began to contribute more, without Ian feeling criticized for his valuable contributions.

Late attenders

A small group teaching session was scheduled to start at 9am every morning. However, a number of members of the group would invariably arrive late for sessions. As it was a small group, this caused considerable disruption. Sometimes the facilitator would wait a few minutes to start the session until a critical mass of students were present. However, this then established a general sense that sessions would always start at 9:15 anyway, which encouraged more students to arrive a few minutes late.

The facilitator addressed this issue in a feedback/review session at the end of term. He discussed the impact of late arrivals on the learning of the group, but also raised the issue of professionalism and respect for the presenter who had put considerable efforts into preparing the sessions. The group agreed that it was important to start the sessions on time, though it was also acknowledged that, on occasions, individuals might be late due to important reasons such as medical appointments, transportation issues, or personal circumstances. The group agreed to contact the facilitator in advance if they knew they would be late. The facilitator reflected on how he could better promote a culture of openness, where students with support needs making a 9am start difficult would feel more able to contact him for support. The group also implemented a flexible grace period for those with such needs. As a result of the discussion, punctuality on the whole improved, and some students with specific support needs reached out to the facilitator directly to discuss accessing support.

Unprepared learners

During a course of small group seminars, it became apparent that a few of the learners were rarely completing the pre-session reading. As a result, they would contribute little to the group discussion relying on other learners who had read the material.

The facilitator raised the issue at a review session midway through the course, and it was apparent that it had been causing some tension amongst the members of the group. It also became clear that some of the learners were finding the volume of reading material overwhelming and the content difficult. This reflected some differences in prior knowledge and experience of the learners, which the facilitator was not previously aware.

The importance of preparing for sessions was discussed, but also of using course material that was accessible to everybody. As a result, some revisions were made to the reading list, and also to the way in which sessions were structured to account for differing levels and experience of the learners.

References

1. Walton H. Small group methods in medical teaching. *Med Educ* 1997;31:459–464.
2. Edmunds S, Brown G. Effective small group learning: AMEE Guide No. 48. *Med Teach* 2010;32:715–726.
3. Knowles M. *Andragogy in action.* San Francisco, CA: Jossey- Bass, 1984.
4. Schön DA. *Educating the reflective practitioner.* San Francisco, CA: Jossey-Bass, 1988.
5. Tuckman BW. Developmental sequence in small groups. *Psychol Bull* 1965;63:384–399.
6. McKimm J, Morris C. Small group teaching. *Br J Hosp Med* 2009;70(11):592–595.
7. Davis M, Harden R. AMEE Medical Education Guide No. 15: Problem-based learning: a practical guide. *Med Teach* 1999;21(2):130–140.
8. Wood DF. Problem based learning. *BMJ* 2003;326(7384):328–330.
9. Dolmans DHJM, Snellen-Baledon H, Wolfhagen IHAP, Van Der Vleuten PM. Seven principles of effective case design for a problem-based curriculum. *Med Teach* 1997;19(3):185–189.
10. Maudsley G. Roles and responsibilities of the problem-based learning tutor in the undergraduate medical curriculum. *BMJ* 1999;318:657–661.
11. Jacques D. Teaching small groups. In: Cantillon P, Hutchinson L, Wood D (Eds.), *BMJ ABC of learning and teaching in medicine* (pp. 19–21). London: BMJ Publishing Group, 2003.
12. Spencer J. ABC of learning and teaching in medicine: learning and teaching in the clinical environment. *BMJ* 2003;326:591–594.
13. Pendleton D, Schofield T, Tate P, Havelock P. *The new consultation developing: doctor–patient communication.* Oxford: Oxford University Press, 2003.
14. Lohman MC, Finkelstein M. Designing groups in problem-based learning to promote problem-solving skill and self-directedness. *Instr Sci* 2000;28:291–307.
15. Elnicki DM, Cooper A. Medical students' perceptions of the elements of effective inpatient teaching by attending physicians and housestaff. *J Gen Intern Med* 2005;20:635–639.
16. Dent JA. AMEE Guide No 26: clinical teaching in ambulatory care settings: making the most of learning opportunities with outpatients. *Med Teach* 2005;27:302–315.
17. Ramani S. Twelve tips to improve bedside teaching. *Med Teach* 2003;25:112–115.
18. McCrorie P. *Teaching and leading small groups.* Edinburgh, UK: Association for the Study of Medical Education, 2006.

Chapter 4

Large group teaching

Jessica Stokes-Parish, Yvette Annan, and Jo Bishop

Introduction to large group teaching

'You will remember some of what you hear; much of what you read; more of what you see, and almost all of what you experience and understand fully.'

KL Moore

In a world of increasing class sizes, maintaining engaging learning models and responding to significant shifts in learner preferences is a challenge. Large group teaching (LGT), often referred to as 'the lecture' is one of the oldest and most widely adopted teaching methods. It continues to prove valuable in terms of its potential reach and its ability to introduce and maximize the efficiency of further learning. It also enables the delivery of teaching in a structured and uniform way. The convening of a large group of learners maximizes opportunities for social learning amongst peers, which adds value to the 'university experience'.

▶ A 'large teaching group' has no agreed definition, but historically, LGT refers to the delivery of teaching to group sizes of 25–30 or more (there is theoretically no upper limit to the size of the group). In many places, teaching during the preclinical years of medicine is delivered via LGT methods alongside other small group teaching methods, as discussed in the small group teaching chapter (➋ Chapter 3). The decision to use LGT reflects the practicality of delivering content to high volumes of learners within time and space constraints. In this chapter, we explore the types of LGT, evidence and theory for LGT, inclusive practice, and finally, we provide practical tips and case studies of ways to engage learners in a LGT format.

The larger the group, the greater the likelihood of variation among its learners in terms of how they may engage with the teaching methods, level of understanding, and previous exposure to a topic. Creating and delivering educational content simultaneously across a large group may mean considering and incorporating a variety of education styles and/or comprehensive introduction of each topic before building on it during the LGT.

What are the different types of large group teaching?

The often-assumed modality of LGT is the lecture in a theatre, with all eyes on the educator at the front. This has long been the traditional method of delivering teaching to medium to large class sizes. Indeed, the term 'lecture' is frequently used interchangeably with LGT.[1]

The appeal to the lecture is the educator to learner ratio, non-resource intensiveness, and en masse delivery; lectures are a cost-effective and efficient way to introduce ideas and concepts to large class sizes such as year groups simultaneously. This is particularly relevant as the number of students in higher education establishments have been steadily increasing over the past two decades. LGT can also introduce applications, concepts, and expert thinking, inspiring students' desire to learn.[2] Well-delivered lectures can serve to provide a foundation on which self-directed and smaller group learning are underpinned, although it may also work in the reverse.

However, LGT is no longer limited to the lecture theatre, and can be materialized through workshops, symposia, or even anatomy lab demonstrations. These other formats allow the educator to group learners together at tables or in pairs, supporting interaction which we will explore later in the chapter (➋ and are discussed in greater depth in the small group teaching chapter, Chapter 3). LGT and collaborative learning between large numbers of learners can also occur in multiple spaces simultaneously and outside of the traditional lecture theatres.

What evidence is there about large group teaching?

Large group teaching has a long history and remains a popular educational style, ● but it has not been found to be superior to others. Donald Bligh extensively examined LGT as an educational tool.[3] He found that lectures were as useful as, but not more useful than other educational methods.

Historically, the LGT style was best suited to imparting information, not promoting higher learning processes. However, used in conjunction with other tools and engagement strategies, LGT can be optimized to achieve depth of learning.

In more recent work, Luscombe and Montgomery highlighted that LGT sessions can be effective if students are actively engaged, as opposed to passively listening, and the way in which educators interact with the learners heavily influenced the learner perception of the learning activity.[4] Gold et al. (2020) demonstrated that case-based learning in an LGT setting (i.e. learners worked in groups with one facilitator in a large lecture hall) worked as effectively as small group learning settings, highlighting that active learning strategies (discussed below) can mitigate the traditional stereotype of the didactic lecture.[5]

There are several ways in which LGTs can be made more student-centred, which we detail in this chapter. For example, large group sizes can allow for efficient discourse between educators and learners and between learners. Educators can use flipped learning, where learners are introduced to some of the teaching material ahead of the lecture. This encourages self-directed learning and maximizes the value and contributions during the LGT. Before we explore these strategies and other considerations, we highlight learning theory that can inform your LGT practice.

Theory that informs large group teaching

Learning theory is an important consideration with regards to evidence-based teaching of large groups. ▶ Ensuring your teaching practice has a firm grounding in theory is one way to engage in high-quality educational practice. You can read about educational theory in depth in ❷ Chapter 2.

Here, we will recap some learning theories covered in ❷ Chapter 2, and introduce new theories (active learning, social cognitive, and visual attention theories) that can inform your LGT and help you to make the most out of the opportunity that you have to progress student learning.

Constructivism

Firstly, active learning theory draws on constructivist learning theory, which describes how learners bring preconceived ideas and experiences to a learning encounter or interaction that inform their construction of knowledge. Within an active learning approach, educators are encouraged to focus on deliberate student participation, exercise mindful watching and listening, and reflect critically on their own practice. This model shifts the position of the educator from the central position of power to a collaborative, adaptive approach. Evidence highlights learners retain more information, have decreased distractions, and increased confidence with teaching material when engaging learning methods are used.[6]

Social cognitive theory

Social cognitive theory, formerly known as social learning theory, is another important theory in reference to LGT. Bandura developed this theory in 1997, and the model itself contains four stages (see Figure 4.1 for details).[7] The model highlights that learners observe and interpret actions, based on their understanding, and then mimic or reproduce the behaviours that they have seen.

In the first stage of Bandura's model, learners must observe modelled behaviours, described as 'attention'. The learner then moves to the second stage, retention, in which they rehearse the behaviours they have observed mentally. In an LGT setting, this might occur through observation of videos, described behaviours, or through a simulated role play. The third phase, reproduction, invites the learner to reproduce what they have observed and rehearsed, further solidifying their knowledge. Finally, motivation refers to the learner's ability to see that they have achieved a goal in reproduction, extrinsically motivating them to continue learning.

Motivation can also refer to positive emotions and reinforcement—that is, the learner feels the satisfaction of completing the learning, motivating them to continue learning. This theory is also relevant when considering behaviours in the learning environment, as social cognitive theory states that behaviours and learning are shaped by the environments and interactions within it. To this end, an educator may consider the following: how does the educator engage with learners, how do other learners engage with each other, and what are the personal factors that might contribute to a learner's engagement with knowledge?

Central to this theory is the idea that learners have the ability to self-direct their own learning. This means that students can recognize their own

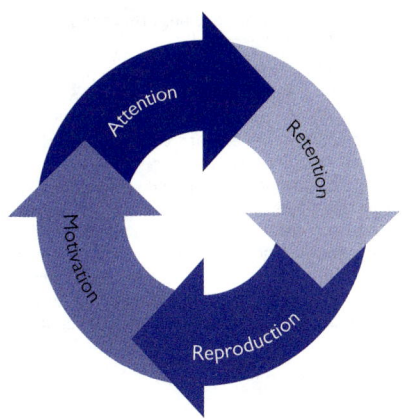

Fig. 4.1 Stages of social cognitive theory. No permissions necessary.

learning needs, set goals, monitor their own progress, and adjust their strategies for achieving understanding. Recognizing that learners have the ability to self-direct within learning means that all educators should consider ways in which to facilitate learning, rather than just dictate knowledge. There is detailed guidance on this in Chapter 3 ➔, but later in this chapter we will also explore ways in which you can acknowledge and promote self-directed learning in a large group setting (e.g. by flipping a classroom, using interactive learning technologies, encouraging peer learning, and connecting the material learned in the lecture theatre to clinical practice).

Visual attention

Another theory relevant to LGT, but one that may not traditionally be considered, is the theory of visual attention. The theory of visual attention suggests that our brains are always working in the background to determine what visual stimuli we should pay attention to.[8] This process helps prevent us from feeling overwhelmed with information (or experiencing cognitive overload) and allows us to filter out unnecessary visual information.

This theory has relevance for LGT from not only an engagement perspective, but also an accessibility perspective (which we discuss later in this chapter). The cognitive processes that determine where we look are considered 'bottom up' (sensory data that influences our thinking) factors.[9] That is, the properties of a stimulus contribute to our attention. Factors that contribute to visual attention include factors such as:

- Colour: Distinct colours can be eye-catching.
- Illumination: Brightness, or the way that light interacts with text or an image on a slide.
- Contrast: High contrast between the background of a slide, and images or text in the foreground can make content not only stand out but can ensure that all content is readable.

- Well-defined edges: clear, sharp outlines of text and images makes content more readable and accessible.

Consider the examples in Figure 4.2. On the bottom, you have a slide with good illumination, high-contrast, and defined edges, on the top, you have a slide that is too light, with poor contrast, and poorly defined edges. Which is more pleasing to your eye? As educators we can apply this theory to our slide design with little additional effort.

Of course, graphic design is a specific and professional skill. We do not anticipate that all educators will feel immediately comfortable with slide design, and educational material design. It can take time to develop slides and material that adheres to good-practice principles in graphic design that adhere to the principles of visual attention theory. There are, however, frameworks you can follow that build on the theory of visual attention and offer clear guidance on how to put the key components of this theory into practice.

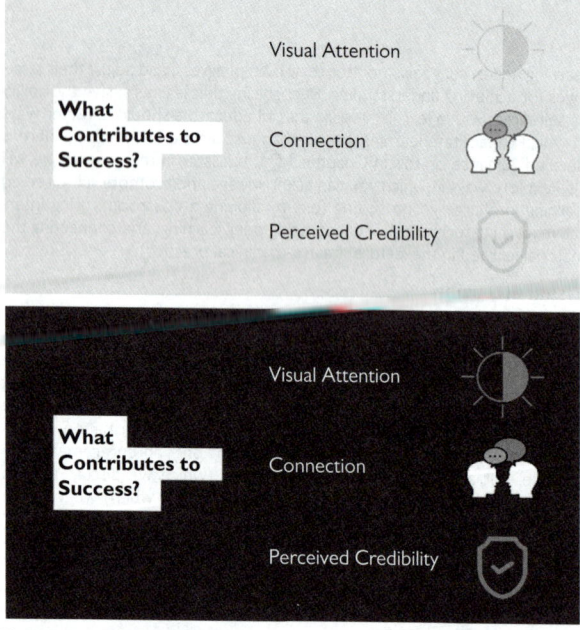

Fig. 4.2 Examples of slides that demonstrate the impact slide design choices can have on visual attention. Above, a slide that is light, with poor contrast, and poorly defined edges. Below, a slide with good illumination, high-contrast, and defined edges. No permissions necessary.

Asif and Burton's graphic design framework (see Box 4.1) offers clear guidance for educators on utilizing good-practice principles in their own instructional design. We have summarized this framework here, for ease of reference, but recommend that interested readers review the framework within the original reference in depth.

Box 4.1 Asif and Burton's framework of graphic design for clinical teachers

The framework includes six principles, which the authors recommend using to create visually appealing graphics that can engage learners and enhance the dissemination of important information. These principles should be considered in a graphic design plan, or blueprint, created as part of the planning of your content, during the design of your educational session or presentation.

The six key principles are:

- **Layout**: The arrangement of items such as text and images and how these objects are positioned in relation to one another. Key considerations include creating a visual hierarchy that guides a reader's eye through a graphic, using whitespace to avoid clutter, and ensuring that your layout is appropriate for your intended medium (print versus digital)
- **Hierarchy**: The use of characteristics such as size and colour to indicate the importance of different elements on a page. Key considerations include using size and colour to create contrast between elements, ensuring that the most important information is most prominent, and using consistent visual cues to indicate different levels of importance
- **Colour Theory**: The study and use of colours, which involves finding combinations of colours which work well together and do not clash. Key considerations include understanding the psychological associations that different colours have (e.g. red for danger, blue for calm), using colour to create contrast and highlight important information, and ensuring that a colour scheme is appropriate for intended audience and purpose.
- **Typography**: The use and arrangement of text elements within a design. Includes type of font, actions such as bolding or underlining text, and spacing between letters. Key considerations include choosing legible fonts, using font size and weight to create hierarchy, and ensuring that spacing between letters and lines creates legibility
- **Simplicity**: Keeping design as simple as possible or using the minimum number of design elements required to convey an intended message. Key considerations include focusing on the most important information, using concise language, and avoiding clutter.
- **Balance**: The even distribution of elements in a graphic or across a slide. Key considerations include ensuring that a graphic is not top-heavy or lopsided, and using whitespace to create balance and avoid clutter.

📖 Asif and Burton, 2021. Comic Sans or common sense? Graphic design for clinical teachers. The Clinical Teacher, 18;6:583-589. https://online library.wiley.com/doi/epdf/10.1111/tct.13417

Inclusivity and accessibility in large group teaching

Widening participation refers to increasing access to learning and offering opportunities for success and progression to all people. Medical education has a long history of oppression and exclusion, and there have been many decades of research dedicated to improving access to the study of medicine, and to improving diverse learners' experiences once within medicine.

▶ All learners benefit from inclusive approaches to education, not just those currently or historically minoritized by medical education, but there are students who may face additional barriers to studying medicine, and for whom adopting universal approaches to design is particularly critical (See Box 4.2).

Given that widening participation is not just about widening access, but also involves ensuring that all learners studying medicine have the opportunities and support they require to flourish, inclusive educational design is critical.

Box 4.2 Access issues for educators to consider; from Health Education England (HEE), evidence brief: widening participation

- Students from ethnically minoritized backgrounds
- Students from areas of socioeconomic deprivation
- Students who have experienced care or are carers
- Students who have ongoing physical and/or mental health needs and possible challenges
- Students with disabilities or additional access needs
- Students with literacy or language differences

Access full document online: https://www.ewin.nhs.uk/sites/default/files/Widening%20Partici pation_Evidence%20Brief.pdf

---

Universal Design for Learning

Universal Design for Learning (UDL)[1] is a concept which educators can consider to reflect on, evaluate, and improve their approach to inclusive instructional design. The principles of UDL can be summarized by considering three key components: engagement, representation, and expression:

Engagement involves promoting session design that optimizes individual choice, reduced distractions, and threats (whether from noise or presentation slides), provides opportunity for varied levels of challenge, which in turn facilitates self-regulation. Taking these steps allows learners to understand why they are engaging, reducing the first hurdle of engaging.

Representation encourages educators to offer a variety of ways to engage with information (visual, auditory, etc.) and to use strategies that clarify and decode information (such as illustrations, verbal descriptions of symbols, and breaking down complex topics)—this enables learners to understand what they are learning.

Expression promotes the use of physical modifications, multiple communication strategies, and providing monitoring and support for learners are essential for how learners learn. Working together, these three domains aim to produce an expert learner who is purposeful, motivated, resourceful, knowledgeable, and goal directed.

All three of these principles lead us to the fact that learning is deeply personal. While learning styles have been largely debunked, learners do have varied levels of learning capabilities, preferences for learning approaches, and more. Principles of accessibility and inclusion can only benefit the whole learner group. However, as the student population increases in size, and access improves, so does the likelihood of encountering students with diverse learning needs, for whom universal design is particularly key to their success.

There is widespread agreement that disabled students needs to be offered opportunities to facilitate access to education. Higher Education Institutions have seen an increased number of learners from diverse backgrounds. These include learners who are neurodivergent, such as Autistic learners, people with attention-deficit hyperactivity disorder (ADHD) and learners with dyslexia. Some people who are neurodivergent may identify as disabled.

In the UK, Higher Education Institutions have a legal duty to make 'reasonable adjustments' to ensure disabled students are not discriminated against (See: Online reference, https://www.gov.uk/government/publications/reasonable-adjustments-a-legal-duty/reasonable-adjustments-a-legal-duty). In the context of LGT, by applying the principles of UDL, educators can take steps to increase the inclusivity of LGT sessions and encompass any specific learning needs.

ADHD, for example, can contribute to impairments in personal, social, and academic functioning, and some individuals with ADHD may identify as disabled. ADHD is believed to affect 4–6% of the general population (though there may be more people with ADHD who are undiagnosed), and so it is increasingly likely that educators will encounter ADHD learners in their learning environments. Taking steps to promote UDL means that educators can create a safe learning environment for all learners (see Box 4.32).

Beyond legal mandates and social expectations, there is significant benefit to Higher Education Institutions and educators engaging and creating diverse learner populations, such as increased social inclusion and widening of the talent pool both for institutions and industry. There is also personal and social economic value that come with widening access for learners if it leads to improved work opportunities.

For example, Deaf nursing graduates have lived experience that can add value to the service they provide to their patients both with and without hearing loss. Moreover, as educators we should see it as our social responsibility to ensure training is accessible to all. Admitting disabled students, or any student with diverse lived experiences, only on the basis that they add value to the learning community or profession, is reductive and misses the broader point of inclusion. Every student, regardless of their background or value added, has a right to education and should be valued intrinsically.

> **Box 4.3 ►► Accessibility tips for medical educators, based on the principles of Universal Design for Learning**
>
> - provide clear, concise, and positive instructions and feedback
> - minimize distractions and communicate that there will be breaks within a session (and when these will be), to allow for movement and refreshment
> - select an adequate font size for presentations (minimum 24 pt)
> - use high colour contrast within presentations
> - reduce the volume of information per slide
> - provide information in different formats for students e.g. written transcripts or materials to complement a presentation
> - use visual cues and creative presentations to reinforce concepts, and to engage
> - provide access to organization tools, and discuss organizational strategies to support the preparation and completion of tasks
> - use a microphone to promote clarity of audio, and allow Deaf students to access hearing loop systems where these are available

Strategies to widen inclusivity in large group teaching

To widen participation, educators should consider a wide range of practical strategies, including technology, alternative engagement modalities, and more.

Educators should record their sessions, where possible, so that they can be later accessed by students who wish to follow the lecture at a different pace. Students may adjust the pace of a lecture to suit their individual needs, and make actions such as pausing and rewinding, or speeding up the recorded speed. While this is considered beneficial for disabled learners, this also provides widened access for students who may have additional responsibilities (such as caring responsibilities), and learners who wish to reengage with LGT for revision or to consolidate learning. In addition to recording, learners may choose to activate closed captions on recorded content. This offers learners more choice in how they learn and removes the hurdles for learners to participate (in line with the principles of UDL).

While closed captions are intended to make live presentations and videos accessible to disabled people, they can benefit all students, as with all design elements stemming from UDL. Many individuals who choose to use captions do so because they find that captions improve their engagement, focus, and comprehension.

Planning large group teaching

Though you are now armed with relevant learning theory, and key considerations in relation to inclusive practice, there is still much planning to do! After all, a good educator prepares well for a productive educational session. There are several principles to consider when planning or modifying a session, webinar, or large group activity to proactively address some of these challenges, outlined later in this section. Box 4.4 presents some key considerations.

> **Box 4.4 Considerations for large group teaching to proactively address possible challenges**
> - What are the rationales for choosing large group teaching for this content? What are its advantages?
> - What are the challenges confronting large group teaching, now and in the immediate future?
> - What teaching methods or strategies can be applied to large group teaching to enhance its impact and effectiveness?
> - What are student perceptions and expectations regarding large group teaching?
> - Which approaches to large group teaching best support student learning success?
> - How do we determine which large group teaching strategies are best suited for a programme, and how should these be approved?
> - Should individual students have options within each subject regarding how they engage with content?
> - Should we distinguish between undergraduate and postgraduate students?

Constructive alignment within curricula

A well-designed session should start with an introduction that may include learning objectives mapped to a syllabus. This will usually then cover series of themes illustrated with examples with or without multimedia.

It is crucial to consider the context and learner when developing the learning objectives and subsequent educational materials. ▶ Bigg's Constructive Alignment postulates that what an educator does should be aligned with the assessment of the subject and the stated learning objectives: ∴ the most effective way that your learner will achieve the intended outcome of the teaching is through aligning the educational activities with those outcomes[10] (see Figure 4.3).

In the context of LGT within a broad educational programme, this would mean understanding of the wider curriculum and what students would be assessed on and the suitability of the environment for the teaching activity and the group (see Box 4.5).

Learner cohort

In the context of a stand-alone LGT the educator would need an understanding of the background of the learner cohort and to align the teaching to objectives of their roles. For example, when providing an update of

Intended learning outcomes

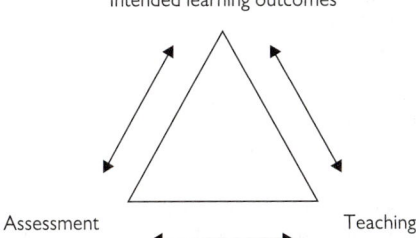

Assessment   Teaching

Fig. 4.3: Constructive alignment of learning objectives, assessment, and teaching. Adapted from Barrow, M. and McKimm, J. (2010); See: ◐ Barrow M, McKimm J. Assuring and maintaining quality in clinical education. *British Journal of Hospital Medicine* (2005). 2010 Apr;71(4):224–8. No permissions required.

Box 4.5 Considerations for planning a large group teaching session so that it is constructively aligned with broader curricula

- **Learner cohort:** Determine the level of understanding the group have—is this an introduction, revision, or more advanced group who will have some prior knowledge and exposure to the theme(s)?
- **Curriculum in context:** Consider the interplay between this session and other sessions more broadly within the curriculum. How will the session enhance and be enhanced by other teaching within the wider course or programme?
- **Learning objectives and assessment:** Ensure that the goals of the teaching session are clear, and that any assessments you use are directly related to these goals.

---

sepsis management based on a new international consensus for early recognition of sepsis, the content and depth of LGT of a team of experienced emergency department consultants would be different to newly qualified doctors working across specialities who may have had limited experience of sepsis management. A diverse clinical team, each with specific roles in diagnosing and treating septic patients, will have varying depth and breadth of training requirements.

Similarly, a 45-minute lecture on medical imaging would differ for second year medical students compared to a lecture for core medical trainees. The approach you would take would be tailored based on the expected outcomes for each level of trainees' specific roles, the type of assessments they will undergo (e.g. undergraduate versus specialist exams), and the practical experiences they are likely to commonly encounter in the near future (e.g. interpreting common clinical imaging expected for their stage of training). If LGT does not align with learners' needs and expectations, then educators run the risk of their session being perceived as irrelevant, and learners disengaging with the content they are delivering.

Curriculum in context

Depending on the subject area or topic, one session alone may be insufficient to achieve all outcomes; an LGT session, or series of sessions embedded within a wider curriculum of activities can orient a large number of learners to their specific learning objectives.

Educator experience

Relevant experience and the background of the educator are also important factors in understanding how to plan to deliver a unit for LGT that is relevant to learners. Often, educators will approach sessions with a wealth of knowledge, which is usually greater than the information that they wish to impart to learners. This can assist in providing a stimulating session and answering challenging questions but can be problematic if the scope of the LGT session expands too far beyond the required learning objectives.

If an educator is a novice educator, or a near peer educator, they may have more recent first-hand experience of similar learning needs that they can use to plan their LGT sessions; but, coached practice and faculty development may be required. This might include orientating new educators to writing clear session objectives, planning an educational session (and its timing), and practical tips on presentation skills.

Some educators are less confident in front of large groups, and ∴ could benefit from public speaking coaching. After all, there is a big difference between an educator who reads the slides versus an educator who engagingly presents their content. If you yourself are a novice educator, it is worthwhile reaching out to more experienced educators in your department or field to ask for advice on delivering LGT prior to your first teaching experience, and if you are affiliated with a university, they often have presentation skills training that you can join.

Engaging learners

The value of an educator who is engaged in relation to both their topic of interest, and also in relation to learners, cannot be overstated. Engagement of not only educators, but also the engagement of learners is critical for successful learning. Engagement can be challenging and, often, has been made more challenging to assess for educators now that we have moved into an era of virtual and hybrid teaching. There are no way 'quick fixes' for engagement, and forcing engagement (e.g. making learners turn on cameras in an online teaching session) rarely helps, and can differentially negatively impact minorized learners. Instead, it is best to plan for learner engagement, and have dedicated strategies within an LGT setting to enhance engagement. We have outlined creative ways in which educators can optimize engagement in LGT settings within Box 4.6.

Box 4.6 Educator ideas to optimize engagement in large group teaching

- **Flipped learning:** A blended learning strategy in which online lectures and audio-visual resources introduced to learners prior to the lecture to maximize the active learning while it takes place
- **Socratic discourse:** Dialogue can be applied in a limited way during the lecture to maintain learner engagement
- **Polling tools:** Use quizzing tools to quickly assess student understanding, or to gather opinions and generate discussions during the lecture
- **Think-pair-share:** A technique to stimulate engagement and discussion—pose a question to the large group and give individual students an opportunity to think through their answer. Then ask students to discuss in pairs, then share with the larger group
- **Active recap:** At regular intervals, pause the lecture and let students summarize their understanding in pairs or small break out groups
- **Guest speakers or perspectives:** Consider inviting guest speakers to deliver lectures, or engage guest perspectives during a lecture, to stimulate engagement, discussion, and provide students with the opportunity to hear from a fresh perspective, or a different perspective. Can be particularly useful to engage patients and forefront patient perspectives and experiences within a large group setting
- **Use multimedia content:** Consider use of videos, music, audio clips, animations, etc., in your slides to make them more engaging. Make sure to consider previous advice on inclusivity to ensure your content is accessible to all
- **Consider practical applications:** Relate your topic to application within clinical practice, or to current social events, to increase the perceived relevance of your content

Pacing

The way an LGT session is paced has a close relationship with how much information will be retained and the quality of the learning experience for students.[1] To maintain the maximal engagement of the group, breaks and activities should be scheduled to maintain focus. Natural breaks can occur during periods of silence when students are encouraged to reflect and apply the concepts being discussed. Sessions of more than 1 hour duration or a series of sessions with cumulative duration of greater than 60 minutes should include scheduled, formal breaks incorporated in the timing.

Psychological experience of large group teaching

Hogan and Kwiatkowski describe the importance of considering the emotional aspects of LGT both from the perspective of educators and learners[11] (⊕ Consider Bandura's mental states of the social cognitive theory, in 'Theory that informs large group teaching'). They suggest powerful feelings of alienation, anger, and envy are experienced by learners in large groups for which they compensate in ways which may be counterproductive to their learning. Educators may also experience anxiety or apprehension which may impact the quality of the presentation. An understanding and preparation to manage these emotions as part of the LGT can be beneficial to the value of the experience.

An example of a psychological experience that may affect both educators and learners is imposter syndrome, or imposter phenomenon. Imposter phenomenon occurs where individuals doubt their ability and accomplishments, and experience persistent fear that they will be exposed as a fraud. ▶ Imposter phenomenon is disproportionately experienced by minoritized learners, as environments within medical school send both overt and hidden biased messages that minoritized people do not belong within medical spaces.

In large groups, where there may be wide ranging backgrounds of learners and, given the increasing sizes of cohorts in higher education institutions; it is likely that imposter phenomenon will be the experience of a proportion of the group. An awareness of this phenomenon and how to reduce its negative effects may improve the educational experience of learners.

Enabling learners to participate in the larger group via a safe space (such as a breakout session or virtual noticeboard/discussion board, see below) is one example of increasing contribution of people experiencing this phenomenon.

Learning environment

We suggest educators consider LGT through a holistic lens, considering the physical environment, the state of the learner and educator, and the outcomes of learning as contributors to the learning activity itself (see Figure 4.4).

Bishop[12] emphasizes that the well-being of the learner and the well-being of educators are critical in ensuring that both students and staff thrive in their institution. To achieve this, Baik and Larcombe[13] suggest using a framework that examines the entire university ecosystem in terms of student and staff well-being and consider good practice in elements of that ecosystem that contribute to well-being.

The 5-point framework for ecosystems that contribute to well-being[13]:

1. Foster engaging curricula and learning experiences
2. Cultivate supportive social, physical, and digital environments
3. Strengthen community awareness and actions
4. Develop students' mental health knowledge and self-regulatory skills
5. Ensure access to effective services

Concentrating on the first action area, 'foster engaging curricula and learning experiences', it is important to note that student mental health and well-being are enhanced when courses and learning experiences offer a range of options—i.e. they are adaptable by design. These adaptable educational

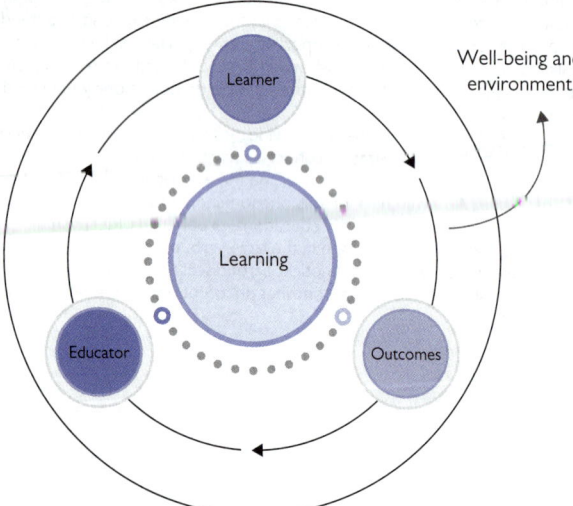

Fig. 4.4 Key factors influencing large group teaching and learning. No permissions required.

settings should also promote social connections, build competence, and foster intrinsic motivation.

Key indicators for success may include, but are not limited to:

- Proportion of students who report having had a positive experience working with their peers (in class or online) to complete learning tasks
- Proportion of students who report a sense of social connection with students and staff in their course (e.g. having made at least one or two friends within their cohort; being confident a staff member knows their name)

Gathering learners in a common physical space can encourage the exchange of ideas and discussion. We suggest that this benefit may arise from establishing shared understandings during active discussions, and that these discussions can even continue outside of the classroom (sometimes referred to as 'corridor conversations'), which enhance students' experiences as learners. Indeed, a key value of traditional LGT within a physical space is the opportunity for an entire cohort of learners to meet and interact. Box 4.7 describes a case example of how a space for medical students to interact and socialize within LGT was created within the formal curriculum of an institution.

Our traditional understandings of student learning, and the need for a physical environment, have, of course, evolved since COVID-19 and the rapid shift to online learning. Throughout, interaction remains a key character, but ideas regarding how this can be achieved successfully are changing.

Box 4.7 Back to base sessions

An example of cohort socialization in action is whereby a medical school schedules a 'back to base' (a return to campus) for all of their senior clinical students who spend their last two year of their training within hospitals, in the community, or on electives. The back to base sessions are scheduled after the completion of two rotations and deliver content to support the students' work-based placements and include sessions around medico-legal considerations, professionalism, as well as prescribing and preparation for being a doctor, for example. The sessions can either take place in a traditional lecture theatre, within a flat collaborative learning space, or online during the pandemic. Feedback from students have stated that they value this opportunity to collaborate with their cohort as they spend limited time with their peers when immersed in practice. The unexpected hidden curriculum has allowed camaraderie, shared experiences, advice on how to best prepare for specialty rotations, along with an opportunity to receive updates and communicate with their home institution. The plan to bring the students back to base was met with resistance originally as it was perceived this would diminish the placement opportunities, to the contrary it has enhanced the students' motivation to engage with additional skillsets and guidance from faculty and peers.

Technology-based strategies

Here, we offer an overview of technology-based strategies in relation to LGT. ⊋ See Chapter 9, on Technology Enhanced Learning (TEL), for an in-depth discussion of TEL and, relating to our discussion above on socialization, on interaction in online spaces, including counterarguments to the need for physical spaces for interaction.

As more students enrol in higher education, leading to larger class sizes, technology offers a way to efficiently teach these large groups. It can be integrated into real-time, or synchronous, classroom sessions and fits well within a standard lecture hall setup. This can make education more accessible to a broader audience, including international students who may be based in geographically distant locations. Additionally, some educational material relating to LGT can be accessed on-demand, allowing students to learn at their own pace in an asynchronous manner.

Remote delivery of teaching

At a time where traditional LGT has or is quickly transitioning to fully or partially online formats, Fong et al.[14] outline the challenges that educational institutions face in implementing online LGT. These challenges include:
1. Cognitive overload of both tutors and learners
2. Technical issues and security risks
3. Mitigating inequity in accessing online learning
4. The need for programme evaluation to ensure sustained improvements to teaching

To address these challenges, they suggest some strategies. These include conducting test runs of the technical platforms before the actual teaching sessions and adopting an iterative development process to online LGT. Educators should also establish clear learning objectives and assess whether online LGT is the right approach for meeting these objectives. If it is, they should then determine whether any adjustments are needed to improve its effectiveness.

Microsoft Teams© and Zoom© can be used for online teaching using Meeting, Webinar, or live event versions, which each provide slightly different functions for invitees, and enable varying levels of learner interaction.
- Meetings are generally used for smaller, more interactive sessions where everyone can speak freely.
- Webinars and Live Events are more suited for larger audiences where the focus is usually on one or a few presenters. These formats allow you to control who can speak, share their screen, or interact in other ways, giving you the ability to manage large groups of learners more effectively.

Both Microsoft Teams© and Zoom© enable exchanges between the educators and the rest of the group to take place via a chat function. This is particularly useful for asking and answering questions, sharing resources like links or files, and even for quick polls or quizzes. Participants can also select a 'raised hand' function to alert the educator that they wish to contribute verbally.

One standout feature on both platforms is the capability to create breakout sessions. This functionality allows the main large group to be divided into smaller groups for more focused discussions or team activities. Breakout sessions can be particularly effective for encouraging student participation, facilitating peer-to-peer learning, and for conducting group projects or exercises.

Real-time online collaborative platforms

There are several online collaborative platforms to break up and enhance the value of a lecture by encouraging participation through polls, free text entry, or other tools.

For example, 'Padlet'© is a real-time collaborative web platform that enables users to add content including drawings, images, and text and share and organize content. An educator can ask for lecture attendees to jot down their answers to a question, for example 'name of one of the four main drug classes of antihypertensives, give an example'. This is a particularly useful way of encouraging participation in remote learning lecture settings. It does so in the following ways:

- Breaks up longer periods of passive learning.
- Encourages participation.
- It can provide a quickfire formative assessment of the group's level of understanding of a topic to inform the educator on how to frame further teaching.
- Enables shared knowledge between learners.

Another useful and popular tool used by educators and students is Kahoot!©, which is an online polling, quiz, and game application. Educators or learners create questionnaires and games to be accessed online in real time by participants through their devices using a unique PIN. It is designed to enable collaborative creation. Poll and quiz results are collected in real time and shared on the presenter's screen. Kahoot can be accessed from any smartphone or device that is mobile internet or Wi-Fi enabled.

We have chosen to describe Padlet© and Kahoot!© but many online collaborative platforms exist. Over time we hope you will explore a variety of platforms and settle on your preferred tools. To find out more about various online educational tools, both collaborative platforms and beyond, we recommend the annually complied 'Top 100 Tools for Learning List'. The most current version of this list is from 2023, but be mindful to search for the most current version: ℰ https://toptools4learning.com/

Digital spaced repetition platforms

In emerging, game-based models, applications are increasingly becoming available for spaced repetition of learning. Quitch © an app-based platform that supports spaced repetition learning whereby students can answer questions related to the content that has been delivered. Frequent quizzes and tests facilitate knowledge recall and understanding.

There are a range of different tools and platforms that can be used to engage learners in LGT, however there are some limitations. The pitfalls of technology, particularly live online teaching include: difficulties accessing links; failure of software; failure of internet connections; technical inexperience; distractions, where learning occurs in busy non-institutional environments; cognitive overload; limited non-verbal cues from learners and educators; lack of immediate feedback; accessibility concerns, loss of social learning.

Social learning within online large group teaching

Loss of social learning is a common concern that educators have when learning moves online. However, university students often express a preference for independent, online study. For example, we have experienced requests that recorded presentations have functionality that enables them to be viewed at an increased speed. However, the shift towards independent and often asynchronous study does not mean that social learning needs to be lost. Careful online learning design can incorporate elements which align with active learning strategies, such as discussion forums, peer review assignments, and breakout discussions to foster community and collaboration between students. In fact, online LGT is often more consciously focused on designing spaces for community and collaboration—given the more obvious distance between participants, educators often prioritize strategies that encourage interaction and engagement.

Communities of Inquiry

Online features that stimulate dialogue and teamwork not only encourage social learning but also serve to deepen cognitive understanding of course material. 'Communities of Inquiry' theory, proposed by Garrison, Anderson, and Archer to examine the potential of computer conferencing can be applied here. See: ➜ *Garrison DR, Anderson T, Archer W. The first decade of the community of inquiry framework: A retrospective. The internet and higher education. 2010;13(1–2):5–9.*

Communities of inquiry are online spaces in which media supports collaborative learning. Communities are structured around the endeavour of learning, or 'inquiry'. The framework considers three domains of learner interaction within online spaces. These domains are referred to as types of 'presence', and include social, cognitive, and teaching presence.

- **Social presence**: The extent to which learners feel a sense of belonging to a community, such as a specific course or programme, while effectively communicating in an environment designed to foster trust, and connectivity, between learners, and between learners and educators. Social presence involves open communication, group cohesion, and affective expression.
- **Cognitive presence**: The extent to which learners can construct and confirm meaning through sustained reflection and discourse. Cognitive presence has four phases:
  1. **Triggering event:** Learners recognize a problem and experience a degree of disorientation
  2. **Exploration:** Learners use different sources and discuss with others to solve ambiguities
  3. **Integration:** Learners reflect on the task, link ideas, and try to come up with solutions
  4. **Resolution:** Learners apply the knowledge created to new situations, testing its fit
- **Teaching presence**: The design, facilitation, and direction of cognitive and social processes for the purpose of realizing personally meaningful and educationally worthwhile learning outcomes. Teaching presence facilitates the establishment and growth of social and cognitive presences.

By proactively designing courses with this theoretical grounding, which include interactive and collaborative elements, educators can essentially create a virtual community of inquiry, helping to mitigate the loss of social cues and immediacy that are often present in traditional classroom settings. Thus, despite the shift towards more independent study patterns, carefully designed online courses can still offer rich social learning opportunities that align with well-established educational theories.

Large group teaching approaches: Tactile strategies

One way to engender intentional engagement is to utilize tactile strategies to engage learners. While the concept of 'learning styles' has been debunked, there are useful tactile strategies that can be embedded in LGT to facilitate deeper knowledge transfer and application. From a theoretical perspective, tactile methods can contribute to the development of long-term memory and better academic performance.

For more information see: ℘ Valcke M, De Wever B. *Information and communication technologies in higher education: evidence-based practices in medical education. Medical Teacher 2009;28(1):40–48;* and ℘ Kumar LR, Voralu K, Pani SP, Sethuraman KR. *Association of kinesthetic and read-write learner with deep approach learning and academic achievement. Can Med Educ J 2011;2:e23–27.*

We outline some examples of how you might embed tactile strategies into your LGT session. Box 4.8 begins this collection of examples by presenting a case study using plasticine in anatomy teaching, presenting our reflections as educators regarding the benefits of such an approach.

Other tactile strategies that you can consider include:

- **Drawing:** Drawing is a commonly used technique in anatomy, where it has been found to improve retention of knowledge. Examples of this include, educators drawing during the LGT, asking students to draw alongside them, or provide drawing as revision pre- or post-LGT. There is mixed outcomes between drawing on paper and drawing on tablets.
- **Movement/dance:** Movement in the childhood classroom has long been associated with learning benefits, such as improved cognitive function and academic achievement. An educator can implement physical movement within their LGT—this might be through group activities, games, or dance to break up the session.

Box 4.8 Case study: plasticine

Learner Cohort—Final year, pre-registration Physiotherapy students
   Objective—Review and revisit anatomy and physiology of skin
   Task—Create a model of the skin using plasticine

This session was particularly challenging as it was 5 hours long. Instead of presenting didactic content, I designed a learning session with various activities to cover the content engagingly. One of these strategies was the use of plasticine. I set a task for the students to recreate a representation of skin in whatever way they chose (drawing, plasticine—some even chose interpretive dance).

This allowed students to consolidate knowledge and break up the session activity. Some students chose to create the anatomical components of skin using plasticine. This allowed them to revise their knowledge of anatomy and reconstruct the layers of the skin. Below is an image of one creation. I hope you will agree this is an impressive model.

Box 4.8 (*Contd.*)

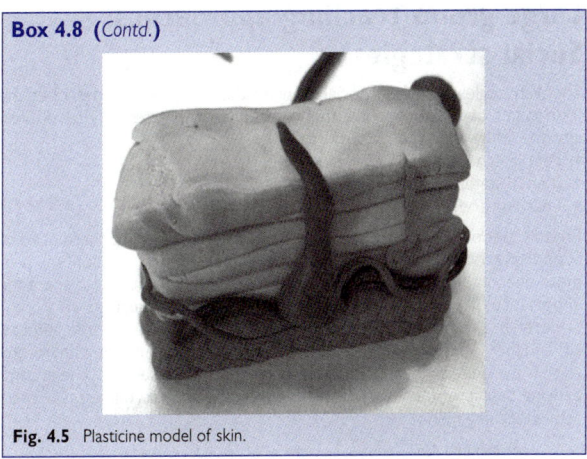

Fig. 4.5 Plasticine model of skin.

- **Designing technological tools, such as infographics:** Another way to keep learners focused may be the development of revision resources such as infographics within the LGT. An educator may instruct the class to create a revision resource for a specific aspect of the session at various points in the classroom. This provides the learner with opportunities to revise, reinforce new learning, and exercise creativity.
- **Cadaver-based activities:** In traditional, LGT anatomy lab sessions, educators might use cadavers as the focal point of discussion for the educational session. This allows the learners to visualize more completely the multi-dimensional aspects of the human body, as opposed to 2D form.
- **Simulations of tasks and procedures:** There are examples of large group case studies whereby the whole class will review an unfolding case—→ see whole of cohort case conference, p. 115. This can also be considered for simulation and procedural tasks, where the skill can be observed by the whole of group and then small groups are encouraged to practise with a facilitator. The whole of cohort can then re-group to review the skills and discuss the 'What if?' scenarios. → See Chapter 5 for more content on simulation within medical education.
- **Board games:** The use of board games can increase engagement by adding a certain excitement to the environment, the play element can support attention, plus many learners thrive with healthy competition. Board games reinforce learning, especially for targeted skills, and can be less overwhelming for some students in that they support students' social and emotional skills (require student interaction, have rules, involve cooperation, often involve collaboration). The benefits for educators are that board games allow observation of students and listening to ascertain mastering of skills.

Large group teaching approaches: Social strategies

Social strategies draw from social cognitive theory.[7] While we described the four stages of social cognitive theory earlier, it can essentially be distilled into the following:

- People can learn through observation.
- Mental states are important to learning.
- Learning does not necessarily lead to behaviour change.

Broadly, people learn by watching others and then imitating these actions. Supporting increased participation by learners with cooperation will promote deep and critical thought by social interaction. We will also share the importance of a safe environment to enhance student learning.

Here we present how in a recent all of university strategy, the authors' (JB and JSP) institute removed the term lecture and replaced it with 'forum' to shift the underpinning philosophy of the education session. The accompanying definition for a forum was published within the university's interactive teaching menu:

' ... an open and active learning experience that includes the whole learner cohort for a subject, where content, ideas, issues, curiosity, and perspectives are explored collectively to promote learner understanding. Forum learners are engaged in interactive and authentic learning.'

The Office of the Provost at JB and JSP's institute launched the new initiative with the support of the university office of learning and teaching who visited each faculty and delivered workshops and provided supplementary material to support the educators with the redesign of their sessions. This supports the principles of social cognitive theory amongst educators, who were sharing and observing role modelling of others' good practices. Interactive education models draw from active learning theory and moves away from the traditional teacher-centred methodology (as described earlier) to engagement of all participants with the educator, each other, and the learning material by using an array of activities and resources. Activities could be for the individual learner, in pairs, or for the group(s).

In the initiative outlined above, the Office of Learning and Teaching developed resources to support large group delivery ('the forum') and utilized the current empirical literature to encourage an array of learner engagement activities grouped as: *Activate, Collaborate, Contemplate, Evaluate, Consolidate*:

- **Activate:** Provocative prompts allow an educator to engage their learner(s) to think more deeply about the content. This can be achieved by an image, video, or text—this could allow a learner to re-evaluate their own thoughts and beliefs with an ethics session for example. This is an effective method to ask important questions and stimulate self (and group) reflection.

- **Collaborate:** Think-Pair-Share allows the educator to pose a question allowing the learner to think of the answer individually, for a pair to work together on it and then an opportunity to share with the wider group.
- **Contemplate:** What if prompts allow the educator to pose questions to the learners from a different point of view, a different lens, and encourages true understanding and sometimes outside of the box thinking.
- **Evaluate:** The "why should I care?" activity encourages educators to ask learners at the end of the session how the topic could be applied later (in their training) or in real life situations.
- **Consolidate:** Is an opportunity to verify their understanding of key concepts from the session. This can be done by allocating a specific time to write down key concepts (beat the clock) and share to the group or in pairs.

We provide a case study in Box 4.9 of a panel discussion for medical students which leverages these principles, to demonstrate *Activate, Collaborate, Contemplate, Evaluate, Consolidate* in-action.

Whole of cohort case conference

Problem-based learning (PBL) is a widely used method that encourages active learning, particularly in small groups. It allows students to direct their own learning journey as they explore clinical cases, ethics, and legal issues. In this process, students also develop crucial competencies relating to communication, leadership, and teamwork. Many educational institutions have also incorporated team-based learning (TBL), a small group teaching method originally introduced in the field of business, to reinforce curricula content. This teaching approach enhances learning by utilizing techniques like knowledge retrieval, peer discussion, feedback, and the application of learned concepts to new situations. ➲ See Chapter 3, on small group teaching and learning, for more detail.

We present this overview of PBL and TBL here to contextualize the method of 'Whole of cohort case conference'. The psychological safety built in small group PBL or TBL settings can be leveraged to hold larger case, or scenario conferences. In these conferences, the small PBL group collaborates with a facilitator to review content delivered by an expert. This conference format supports students' learning experience by leveraging the benefits of both small and large group instruction. It increases student engagement with large group content and allows them to consider alternative perspectives that their peers or facilitators may raise. This is a useful, and little-used strategy that can be implemented throughout a curriculum that has spaces for established PBL and TBL sessions.

Box 4.9 Case study: The panel discussion

Learner cohort—Medical students in their first year of pre-registration training

Objective—Observe and reflect on the experiences of an older person in an aged care facility.

Task—Engage in a panel discussion LGT activity.

The curriculum team designed a replacement education session as students could not attend an aged care facility during the pandemic. Firstly, they filmed a simulation of hospital admission of an elderly patient following a fall, during the simulation the patient was examined and reviewed by several allied health professionals with the final part of the video highlighting a multidisciplinary team meeting to discuss discharge options. The first-year medical student cohort were asked to view the 20-minute video as a group (half cohort ~ 100 students)**—Proactive prompt activity**

The second part of the session involved the students being introduced to the panel which included a moderator, the elderly patient, Mrs Green (an actor), a community General Practitioner, a nurse, and an aged care researcher.

The moderator poses a question to the group around 'which allied health professionals supported Mrs Green and what were their roles?'—**Think-Pair-Share activity**

The moderator then stimulates dialogue with each panel member including Mrs Green and allows considerations of what a discharge following a hospital admission would look like, back to the home independently or with support or to an aged care facility. The cohort are asked to consider this and the likely outcomes—**What if activity**

At the conclusion of the session the moderator asks the students how they might apply this session in their learning—e.g. **why should I care** about the activity? This is a great opportunity to encourage the benefits of teamwork for better patient outcomes and the role of each allied health professional in the team.

The video showcases high level of communication skill and pathophysiological and pharmacological knowledge that they haven't covered yet—this reinforced their curiosity in learning.

The students are presented with a revision question at the end of the week to consolidate their individual learning for the session which is prepared by the lead educator—Quitch© (see below)

Of note the students often believe that Mrs Green is a real patient, and the simulation is maintained until the debrief in their small group learning environment later in the week. Although students can now attend their aged care placements the curriculum team have maintained this session.

The session exemplifies an opportunity of co-delivering of material to a group of students as well as 'chunking'—the breaking up of delivery of content to allow learner interactions using an array of activities.

It also delivers content in a meaningful way, with depth and an opportunity for experiential learning and application in the future.

Evaluation of large group teaching

With any educational intervention, a process of evaluation should be undertaken. Evaluation is particularly important for LGT when the cohort of learners is relatively large; there may be a broad variation in approaches to learning amongst the group and there is limited opportunity for one-to-one interaction between educator and learner to receive direct feedback.

Determining how well learners can engage and draw from LGT through formative assessment and qualitative feedback will provide valuable information regarding how to refine it. This will involve determining specifically what learners require and if the LGT has any deficiencies in that regard, how useful and interesting they find the teaching, and how much learners are benefiting overall as a group. To do this, educators can: 1) embed just-in-time surveys at the end of an educational session (for quality improvement), 2) review end-of-semester student evaluations, or 3) conduct deliberate focus group evaluations on a series of educational sessions, or on an educational programme. Questions that surveys or focus groups may cover might include topics such as alignment with the curriculum, perceived engagement, rating the engagement of the educator, or rating of/comments on the educational activities within the session. ❥ For more information about evaluation of teaching methods, please see Chapter 8.

◖ A word of caution with anonymous student evaluations, however, as it is well documented that students frequently comment on irrelevant aspects of education, such as educators' dress sense or hair styles. Evaluations are often biased against minoritized people (e.g. racialized people, women, disabled people). When these evaluations are used to evaluate the effectiveness or impact of a teacher at an organizational level, or when they factor into progression and career decisions, this exacerbates existing inequities in medical and medical education careers.

Further reading

❥ Barrows HT. *Problem-based learning. An approach to medical education.* New York: Springer, 1980.

♫ National Teaching Fellow 2017: HEA to Z (n.d.). Flipped learning. Advance HE. https://www.advance-he.ac.uk/knowledge-hub/flipped-learning

References

1. Cantillon P. Teaching large groups. *BMJ* 2003;326:437.
2. Sumera A. Large group teaching, an effective and efficient teaching methodology. *Asian J Sci Res* 2014;4:1–5.
3. Bligh D. *What's the use of lectures?*, 5th edn. London: Intellect, 1998.
4. Luscombe C, Montgomery J. Exploring medical student learning in the large group teaching environment: examining current practice to inform curricular development. *BMC Med Educ* 2016;16:184.
5. Gold JM, Collazo RA, Athauda G, Obeso VT, Toonkel RL. Taking CBL to the lecture hall: a comparison of outcomes between traditional small group CBL and novel large group team-based CBL teaching method. *Med Sci Educ* 2019;30(1):227–236.
6. Miller CJM, McNear J, Metz MJ. A comparison of traditional and engaging lecture methods in a large, professional-level course. *Adv Physiol Educ* 2013;37(1):347–355.
7. Bandura A. *Social learning theory.* Englewood Cliffs, NJ: Prentice-Hall, 1977.
8. Posner MI, Snyder CR, Davidson BJ. Attention and the detection of signals. *J Exp Psychol* 1980;109(2):160–174.
9. Bradley MM, Houbova P, Miccoli L, Costa VD, Lang PJ. Scan patterns when viewing natural scenes: emotion, complexity, and repetition. *Psychophysiology* 2011;48(11):1544–1553.
10. Biggs J. Enhancing teaching through constructive alignment. *High Educ* 1996;32:347–364.

11. Hogan D, Kwiatkowski R. Emotional aspects of large group teaching. *Hum Relat* 1998;51:1403–1417.
12. Bishop J. Bouncing forward: mental wealth for all. *Med Sci Educ* 2022;32:9–14.
13. Baik C, Larcombe W. *Enhancing student wellbeing*. 2016. http://unistudentwellbeing.edu.au
14. Fong JMN, Tsang LPM, Tan NCK, Salcedo D, Tan KSW. Effective online large-group teaching in health professions education. *Korean J Med Educ* 2022;34(2):155–166.

Simulation

*Thomas Simpson, Gabriel Reedy,
and Chaoyan Dong*

Introduction

Traditionally, 'see one, do one, teach one', had been used widely in medical education—especially surgical education. This model did have its advantages and many excellent doctors were trained in this way. However, this experiential learning approach relies on a longitudinal, often one-to-one trainee/trainer relationship, and with increasing medical student numbers, it has become impossible for individual trainees to be attached to individual mentors.

Further, trainees may expose patients to potential harm because they do not have the required experience, knowledge, and skills to treat patients independently. Even so, resident doctors and junior nurses have historically cared for patients in complex and dynamic clinical settings with limited supervision from experienced clinicians due to the pressure of clinical service delivery. Legal restrictions on medical trainees' direct contact with patients have become more common, associated with increasing attention to patient safety. Because trainees learn by practising on real patients, trainees are concerned about the issues as well. Research has shown that residents do not feel comfortable to perform procedures safely by themselves on real patients.[1]

Historically, trainees have been assigned a certain number of procedures to perform under supervision before being allowed to perform them independently. Although doctors may have completed this predetermined *number* of procedures by the end of their postgraduate training programmes, they may not have developed sufficient proficiency to perform the procedures independently and safely—let alone the mastery necessary to train others in due course. Indeed, many resident doctors report a lack of confidence in the performance of invasive bedside procedures.[2] However, this is not entirely due to the relative avoidance of these procedures throughout training, but also because of advances in clinical practice; For example, general surgery has gradually moved away from open surgeries to less invasive procedures, while other procedures are replaced by novel therapies or restricted to experienced practitioners as seen with the increasing use of radiologically guided interventional techniques. This suggests the importance of innovative or alternative training approaches so that medical students and residents can build these practical skills before they enter the relevant clinical setting, and the need for a dynamic training approach that can support a dynamic and constantly evolving practice.

In the traditional 'see one do one teach one' model, the trainees are completely dependent on the teacher's knowledge base, technical expertise, and the opportunistic encounter of clinical cases. Therefore, if the teacher is unable to perform a procedure effectively, errors or complications will likely be propagated. For rare but important clinical cases or crises, it has historically been difficult for doctors to rely on the serendipity of these occurring during their training.

In addition, competency-based education has become dominant in medical education. Among many others, the Accreditation Council for General Medical Education (USA), CanMeds (Canada), Scottish Doctor, and Tomorrow's Doctors (UK) have defined core competencies for postgraduate medical education, including patient care, communication, professionalism, in addition to medical knowledge. Some of these competencies cannot be taught and assessed by the 'see one, do one, teach one' model. Instead, alternative teaching models, such as simulation, are more effective in teaching trainees in the clinical setting.

For medical students, similar professional competencies have also been defined, because undergraduate medical education (UME) must prepare students to achieve these competencies before entering their postgraduate training years. To promote trainees' clinical skills acquisition during medical school, the Association of American Medical Colleges has advocated a variety of teaching formats including lectures to explain the theoretical underpinning of skills, workshops to learn to apply knowledge with peers, simulation for students to practice on task trainers and mannequins; patient care experiences under supervision, and longitudinal patient care experience for students to learn about the experiences of patients before and after treatment episodes. Benefits of using a range of instructional methods include accommodating various learning approaches, providing opportunities for repetitive practice with observation and feedback, encouraging progress growth and development of the desired skills, promoting active learning by allowing trainees to apply and practice these skills in different settings, and introducing trainees to skills experiences in diverse specialties.

Simulation has been adopted in both undergraduate and postgraduate medical education. Simulation has been shown to prepare medical students to master practical skills before they start work. Simulation also can train senior trainees to manage crisis situations in clinical settings so that those doctors learn to recognize adverse events and react to them quickly and safely. With simulation, trainees' progress in passing required milestones can be assessed.

Having evolved from a niche teaching method for specific skill acquisition to a potentially fully immersive method of training for all manner of complex clinical scenarios, simulation has broadened its scope significantly in the last decades. Beyond education and training, simulation can also assist in diagnosing latent threats, responding to and recovering from adverse events, and as a method of exploring and improving team culture and practice. In this chapter, the foundational principles of simulation are introduced, and practical advice for designing and delivering simulation training is offered.

Practical skills training

Practical skills training has seen a huge shift over the years, from an art form learned on the job, to a skill that can be mastered through evidence-based approaches to teaching using increasingly sophisticated training tools.

The 'best' approach is still a matter for discussion, however the core principles of practical skills training are increasingly well established. Whether you choose a four-step approach to instruct and run your session in a dedicated clinical skills laboratory, or implement a two-step approach on a busy hospital ward (see ➋ Techniques for practical skill teaching, below), there are four key principles that should inform your teaching:[3]

- **Observational practice:** Combining the practice of a skill with the observation of others practising a skill, for example by working in pairs, has benefits both in terms of enhanced learning and cost
- **Self-controlled practice:** Allowing learners the time to practice free of external controls on conditions enables them to achieve mastery at their own pace
- **Feedback:** Feedback on skill performance must be carefully judged. Evidence suggests that positive feedback has significant positive effects on learning. Negative feedback or feedback which suggests that the trainee is performing at an average or below-average level can significantly inhibit motor learning. Errors in performance to standard may best be dealt with through exploring a trainee's awareness of the error and response to it, rather with critical feedback. In tandem with self-controlled practice, allowing trainees to choose when to receive feedback on their performance has also been shown to be beneficial
- **External focus of attention:** Interestingly, giving instructions which lead to a focus on external objects (e.g. implements, tools, surfaces) rather than internal structures (hands, fingers, feet) produces significantly faster learning of skills. This is presumed to be due to the triggering of automatic and unconscious motor control strategies, adapting existing movements to the task at hand. Directing candidates to consider their hand or finger placement requires a cognitive and active control of movement, disrupting the flow of automatic movements.

Any approach which can maximize these four elements should enhance learning. Practising in a dedicated skills lab makes it easier to employ these principles. Evidence shows that learning according to 'good practice' in a skills lab outperforms that in traditional clinical training, both on immediate assessment of learning, and on follow-up retention tests.

Techniques for practical skill teaching

Peyton's four-step technique:

This is a widely used and well-recognized approach to teaching practical skills.[4] The four steps are:

- *Step 1) Demonstration*: The trainer demonstrates the skill at normal pace without any commentary. The learner watches.
- *Step 2) Deconstruction*: The trainer repeats the performance, describing all necessary sub-steps. The learner is able to ask questions.
- *Step 3) Comprehension/Formulation*: The student instructs the teacher through each sub-step to complete the performance.

- *Step 4) Performance*: The student performs the complete skill themselves.

Advantages:

A widely used and easy to remember technique which can be used for both practical skills such as intubation and team-based performances such as cardiac arrest team training.

Disadvantages:

It is criticized for being a time-inefficient technique. Some trials have called into question the need for all four steps, as many trials have shown equivalence between this approach and others with fewer stages. The complexity of the skill in question may be a significant factor in the utility of the approach, with very simple and very complex tasks perhaps needing a different approach. It was also originally designed for situations with a 1:1 trainee to trainer ratio.

Modified Peyton's technique for small group teaching

This modification encourages each trainee to complete all stages while also utilizing the performances of multiple trainees as an opportunity for further observations and feedback.[5] Steps 1,2,3 etc. refer to the original Peyton's Four stages:

- *Part A: Demonstration and Deconstruction*: The trainer performs Steps 1 and 2 of Peyton's Four-Step Approach to all trainees
- *Part B: Comprehension, Trainer's Performance and Observation*: The trainer performs Step 3 following the instructions of Trainee 1, while all other Trainees are observing
- *Part C: Comprehension, Trainee's Performance and Observation*: Trainee 1 performs Step 3 following instructions of Trainee 2, while the other Trainees are observing
- *Part D: Tutor and Peer Feedback*: Trainee 1 receives feedback by Peer Trainees, followed by Tutor feedback
- *Part E: Circulation*: Parts C and D are repeated in turn until the last Trainee has performed Step 3 following the instructions of a Trainee
- *Part F: Completion and Conclusion*: Finally, the last Trainee performs Step 4, followed by Peer and Tutor feedback.

Two-step technique

Where skills are considered simple and easier to master, with fewer sub-steps in their performance, it may be more suitable to utilize a more streamlined approach. The two-step technique has been demonstrated to be as effective as the four-step technique in the teaching of simple physical skills, such as Laryngeal Mask Airway insertion.[6]

- *Step 1) Demonstration*: The trainer demonstrates the skill while describing what they are doing.
- *Step 2) Performance*: The trainee performs the skill, with feedback from the trainer as necessary.

Acquisition of simple skills can be achieved with this technique. There may be a small but significant deterioration in retention of skills using this technique and so it may be less appropriate for rarely encountered skills.

Ongoing learning and skill deterioration

It is well-recognized that acquisition of clinical skills in a training environment does not, by itself, produce long-lasting retention of those skills. Skill fade is most marked in the first few months after training, especially in the absence of continual practice, but decline continues indefinitely. This is obviously a greater problem for skills which are infrequently encountered and is potentially problematic if skills are both rare for an individual and high-risk (e.g. emergency tracheostomy).

One solution is to encourage post-training exposure to skills in the real clinical environment through linking certification in the skill to both attendance on a course and episodes of observation and performance in clinical practice. One example of this includes the Royal College of Radiology's recommendations for Ultrasound Training for medical and surgical specialties. This stipulates attaining a core knowledge base, as well as competencies and skills to be acquired over a longer timeframe, recorded in a logbook to be countersigned by an appropriately experienced supervisor and trainer.

Use of a logbook, with named supervisors and an approach based on Entrustable Professional Activities (see ➲ Supervising Clinical Skills in practice), is likely to produce the strongest acquisition and retention of clinical skills in the majority of trainees.

Simulation

Gaba[7] stated that 'Simulation is a technique, not a technology, to replace or amplify real experiences with guided experiences, often immersive in nature, that evoke or replicate substantial aspects of the real world in a fully interactive fashion'.

This definition from Gaba highlights that simulation encompasses a range of learning activities—such as tabletop exercises discussing cases, part-task trainers, virtual or augmented reality-based training, utilization of actors or standardized patients, and high-fidelity scenarios with human-patient simulators, or manikins.

Many learning techniques utilize elements of simulation, however, for the purposes of this chapter we will be focusing mainly on simulated patient actor- and manikin-based full patient simulation, as these approaches to simulation are particularly prevalent in medical training.

Simulation is not a new teaching modality. Resusci–Anne models have been in use since the 1960s and the use of obstetrics 'phantoms' to train midwives and doctors dates back as far as the 1600s. Modern simulation has become associated with two key movements in healthcare: the patient safety movement, and increased attention to the learning and application of so-called 'non-technical skills'.

Simulation allows learners to practice and develop skills in an environment where patient risk is mitigated (because patients are removed from the scenario), with the potential to increase individual competence without exposing patients to the risks of being treated by students or trainees. Simulation also enables the testing of systems in clinical environments, identifying latent threats to patient safety.

Fidelity in simulation

Fidelity is a term much used in simulation and refers to the degree to which the simulator replicates reality. Historically, the term 'high-fidelity' is used to describe simulation activities which most closely resemble reality as perceived by the educator and is often associated with full patient simulators or when actors or simulated patients are used. However, while fidelity has often been conceived as a one concept, there are domains of fidelity it is important to consider.

Lavoie[8] offered the following four types of simulation fidelity:
- Environmental fidelity
- Equipment fidelity
- Psychological fidelity
- Sociological fidelity

Environmental fidelity

This incorporates the visual, motor, and sensory clues of the training environment, such as noise, smell, and touch. In-situ simulation is considered to possess a very high level of environmental fidelity, because the workplace and the training environment are the same. Greater environmental fidelity improves the chances of identifying latent threats to performance inherent in that specific environment. However, recreating these can be challenging, time intensive, and not always necessary or appropriate, depending on the learning objectives.

Equipment fidelity

The equipment used, both clinical items and the training tools, can impact the fidelity of your training scenarios. Using genuine clinical equipment creates the highest possible fidelity, but may have cost implications, especially with regards to consumables. In many centres, viable kit is 're-used' in ways that would not be appropriate in the clinical environment to balance fidelity with cost and unnecessary waste.

Procuring equipment for training and simulators should be guided by both the utility of the item, and the cost of ongoing replacement parts and technical support. Given the demands of the environments in which these items are used, damage and malfunction are common.

Psychological fidelity

This is the degree to which the trainee perceives the simulation as real, both in terms of its content and the emotional responses that are triggered. Some consider this the degree to which participants are able to 'suspend their disbelief', reflecting participant engagement and learning. While specific methods may increase psychological fidelity, this is ultimately a reaction by the participants rather than a design element imposed by the designers.

Sociological fidelity

This newer concept reflects the degree to which a simulation replicates the social aspects of clinical practice. In the increasingly inter-professional training environment, attention to this form of fidelity is vital. Its presence creates sociological experiences with genuine clinical team interactions. Its inclusion can reveal challenges in healthcare, including collaborative working, professional identity, inter-professional tensions, and hierarchy. Sociological fidelity can increase the level of participant immersion resulting in visceral and emotional engagement.

All types of fidelity can be achieved, but at a cost. It is commonly assumed, but as yet unproven, that higher fidelity simulation (highly realistic and interactive simulation) produces greater benefits to learners. While high levels of fidelity may superficially seem like the preferable approach, low-fidelity (lower levels of realism and interactivity) may have significant advantages in terms of cost and accessibility. Evidence suggests that optimizing aspects of fidelity appropriate to learners' background, skill-level, experience, and the task at hand creates the most effective simulated learning environment.

Examples of lower fidelity simulations include part-task trainers, but also clinical vignettes for role-plays or tabletop exercises as are used in major incident preparation. While these may lack realism, they offer advantages in terms of cost and simplicity, and they are ideally suited to learning the skills for which they are designed. In many studies, learning from low-fidelity simulations is comparable to that from high-fidelity simulations.

Focusing on methods to achieve psychological and sociological fidelity, over equipment and environmental fidelity, might produce greater learner benefit without requiring expensive equipment and facilities.

▶ The important question to ask is, 'in what ways is the fidelity of your simulation essential in enabling your trainees to meet their learning objectives?' If it is not clear how a more complex or technologically-enhanced simulation would offer benefits over a simpler simulation, it may be beneficial to use a low-fidelity approach.

Fidelity across disciplines

▶ Importantly, fidelity is not perceived equally by all individuals. There is some evidence that there are meaningful differences in perception of fidelity between different disciplines, depending on the focus of the simulation. For example, doctors are likely to respond well to clinical elements of the fidelity (i.e. does the scenario match what would happen in real life in terms of pathology, physiology etc.) whereas nursing trainees, for example, may be more responsive to how much the patient seems like a real human being. ∴ Focusing on either element to the detriment of the other may impair learning on a multi-disciplinary course.

Simulation for teaching and assessment

Simulation is a valuable modality that has been, and continues to be, applied in a variety of ways. With the advancement of simulation technology in the clinical sciences, simulation is now commonly used in teaching medicine, nursing, and allied health professions. Within these professions, simulation has been used to teach psychomotor skills, decision-making skills, clinical processes, non-technical skills, and individual and team skills. From a teaching and learning perspective, simulation can be used as a teaching tool, an assessment tool, a formative feedback tool, and as a research instrument to gather outcomes and impacts of education. Perhaps the most important thing to consider, however, is the distinction between using simulation to create a learning environment or using simulation to assess. The distinction is crucial, because learners approach assessments and learning experiences with different goals and will thus participate in both the scenario and debriefing differently.

Simulation for assessment is generally when a decision about progression is made as a result of the simulation, or when a judgement about a candidate's or team's performance is recorded in a way that may later impact their professional practice. The confusion sometimes arises because simulation provides a valuable opportunity for formative assessment; that is, it can help trainees to improve their skills through practising and debriefing their performance, often including feedback from their colleagues, peers, and supervisors.

Simulation can also be used for high-stakes assessment, for example, selection of medical students, or selection for postgraduate training. High-stakes assessment using simulation in many professions and disciplines, including board exams in anaesthesia, licensing exams for paramedics, and advanced nursing licensure exams. These high-stakes assessment simulations cover areas such as communication, teamwork, procedural skills, management, coping under stress, ethical reasoning, error disclosure, and informed consent.

A common use of simulation for assessment is the Objective Structured Clinical Examination (OSCE). In an OSCE, students rotate through a series of stations designed to simulate common patient interactions that resident doctors are expected to be able to show competence in. Students may take a history, conduct a physical examination, order and interpret investigations, initiate management plans, and communicate with patients. The OSCE has shown to be a valid and reliable method of assessment across a wide spectrum of learners. Other, similar formats have also been developed such as the Objective Structured Teaching Exercise (OSTE) used for faculty development, and the Objective Structured Assessment of Technical Skill (OSATS) which is commonly used in surgical training as the basis for assessing competence in specific procedural skills.

Remember to try and be clear with yourself, and with your learners, about whether you're using simulation for assessment purposes. If participants believe that they are being assessed, or judged on their performance, they may experience more stress, may be less likely to stretch themselves to develop their practice, and may be less likely to explore their underlying feelings and reactions to the scenario in debriefing.

Simulation with a focus on learning needs to be equally clear and explicit, so that participants can feel comfortable and take risks that help them to learn and grow.

Low-resource simulation

Typically, simulators in healthcare are quite expensive, which is a potential problem for many schools and hospitals with limited resources. In fact, it is one of the major barriers to implementing simulation-based education. Therefore, low-cost simulators are of interest for many working in resource-constrained environments. The high cost of many simulators is normally associated with their technological sophistication, which is required to create a higher level of physical fidelity. High physical fidelity may enable trainees to engage as if the patient care setting is real, but also enables them to practice skills on a simulator that more closely reflects the physical characteristics of a live patient.

The first consideration for low-cost simulation, then, is to determine exactly what the learning outcomes are for the scenario. In the case of non-technical skills learning, for instance, an embedded practitioner, simulated patient, actor, or other trained volunteer may provide a very high level of fidelity at a very low cost. For learning specific technical skills, part-task trainers are valuable and relatively less expensive than full-body mannequins. Kneebone and colleagues[9] suggested an approach called Distributed Simulation to create an extremely high-fidelity experience, with relatively low cost and flexible application. Avoiding the need for a bespoke simulation centre by embedding the simulation in a real clinical context, 'in-situ simulation' (see ➲ In-Situ Simulation below) can improve psychological fidelity at a minimal cost, and thus further facilitate learning. Other examples of low-cost simulation solutions include:

- Using pigs' feet or inexpensive synthetic skin for suturing techniques
- Using cardboard or plastic eyeglasses to simulate visual loss from glaucoma, macular degeneration, and retinopathy
- Laparoscopic home box trainers
- Low-cost simulators for managing postpartum haemorrhage

In some cases, industry providers and users in resource-constrained settings have partnered to explore the possibilities and develop simulators for resource-constrained environments. In addition, some simulation educators have been inventing and using their own home-made solutions (e.g. ADAMgel—see ➲ Practical Tips section below). Local, regional, national, and international simulation education organizations are excellent sources of information in this area.

What is a simulated patient?

Simulated patients (SPs) are individuals who portray a specific clinical case in the same way over multiple encounters with different learners and can be represented by standard role-playing. SPs present existing disease processes and a history consistent with the disease for students to learn and practice or to assess their skills. SPs commonly provide feedback after such encounters and are trained to do so.

Many different terms exist for SPs and they may have different characteristics depending on learners' needs; 'Patient actors' may portray a patient with some clinical accuracy and may or may not perform their roles in a highly standardized way. 'Patient educators' are usually patients who are trained to teach, while professional actors may also participate in simulation. Nestel and Bearman,[10] contains a comprehensive exploration of the concepts, issues, and considerations involved in using patients and actors as part of a simulation, where the aim is often to add realism in the patient story or the scenario using real stories from real people. These individuals are often encouraged to be flexible in their performance and response depending on the activities of the clinician. A standardized representation of a patient can create a repeatable experience for clinicians to assist in their learning and assessment. SPs have become more professionalized and in recent years standards have been established for their training and ongoing professional development.

SP core competencies

SPs should demonstrate the following competencies to simulate medical problems and conditions:

- **Professional conduct:** SPs are required to demonstrate professional behaviours that guide their actions, including being reliable and carrying out committed activities as planned, being able to monitor and respond to one's own and others' emotions, and being able to communicate to others as described in the patient scenarios.
- **Acting:** SPs should be able to learn patient roles and credibly simulate a patient's conditions.
- **Documentation:** SPs should be able to memorize the checklist items if the scenario is related to history-taking and physical examination skills, observe the learner during the encounter, and document based on the checklist what the trainees have done.
- **Assessment:** SPs interact with the trainees, so are in the best position to assess the trainees in the exam room, for example, in how they demonstrate communication skills.
- **Feedback:** Since SPs may assess trainees' communication skills, it is important too that SPs are involved in any feedback. This requires SPs to come out of the roles quickly and to comment on the trainees' performance during the session in a psychologically safe way for trainees. This can be a difficult competency for SPs to acquire.

Application of SP

SPs have been used in a wide variety of training, education and assessment settings including:

- Evaluating learners' clinical and conversational skills in the context of an actual patient encounter.
- Improving communication skills between clinicians and patients and medical trainees' skills in history-taking and preventive medicine skills.
- SPs have demonstrated effectiveness in licensure and certification testing.
- SPs have also been integrated into nursing education curricula.

Advantages of using the SP approach[11]:

- SPs are able to provide cases for just-in-time training.
- They are more reliable, and more tolerant of multiple student interactions, than real patients.

- Depending on the scenarios, SPs can allow students to follow-up with patients as a condition develops or changes over time, even in a compressed time frame of examination.
- SP encounters allow students to learn about situations they may not be able to manage alone in a real clinical setting, or where the use of a real patient may be inappropriate.
- SPs can reduce the need for supervision of medical students by physician faculty during clinical encounters.

SP selection and training

SPs need to be carefully selected; Consider asking about their motivations and their understanding of the SP role, and their previous experience working with clinicians or trainees. Debriefing and feedback activities require maturity, emotional intelligence, and discernment, and so may not be appropriate for every SP.

Once SPs are selected, training should be provided to prepare them for both working in scenarios as well as for providing effective feedback. Role portrayal guidance and practice with feedback (ideally from learners as well as other, experienced SPs) should be provided. If SPs are engaging in debriefing, then explicit training on debriefing, including models of debriefing and practice sessions should also be offered. Opportunities for SPs to work with and learn from each other can benefit both individual SPs and your programme as a whole. Remember, SPs are part of your simulation team.

When portraying a standardized patient condition for learners, SP training must be thorough and rigorous. This ensures a consistent performance for learners. At a minimum, SP training should include:

- Familiarization with the physical environment, the learner population, and the assessment regime or learning goals
- Familiarization with the case, including any background scenario details
- Learning to use the checklist
- Putting it all together (performance, checklist, feedback)
- Rehearsal or practice with guidance and feedback

You should closely support SPs—even experienced ones—through this process, introducing them to the checklist and the guide to the checklist, and watching and discussing a learner/SP encounter on video if possible. Feedback from learners and experienced SPs is invaluable in training and development. If appropriate, SPs should participate in a progress interview of the entire case, with the trainer assuming the role of the medical student interviewer.

Supervising practical skills in simulated clinical practice

Historically an approach of 'See one, do one, teach one' was used to supervise practical skill acquisition in the clinical environment, based within an apprenticeship approach. It still permeates some specialties but is generally regarded as unsatisfactory both in terms of learning for the trainee, and for patient safety. However, adaptations of this approach may be more beneficial, and an enhanced version might be: 'See many, learn from the outcome, do many with supervision and learn from the outcome, and finally teach many with supervision and learn from the outcome'. This approach aligns with the new concept of Entrustable Professional Activities.

Entrustable professional activities

An entrustable professional activity (EPA) is an independently executable, observable and measurable clinical skill, ability, or facet of competence, both in terms of its process and its outcome.[12]

EPAs provide a link between the competency-based approach to clinical training and the real-world training and assessment of practical skills. While competencies are descriptors of individuals, EPAs are describing the work unit related to that competence. EPAs may require proficiency in several competency domains and therefore are a more authentic reflection of a clinical encounter's complexity. So rather that assessing single skills such as 'suturing' or 'chest compressions' examples of EPAs might include 'perform an appendectomy', or 'manage a cardiac arrest team'.

Considering practical skills in terms of EPAs and ensuring that those EPAs form a logical sequence with increasing levels of difficulty, risk, and sophistication enables the development of a realistic and achievable practical skills curriculum. It also creates clear expectations for trainees and supervisors about what is expected of them in terms of performance and assessment.

Assessing trainees against the established EPAs can produce 5 levels of required ongoing supervision for that EPA:

- Observation but no execution, even with direct supervision
- Execution with direct, proactive supervision
- Execution with reactive supervision, i.e. on request and quickly available
- Supervision at a distance and/or *ad hoc*
- Supervision provided by the trainee to more junior colleagues.

A full programme should include no more than 20 to 30 EPAs which lead to formal acknowledgement of a decreased need for supervision. Table 5.1 and 5.2 contain illustrative EPAs and detail the elements of an EPA, respectively.

Table 5.1 Examples of EPAs (adapted from Ten Cate, 2013)

Illustrative EPAs	Medical Knowledge	Patient Care	Interpersonal Skills—Communication	Professionalism	Practice-Based Learning—Improvement	Systems-Based Practice
Appendicectomy	✓	✓				
Executing patient handover	✓	✓	✓			✓
Designing therapy protocol	✓				✓	
Chairing multi-disciplinary meeting		✓	✓	✓		✓
Requesting organ donation		✓	✓	✓		
Chronic disease management		✓	✓	✓		✓

Table 5.2 Table demonstrating elements and consideration of designing an EPA (adapted from Ten Cate, 2013)

Element of EPA	Notes
Title	Make it short and avoid words related to proficiency or skill. Ask yourself: can a trainee be scheduled to do this? Can an entrustment decision for unsupervised practice for this EPA be made and documented?
Description	To enhance universal clarity, include everything necessary to specify the following: What is included? What limitations apply? Limit the description to the actual activity. Avoid justification of why the EPA is important, or references to knowledge/skills.
Knowledge, skills, and attitudes	Which competency domains apply? Which sub-competences apply? Include only the most relevant ones. These links may help build observation and assessment methods.
Required knowledge, skills, and attitudes	Which knowledge, skills, and attitudes are necessary to execute the EPA? Formulate this in a way to set expectations. Refer to resources that reflect necessary or helpful standards (e.g. books, a skill course, etc.)
Information to assess progress	Consider observations, products, monitoring of knowledge and skill, multi-source feedback.
When is unsupervised practice expected?	Estimate when full entrustment for unsupervised practise is expected, acknowledging the flexible nature of this. Expectations can shape curricula.
Basis for formal entrustment decisions	How many times must the EPA be executed proficiently for unsupervised practice? Who will judge this? What does formal entrustment look like (e.g. documented, or publicly announced?)

How to set up a simulation training day

The most important consideration when setting up a simulation training day is whether simulation is the correct modality (approach to training), and how best to use it. Having decided that simulation is appropriate, it is then important to be clear about your learning objectives for the day and the best ways to achieve these.

A successful simulation training day requires:

- Involving subject-matter and simulation experts and engaging them as stakeholders and faculty
- Setting up a run-through of the course, where the course can be rehearsed in its entirety, allowing issues to be identified and resolved prior to delivery
- Ensuring that the course legacy is considered from the start, developing supporting materials such that it can be delivered in the future even without key faculty present

Faculty

A variety of faculty will be needed to help you create and sustain a successful simulation training day.

A subject matter expert faculty can support the development of subject-specific training, giving credibility to the intellectual content of the course. However, be aware that expert faculty may not always be experienced in either teaching in general, or in simulation specifically, and may need support to understand the features and limitations of the modality.

Simulation faculty will bring their experience of running simulation-based training and debriefing; however, they may not feel so confident with the specific subject matter content of a particular training day. Therefore, plan on a balance of experienced simulation experts and subject matter experts. It is important, where possible, to ensure that your faculty mix reflects that of your learners. Inter-professional training is often performed by uni-professional faculty. In encouraging open reflection and the establishment of a safe space for debriefing, it is extremely helpful to have an inter-professional faculty who are able to role model an inclusive and collaborative learning environment. Also consider the experience of your simulation faculty. A balance of experienced and novice debriefers can produce learning for both learners and faculty. We recommend, where possible, that all faculty attend a 20-minute pre-briefing prior to any simulation training day to establish these roles and boundaries of responsibility.

Participants

It is vital to consider who your participants are, and how they will find out about your course. The routes by which participants come to your training day can have significant impacts on how it is perceived. While compulsory training has potential advantages in terms of guaranteed attendance, it can significantly impact the response of trainees to the unique stresses of a simulation training environment. Trainees may be more nervous about volunteering—both in scenarios, but also in sharing their thoughts in debriefing. Remember, simulation is not a modality that is appropriate for everyone. With voluntary courses, there is the stress of ensuring that people attend. Contacting your local training administration colleagues responsible for different professional groups can be beneficial in getting your message out. Ensuring attendance, even with mandatory training, can be challenging for many reasons. Many centres still have relatively high rates of registered participants not attending. Measures to reduce this, such as requesting deposits for courses, or outright payment in advance, can ensure better attendance rates, but may put off some potential trainees.

Organizing a training day for an intact team of colleagues, or for individuals in a mixed group, can mean different things for you as well as for participants. This can significantly alter the ease with which people perform and discuss their experiences in debriefs and may need to be carefully managed, particularly when senior members of teams, or those in management positions, are present.

Embedded practitioners/plants

The role of embedded simulation practitioners (previously called plants, or confederates) in scenarios is important to consider when planning a training day. They can assist in ensuring a scenario runs smoothly, and that participants do not get stuck or fixated on various aspects of a scenario. They also have a significant role to play in enhancing the fidelity of the environment, by providing relevant information (e.g. the skin temperature of a manikin). Finally, they can prevent damage to training equipment by ensuring that participants adhere to the limitations of the equipment.

As such, this role is important to the running of the scenario from both a learner and a faculty point of view. In our experience, it can be a role allocated to junior members of the faculty team, or by trained actors. Also, there is sometimes a temptation to introduce a degree of unreliability or difficulty into the performance of an embedded practitioner to make a scenario more complex. We highly recommend that the role be given, where possible, to those with experience in the scenario. Guidance to novices is vital; ● introducing undermining, unreliable, or difficult behaviour in the plant is something we strongly discourage, as it can negatively impact the learning environment.

Technicians

Motivated and capable technicians are important to the running of a simulation centre, let alone a training day. Involving them at the design stage of a simulation-based training programme can help to identify early what equipment is needed and how it might be used.

Establishing what can and cannot be done with the available simulation equipment is important. While manikins are fairly durable, accumulating damage and stains can leave them unsuitable for teaching, requiring repair. If your centre doesn't have the capacity to tolerate regular rotations of equipment, then your technicians will need to let you know what you can and cannot do.

Involve technicians particularly in your run-through and pilot courses to clarify these matters, and to identify gaps in the available equipment or the environment.

We advocate that all simulation training days be accompanied by a technician to guide each scenario, enabling them to rapidly set up the clinical scenarios as well as any accompanying props.

Pre-briefing

A pre-briefing on the day of the course is vital to the success of a training day.

Establishing the experience, expertise, and enthusiasm of the faculty present for the various roles and responsibilities is beneficial to all involved.

We recommend that the pre-briefing include the following:

- Clarify who is doing what throughout the day.
- Establish who is performing debriefing and which stages of debriefing they are performing (depending on model).
- Where possible, allocate more experienced debriefers to observe less experienced debriefers with the remit of giving feedback 'debrief of the debrief'.
- Establish ground rules for interruptions of debriefing. This can be a significant problem with some faculty members, and results in a faculty-heavy conversation, with many contributions back-to-back (known as 'and another thing … ' in our centre). This can overwhelm the debrief, removing the learner-led and reflective aspects of the conversation.
- Run through the scenarios, to establish learning points. Involve the technicians to ensure that the equipment needed is ready and working on the day. Last-minute improvisation is often required but can be avoided through prudent checking in advance.
- Allocate roles for each scenario: Embedded practitioner, Voice—patient, Voice—Phone, Scenario Lead, Debriefers.

Psychological safety

One of the most important considerations in the way you set up your simulation training is to enable your learners to feel safe in the training environment. This will encourage them to engage actively in all aspects of the process and also minimize the threats they may perceive when performing in scenarios in front of fellow trainees, therefore allowing for productive debriefing to take place.

Psychological safety can be established by the selection of appropriate faculty, the consideration of trainee contexts and prior experience in simulation, and finally the scenario itself: both as it is written, but also in how it is run and supported by the faculty.

At the beginning of any simulation training, you can positively impact on psychological safety by clarifying the following:

- Expectations of performance
  - 'We only expect you to be your normal professional self'
- Level of judgement or assessment which will be taking place
  - 'This is a formative experience only, for you to learn, and in which you are safe to make mistakes'
- Ground rules for confidentiality and mutual respect
- Establishment of a 'fiction' contract
  - 'We have tried to make this as realistic as we can, and we ask you to try to suspend your disbelief and to treat this as you would a real clinical scenario'
- Dealing with logistical issues clearly
- Giving a clear briefing of what to expect in the environment and in the scenario

- Meet the manikin sessions allow trainees to get comfortable with the kit, the environment, and the capabilities and limitations of both
- Providing trainees with sufficient information before they enter a scenario, as they would have in real life.
- We use a 'ward-handover' style sheet on some courses which details a number of patients, including those they will see that day, utilizing a familiar tool from the clinical environment to convey information to trainees which we hope allows them to feel more comfortable on entering a given scenario.
- Conveying a commitment to respecting learners, seeking their perspective, and endeavouring to understand it
  - Emphasize the contribution of the trainee
  - Emphasize that mistakes are welcomed as a source of learning for all
  - Express positive regard for your trainees regardless of their performance. 'Nobody gets out of bed to go to work and do a bad job, so what is happening that is impairing performance?'

Debriefing

▶ Debriefing is arguably the most critical phase of any simulation-based training event. Evidence suggests that simulation-based training without debriefing is ineffective.[13] There are many considerations to take into account when approaching this phase:

- Are you intending to give directed, critical feedback to participants based on their performance, or to create a reflective space for them to consider their own assessment of the experience?
- Will the debrief be focused on technical skills (intubation, CPR effectiveness etc) or non-technical skills (leadership, teamwork, management of stress)?
- Will you aim for a non-judgemental approach to the performance of your participants or allow your own views to guide the process
- Will you be aiming for an instructor-led approach, or would you prefer the debrief to be guided by the participants?

The answer to these questions will help to guide you towards an appropriate debrief style and model.

Simulation is ideally suited to improving the performance of clinicians working together in teams. If your goal is to correct specific aspects of learners' clinical practice, you need to plan on giving directed and corrective feedback to participants about their performance in a simulation. That implies a different approach, and one that is unlikely to encourage reflection on overall performance. This kind of feedback may only improve the trainee's ability to manage the same challenge in a simulated environment rather than their performance in their wider clinical practice. It may also damage the psychological safety of the training environment for individual participants, and the group as whole, if the feedback is too critical and faculty-led.

The Debriefing Assessment for Simulation in Healthcare,[14] establishes six elements of effective debriefing and can be used to assess the quality of debriefing practice. The six elements are:

- Establishes an engaging learning environment
- Maintains an engaging learning environment
- Structures the debriefing in an organized way

- Provokes engaging discussions
- Identifies and explores performance gaps
- Helps trainees achieve or sustain good future performance

Regardless of the model or approach to debriefing you choose, a focus on these six elements and their subdomains will increase the likelihood of an effective debriefing conversation.

Debriefing models

The following are recognized debriefing models that can be used to support novice faculty as a script, but also help more experienced faculty to develop other approaches. We recommend that you become confident in a single model before attempting to use other models, so that you always have a method to fall back on. For further reading and references relating to each of these models, please see 'further reading' at the end of this section.

Plus/Delta

Originally developed in the military, Plus/Delta (often abbreviated as $+/\Delta$) is a widely recognized method of simple but effective debriefing. The approach is embodied in the following questions:

- What went well? ('Plus', represents 'positive' outcomes from the simulation)
- What would you differently if you had the chance to repeat the scenario? (Delta, represents 'change')

Advantages: Useful if time is limited (e.g. in-situ). Asks learners to produce suggestions for specific changes to practise.

Disadvantages: Superficial reflection. May not challenge deeply-held assumptions which led to performance gaps in the first place. Focus is primarily on the participant, may not translate to group performance. The Delta part is often incorrectly performed or perceived as 'what went badly?'. This is not an intended output from the model, which should instead focus on planning for improved performance.

Description-Analysis-Application (DAA)

This is a three-phase approach, introduced by Steinwachs:[14]

- Description of the events of the scenario, from the point of view of participants and observers (i.e. 'What happened in there?').
- Analysis of the underlying reasons for the events occurring in the way that they did (i.e. 'Why?').
- Application of the learning from the analysis phase back to routine clinical practice (i.e. 'Now What?').

Within the DAA framework, there are a number of notable debriefing models worth considering:

Debriefing with good judgement and advocacy inquiry

Arguing that it is impossible and unhelpful for faculty to fully suspend their judgement on candidates' performances in simulation, this approach suggests that debriefing is most effective when facilitators use their perspective to help trainees uncover their own underlying emotions and ways of thinking.[16] As a debriefer, this means maintaining a stance of curiosity about what participants are thinking and feeling, and keeping in mind that learners are capable and are trying to improve their practice.

A simple conversational approach helps debriefers to express their expertise and point of view in ways that invite the trainee to consider and explain their own underlying thinking and emotion.

This is achieved through a three-part conversational approach: I saw, I think, I wonder.

- First stage: restating an observed action or behaviour
  - 'I noticed that when you did or said ... '
- Second stage: advancing your point of view as a debriefer
  - 'I thought that this might result in ... '
- Third stage: Inquiry
  - 'I wonder what you think about that?'

Expressed in this way, faculty expertise and points of view can open an invitation to participant reflection, while also allowing them to disagree with the faculty opinion.

Advantages: Structured, allows for faculty viewpoints to be expressed, enables tackling of observed performance gaps, explores assumptions

Disadvantages: Requires expertise to use, can lead to faculty-led debriefs rather than learner-led

The Debrief Diamond

A debriefing method which utilizes a DAA structure, but which aims to support a more learner-led debriefing and provides clear prompts for learners and novice debriefers. Reflection is triggered through an enquiry into emotional responses to scenarios. Emotional responses are conceptualized to be a result of the concordance between an individual's internal assumptions or frames and their assessment of performance in a scenario, either as participant or observer. Exploring emotional responses aims to surface these internal assumptions, allowing discussion and exploration and leading to new insights for the individual or group.

Advantages: non-judgemental, useful in multi-disciplinary faculty and participant training, learner-led, involves whole group

Disadvantages: requires longer debriefing time, initial challenge of using emotions to guide analysis, faculty issues such as observed performance gaps, may not be addressed.

PEARLS/TeamGAINS

These are more complex debriefing methods that encompass a variety of debriefing techniques. These need to be selected depending on features of the scenario and the debrief such as time, rationale for feedback and focus of the debrief (technical/behavioural/cognitive). Both incorporate already discussed techniques such as +/Δ and advocacy/inquiry. PEARLS also gives guidance on directive feedback and teaching. TeamGAINS incorporates more complex debriefing techniques, such as guided team self-correction and systemic-constructivist techniques.

Advantages: Comprehensive, flexible methods for different debriefing scenarios

Disadvantages: Complex and require confidence in multiple techniques, particularly TeamGAINS, which may be challenging for clinicians to implement without significant support/training.

Further reading on debriefing models:
- Plus/Delta
  - ➲ Gardner, R., 2013, June. Introduction to debriefing. In Seminars in perinatology (Vol. 37, No. 3, pp. 166–174). WB Saunders.
  - ➲ Cheng, A., Eppich, W., Epps, C., Kolbe, M., Meguerdichian, M.
  - ➲ Grant, V., 2021. Embracing informed learner self-assessment during debriefing: the art of plus-delta. Advances in Simulation, 6(1), pp.1–9.
- Description-Analysis-Application (DAA)
  - ➲ Steinwachs, B., 1992. How to facilitate a debriefing. Simulation & gaming, 23(2), pp.186–195.
- Debriefing with good judgement and advocacy inquiry
  - ➲ Maestre, J.M. and Rudolph, J.W., 2015. Theories and styles of debriefing: the good judgment method as a tool for formative assessment in healthcare. Rev Esp Cardiol (English Edition), 68(4), pp.282–5.
- The debrief diamond
  - ➲ Jaye, P., Thomas, L. and Reedy, G., 2015. 'The Diamond': a structure for simulation debrief. The clinical teacher, 12(3), pp.171–175.
- PEARLS
  - ➲ Bajaj, K., Meguerdichian, M., Thoma, B., Huang, S., Eppich, W. and Cheng, A., 2018. The PEARLS healthcare debriefing tool. Academic Medicine, 93(2), p.336
- TeamGAINS
  - ➲ Kolbe, M., Weiss, M., Grote, G., Knauth, A., Dambach, M., Spahn, D.R. and Grande, B., 2013. TeamGAINS: a tool for structured debriefings for simulation-based team trainings. BMJ quality & safety, 22(7), pp.541–553.

Debriefing on non-technical skills

While technical skills can be observed and critiqued by clinical faculty with experience in those skills, and this can be the basis for debriefing, non-technical skills similarly require more specific expertise in order to create a valuable learning environment. While giving feedback on the quality of a candidate's observed situational awareness or handover can be helpful to that individual, higher level faculty need access to knowledge and teachable content related to non-technical skills.

Simply describing an observed non-technical skill as 'good' or 'poor' may not enable a learner, or the group of learners as a whole, to productively consider their own practice and develop strategies for improvement.

A few basic theoretical models, tools and resources can assist novice debriefers in exploring non-technical skills and pointing trainees towards ways of improving their performance. Exploring the theoretical models of good performance and discussing barriers to the delivery of good performance in the real world can be fruitful ways to discuss broader clinical performance following a scenario. This approach can also reduce the focus on the performance of an individual in a specific scenario.

Signposting established tools, such as Closed-loop Communication or SBAR handover, as the basis for suggested improvements in non-technical skill performance may support more effective behavioural changes in the long term.

The following non-technical skills are taken from the Crew Resource Management framework by Crichton, O'Connor, and Flin,[17] which was developed in aviation training and translated to healthcare training. The models and tools suggested are ones which have been informative to the author's own development as a debriefer, however there are many other models available, and each has its adherents and critics. Therefore, this is not a prescriptive list but a starting point to assist your initial forays into the non-technical skills literature.

Situational awareness

A model of situational awareness which can help trainees to understand the processes involved is the GUT model. This describes the three phases of establishing situational awareness as: Gathering information; Understanding; Thinking ahead.

An approach to improving situational awareness is called Sharing the Mental Model. This focuses on the systematic vocalization of information by all members of a team within a scenario to ensure that all members are aware of each other's 'mental models'. This improves situational awareness by surfacing all the available information for the group as a whole and the leader in particular. Team vocalizing, coordinated by the team leader and based on the ABCDE approach can be a particularly useful way to do this in an acute clinical scenario.

Decision-making

There are many models of decision-making which can inform a fruitful discussion. Daniel Kahnemann,[18] proposes two 'systems' for decision-making: System 1 is fast, automatic, intuitive, pattern-recognizing, prone to biases; System 2 is slow, effortful, logical, conscious. Each of these systems are useful in clinical practice and have advantages and disadvantages which are worthy of exploring.

A model to support a more logical approach to complex or difficult decisions is FORDEC. This emphasizes a stepwise approach to considering the Facts, Options, and Risks and benefits following which a Decision is made, Executed, and Checked for effectiveness. This process will engage System 2 thinking, in theory producing a more logical decision with less bias.

Communication

Effective communication is a common topic of conversation within debriefs and there are many aspects which can be explored. Discussing the four basic styles (Passive, Aggressive, Passive-aggressive, and Assertive) and considering the advantages and disadvantages of each may be fruitful. Two tools which can support effective communication are Graded Assertiveness and Closed-Loop communication.

Graded assertiveness is a useful approach to voicing concerns and may enable more passive individuals to speak up to more assertive and even aggressive individuals. It is also a useful approach for communication within a hierarchical system to support more junior members in expressing their ideas.

Closed-loop communication is designed to ensure that misunderstandings are avoided when information is transmitted between individuals and is particularly useful when tasks are being requested. It emphasizes the importance of; appropriate formulation of information prior to transmission; effective transmission; checking of receipt of information; appropriate understanding of information; ability to act on information and, in order to close the loop, a process to report back when required activity has either been completed or when problems have arisen.

Whereas a request such as: 'Can someone check the blood glucose please' may or may not result in the blood glucose being tested, a closed-loop request is more likely to result in the task being completed effectively, such as:

> 'Could you (directed to a specific person), please do a blood glucose test because this patient may be dangerously hypoglycaemic. I need the results urgently so please tell me immediately when you have the result or if you're not able to do the test for any reason. Can you repeat this back to me and confirm that you are able to do this task.'

Team working

Teamwork is a complex phenomenon involving the full range of non-technical skills. There are numerous models and theories relating to teamwork which can be a useful basis for discussion.

One specific way to encourage learners to consider their teamwork behaviour relates to the concept of followership. Enhancing followership behaviours is the responsibility of the leader but an awareness of the benefit of these behaviours can be a productive conversation.

A technique used with some success in our debriefs is to ask the group to describe their ideal leader. Having collated their responses on a whiteboard, we then ask them which of these qualities they would wish to see in a team member. Recognition that the same qualities are required can help to break down the perceived gap between leader and team member and empower all team members to be more active. As a specific tool, graded assertiveness, as discussed in the section above on communication, can also be very useful to enable discussion within a team regardless of hierarchy or communication styles.

Leadership

As with team working, leadership is a complex phenomenon to discuss. There are many different ways of approaching this conversation and each has merits. The simplest approach is to discuss the 'ideal' leader as envisaged by the group of learners, and to discuss the barriers which prevent ideal leadership in the clinical environment.

Models of leadership developed specifically for healthcare environments include the NHS Healthcare Leadership Model, which has 9 domains relating to ideal leadership behaviours.[19]

A further approach can be to discuss the different styles of leadership which we may encounter or display ourselves. Considering the advantages and disadvantages of each and how they may be used in different scenarios can be a helpful way to emphasize the flexibility required of an effective leader.

While there are different ways of categorizing leadership styles, commonly recognized styles include: Authoritarian; Paternalistic; Democratic; Laissez-Faire; Transactional; and Transformational[20]:

- Authoritarian—likes to be in control, no consultation with those working with, gives orders, and expects others to obey instructions. Helpful if needing to complete urgent tasks quickly. Can result in resistance due to lack of consultation with team members.
- Paternalistic—similarly to the authoritarian leadership style likes to be in control and takes responsibility for most, if not all, decisions, but attitudes to others in team is more caring. Though employees feel more valued, they may still be frustrated by little autonomy in decision-making processes.
- Democratic—actively encourages team member participation in decision-making through sharing of relevant information, and consultation of group thoughts / suggested actions. Though decision-making is slower, team buy-in to any changes made, or actions taken, is higher.
- Laissez-Faire—little-to-no direction from the person responsible for leading the team. Team members are free to make their own decisions. Useful for highly skilled or expert teams of peers but can lead to a lack of coordinated effort and accountability. High levels of team communication, and regular group feedback are necessary for this approach to succeed.
- Transactional—leaders motivate team members with the offer of rewards for successful performance and, sometimes, punishments or penalties for poor performance. Allows for close monitoring of team member work, but little employee input in decision-making processes so can lead to similar creation of frustration and discontent as with some of the other leadership styles, above.
- Transformational—leaders motivate team members by inspiring them to follow and pursue their values, morals, ideals, and needs. Useful in environments with high levels of change and innovation, can transform f culture. Requires consistent communication and feedback. Transformational change can be risky, and heavy drives for change can lead to employee burnout.

Managing stress

The impact of stress on performance of technical and non-technical skills is a key contributor to observed performance, both good and poor, and is something which simulated scenarios can surface due to the nature of the modality.

A model of the relationship between stress and performance is the Yerkes-Dodson Law, which identifies the impact of different levels of stress, highlighting that both high levels and low levels of stress may impair optimal performance, through overload or apathy.

Stress management requires both an acknowledgement that significant stress is present and affecting performance, and also active steps to manage that stress. Actively engaging learners in a discussion of their own symptoms of stress can assist in discussing how to acknowledge that stress is occurring.

Simple techniques for managing acute stress include deliberate controlled breathing, which reduces physiological symptoms of stress. Gaining situational awareness using a structured approach such as ABCDE may enable stress within an individual and a team to be reduced.

Chronic stress may require more complex interventions and surfacing this in a debrief, while challenging, can be a very powerful moment. Directing learners towards appropriate support outside of the training environment is vital, so it pays to know what support is available within the local organization.

Other models of non-technical skills

The Circle of Care, described by Wilson and Jaye,[21] is an alternative approach to considering non-technical skills relevant to healthcare professionals. In this model, non-technical skills are relabelled as Human Factors Skills for Healthcare, as they are considered to underpin the delivery of all skills in the clinical environment. This addresses the false distinction between technical and non-technical skills, most obviously problematic in mental health scenarios, where the technical skills are also the non-technical skills.

The Circle of Care adds further Human Factors Skills domains, including learning from success and error, and appreciation of the person. This model was developed in collaboration with arts-based educators and aims for a more holistic view of human factors skills in healthcare, and their importance in performing tasks in medicine across all types of healthcare delivery.

Writing scenarios

● The first advice on writing scenarios is, don't do it!

By collaborating with colleagues and other centres, you may discover that the scenario you need is already written. There are many online banks of developed simulation scenarios, including the Sim-One Scenario ExchangeTm (SimulationCanada) and Mededportal (American Association of Medical Colleges), which provide free access to a wide variety of peer-reviewed simulation scenarios. These can be easily adapted to reflect local population demographics and treatment protocols. If you do need to write a new scenario, there are many guides available online alongside templates for documenting the various required elements.

Cognitive load theory is useful to keep in mind when planning and writing simulation scenarios, or indeed when designing any learning environment. The theory holds that people have limitations for processing information, and that this limit is highly contextualized to various aspects of the learning environment and the learner.

An ideal learning environment challenges a learner in appropriate ways that help them develop but does not overload a learner with too much detail or complexity. Cognitive load is made up of intrinsic load (which is how inherently difficult the task is) and extraneous load (how aspects of the design of the learning experience contribute to making it more difficult for learners). The cognitive load of a task depends on the learner—specifically their experience and knowledge. The same task may be much harder for a student to accomplish than for an experienced practitioner, for example. A good scenario design provides the opportunity for a simulation educator to tailor the learning opportunity to a students' ability level, either making it more or less challenging, as need be. A helpful analogy is to consider how good bedside teaching provides opportunities for those at all levels to learn something and how this is achieved.

Good practice in scenario design is to:
- Design a core scenario that allows for multiple potential learning outcomes depending on the level and experience of a learner
- Think about what 'good performance' would look like for different levels of learner and across different disciplines. Ensure that they would be able to enact that within the scenario
- Allow less experienced participants to achieve less within the scope of their practice
- If your training day has very specific learning objectives there is no harm in re-emphasizing these before the scenario. For example, in a simulation course focused on sepsis, we remind our participants before the scenario to ensure they complete the Sepsis 6, the six key immediate clinical interventions which have been shown to reduce mortality from Sepsis. Failure to achieve these interventions despite this reminder can then be more openly addressed in debriefs following scenarios where there have been issues.

Key tips and pitfalls:

- Be clear in your learning objectives for the scenario, both clinical and non-technical.
- Do not be tempted to add extra elements of complexity which do not contribute to your learning objectives simply for the sake of it. A narrower focus can support significant learning towards specified objectives as well as feeding into a more focused debrief.
- Even simple tasks such as attaching monitoring devices to the manikin can significantly slow the progression of a scenario, as these seemingly simple tasks require greater cognitive effort for trainees in an unfamiliar environment. Carefully consider the state-of-play you want at the start of your scenario to ensure that the maximum focus is on the core learning objectives.
- Ensure that you have developed appropriate supporting information (ECGs, Radiographs, Blood test results) and patient notes as these contribute to the fidelity of the learning experience.
- Spend some time developing the 'backstory' to a scenario, the patient, and other characters involved. This will inform any individuals taking on roles within the scenario. The better the characterization, the better the fidelity, regardless of the modality used.
- The speed at which a scenario progresses may not reflect reality. This is more noticeable in centre-based training, where you have control of the environment and equipment and can set the cues. In general, these scenarios progress at a much faster pace than they would in real life.
- In-situ scenarios can progress much more slowly because you are constrained by the equipment and environment to conform to usual practice. Therefore, in-situ, if you want to speed the scenario up, you may need to sacrifice some fidelity, or explicitly step in to do so.
- A useful source of inspiration for new scenarios can be your local clinical incident database. Use this to identify themes in practice rather than copying specific individual cases and take all steps to protect both patients' and colleagues' identities.
- Participants in scenarios are often 'expecting the worst'. Having scenarios where this does not occur can reinforce the importance of good practice and management in all clinical care situations (not just crises).

Table 5.3 illustrates a template which could be used to create a simulation scenario and consider the resources required to conduct it.

Table 5.3 Suggested overview template for a simulation, as used at the Simulation and Interactive Learning centres at Guy's & St Thomas' NHS Foundation Trust, London, UK.

Patient Name: Patient Age:		
Major Problem Learning Objectives	Medical e.g. Sepsis Medical/Clinical e.g. Recognition of Sepsis; Delivery of timely antibiotics	Suggested Non- Technical Skill Learning objectives: Leadership of clinical team; Appropriate escalation; Effective handover
Narrative Description	Story: Past medical history: Drug history: Allergies: Social history:	
Staffing	Faculty Control Room: <1xtechnician> <1xdebriefer> Faculty Role Players: <Nursing assistant>	Candidates <1xnurse,1xNursing Assistant,1xDr> or <1xAllied Health Professional,1x Nurse,1xDR>
Case Briefing	To All Candidates Nurse- Allied Health Professional- Nursing assistant-	To Role Players
Manikin preparation		
Room setup		
Simulator operation	Patient voice x1 <Manikin operator x1>	
Props needed		
Notes to faculty		

Roles

▶ One 'cardinal rule' of simulations is to avoid, where possible, placing people in roles they would not normally take. Do not expect your learners to 'act' in a role they would not normally take. Principally this relates to disciplines (i.e. asking a nurse to pretend to be a physiotherapist), but some learners will also struggle to play a different level within their own discipline. This limits the potential applicability of the learning for those who are working outside their normal (or future) scope of practice.

- When preparing your scenario, try to incorporate flexibility of roles such that they can be adapted for attendance by different professions.
- If you do set up 'role-play' within your training, provide as much information as possible on each role for your learners, and explain the potential benefits in taking on the role (e.g. empathizing with other clinical colleagues, creating a learning opportunity for their peers, etc.)

Table 5.3 illustrates a role guide template for an individual taking part in a simulation.

Table 5.4 Suggested template for a simulation role, as used at the Simulation and Interactive Learning centres at Guy's & St Thomas' NHS Foundation Trust, London, UK.

Role guide for: Patient/Relative/Clinical staff/other (Delete as appropriate)	
Role:	Name:
Role played by (details)	Actor Manikin
	Faculty/Embedded Practitioner
Scenario Description	Story: Past medical history: Drug history Allergies: Social history:
Instructions to actor/faculty/ embedded practitioner	e.g, You are an 80 year old female with a hot, swollen knee which has been causing you pain for the last day. Your mobillty is reduced and you are very worried as you have a dog at home and you don't know who is going to be able to look after it.
Suggested quotes prompts	e.g, I'm so much pain, my knee really hurts … I'm worried about my dog, he doesn't like being on his own ….
Clinical knowledge required for rolCostumee	Nil
Costume	
Props	

Equipment

The equipment available for use in practical skills training is increasingly technologically advanced and realistic, allowing for recreation of a wider variety of clinical situations. At the same time spending on this equipment can consume significant amounts of money in what may be limited budgets and there may be other options to consider.

Human–patient simulators/manikins

These are advanced computer controlled life-size manikins, which simulate clinical signs, such as breathing, pulses, and heartbeat. The most expensive manikins can produce exhaled CO_2 to assess success of intubation or be used for procedures such as chest drain insertion.

However, the expense and complexity of these manikins, as well as their necessary complexity may not be warranted for a centre offering training in more routine clinical care, especially if there is a high throughput of trainees. The more complex a manikin, the greater the requirement for expertise in their use and the more ways in which they can be broken.

Most manikins now support wireless functionality, however certain models still use cable connectivity and this needs to be considered in ensuring both usability and safety (cables are a significant trip hazard).

Using manikins also requires a designated control area, with visibility into the clinical training area and support for audio-visual equipment. Storage space is also required, and so investing in moving and handling training for staff who routinely move this equipment around is recommended, as they are both heavy and cumbersome to manipulate.

As well as the adult multi-function manikins, there are a variety of other models available with specific functionality, including maternal birthing simulators, specific airway training simulators. A range of age-appropriate manikins is also available for training on neonatal and paediatric scenarios.

Maintenance

Manikins require ongoing care to ensure good function. Consumable parts, such as skin and vein sets for arms, require budgeting, particularly if your trainees are encouraged to perform cannulation and venepuncture during scenarios.

Most manufacturers offer extended warranty deals and are usually able to offer visits and repairs on site unless the damage is significant. These are often well worth the cost.

The surfaces of manikins can become quite unsightly if not cared for appropriately. The following are common pitfalls and advice:

- Never write on the manikin in biro, this will be very difficult to remove.
- Check the manufacturing advice for what ink can be used and on what areas.
- Areas of hard plastic (usually the legs) are amenable to greasepaint for moulage and can be effectively cleaned using WD40.
- Areas of silicon-based covering (more skin-like) will stain with greasepaint and will also retain adhesive from dressings, leading to an accumulation of unsightly patches. Use water-based paints (children's face paints work well) for moulage.
- Where adhesives are used, products such as 'Sticky-stuff remover' can be used to maintain the condition of the surface.

It is vital that any faculty using the manikins, especially if they are operating in-situ or without technician supervision, are aware of their appropriate usage and care. We advise that faculty spend some time training with technicians to develop a basic level of skill in operating the manikin as well as covering the basic 'dos and don'ts'. This can form part of continued faculty development, and it may even be worth creating a certification process for this if you have a large faculty.

Audio-visual equipment

To involve all individuals enrolled on a course within the scenarios, a mechanism by which non-participants can observe the scenarios is key. At the simplest level this may include an observation room separated from the clinical training environment by a window.

However, most centres operate some level of audio-visual system both to allow multiple angles of observation, as well as streaming to different sites (e.g. control room and observation room) and for recording and playback. These recordings can be used as a training device and may be useful for faculty development, programme review, and research.

▶ Movable cameras and active management of camera angles produce better results for observers, however, in our experience the greatest challenge is sound quality. Invest in good quality microphones and try to set up your system with an experienced technician. We prohibit untrained faculty from adjusting the settings on audio equipment in order to maintain the best quality sound output.

Audio-visual equipment companies can provide comprehensive solutions, but with the advantage of functionality comes a significant cost. It is possible to set up your own system using network-video recorders and radio microphones as well as telephone recorders, however this will require technical expertise to both install and maintain.

Part-task trainers

The equipment available for use in practical skills training is increasingly technologically advanced and realistic, allowing for recreation of a wider variety of clinical situations. Unfortunately, acquiring this equipment can consume significant amounts of money in what may be a very limited budget, and therefore alternative options might need to be considered:

- Technological solutions: Increasingly realistic, complex, and expensive models are available for many tasks. Robotics devices incorporating virtual reality and haptics (touch feedback) are also increasingly popular. There is significant expense in both initial outlay and maintenance.
- Animal tissue solutions: For some tasks there are animal models available from specialist companies. These include sheep thoraces for chest drain insertion, porcine intestine for basic surgical skills and pigs' blood, which we have used on our Extracorporeal membrane oxygenation training days. These are cheaper solutions and are disposable so can sustain damage. However, they require attention to their appropriate storage and disposal and there may be issues for pregnant or observant religious residents.
- Do-it-yourself solutions: The internet is a good source of recipes for home-made gelatin-based models for practising skills on, particularly for training in basic ultrasound skills. One particular product called

ADAMgel can be made from regular kitchen ingredients and can be adapted for multiple different uses.

ADAMgel (aqueous dietary-fibre antifreeze mix gel)

ADAMgel is a stable elastic polymer gel formed from a combination of a dietary fibre supplement and antifreeze, producing an excellent tissue surrogate and ultrasound medium. As most common antifreeze compounds are humectants and antimicrobials it is also resistant to infection and desiccation.

The concentration of Ispagula used is 2–10% depending on function needed. Anything that facilitates the release of gels from the husk—grinding/simmering/recycling—will increase strength.

Antifreezes used for ADAMgel preparation are:
- mono-ethylene glycol 15–100% (ordinary antifreeze)
- mono-propylene glycol 12–75% ('green' antifreeze, food, and medicine additive)
- glycerol 5–30% (vegan-organic antifreeze. This does need an additional preservative)

Varying antifreezes and combinations produce subtle differences to the texture and properties of the gel. Increasing concentration improves water retention and makes it a more jelly-like, and less porridge-like, consistency.

The water used to prepare ADAMgel can be any non-extreme pH and salinity. Calcium improves gel strength by promoting crosslinking.

Basic 'Recipe':
- mix 100 g ground isphagula husk with 200 ml antifreeze of choice then add 800 ml water and microwave until it boils.

➲ For more information on the properties of ADAMgel, see Willers et al.[22]

Technicians

Technicians are a vital part of your centre. Most technicians have no prior training or background in clinical medical so may need explanation of terminology. With time and support they can become experts in simulating deteriorating physiology for scenarios. Their involvement from an early stage of new courses can ensure the smooth running of your programmes through the preparation of appropriate kit, provided sufficient time is provided in advance to make any special preparations.

Career progression of technicians can be an issue but there are routes to support their development. Most national and international simulation associations have technician specific sections, as well as offering bespoke training and opportunities at conferences such as SimGHOSTS. Other opportunities for training include Moulage courses, as well as ensuring they are invited to appropriate equipment training within your trust, enabling them to keep your training equipment up to date in line with the wider trust.

There is also the possibility for your centre, and your technicians, to assist in trialling new equipment for your trust, such as new 'crash' (cardiac arrest equipment) trolleys or defibrillators.

In-situ simulation

'Simulations that occur in the actual clinical environment and whose participants are on-duty clinical providers during their actual workday' (Patterson,
Blike, and Nadkarni,[23]).

In-situ simulation is a particular application of simulation training that
seeks to explore the ability of staff to perform both technical and non-
technical skills in their actual clinical work environment. It has numerous
advantages and challenges, which make its use both difficult and rewarding.
Advantages:
- Uses intact clinical teams, increasing sociological fidelity
- Trainees operate in their real clinical environment, enhancing
  environmental fidelity
- Real clinical equipment is available for use, increasing environmental/
  equipment fidelity
- All of these features can significantly enhance psychological fidelity
- Tests individuals, teams, and systems, allowing identification of active
  and latent threats

Latent threats are defined as errors in design, organization, training, or
maintenance that may contribute to medical errors and have a significant
impact on patient safety. They are often not apparent until surfaced through
real events. If those real events are based on simulation exercises rather
than actual clinical care, latent threats can be identified and addressed before they emerge in patient care, thus increasing the safety of the system. In-
situ simulation can, in this way, enhance patient care, outcomes, and safety
through promoting change.

🛑Disadvantages
- Requires commitment of clinical staff, potentially decreasing available
  staffing for patient care
- Maintaining psychological safety can be more challenging
- Perception that bystanders, especially patients and relatives, may be
  distressed to witness a simulated crisis event or an event that exposes
  latent errors
- More challenging to debrief, particularly around non-technical skills
- Scheduling in-situ simulations can be challenging. Ad-hoc exercises often
  suffer from a lack of prioritization, whereas timetabled events may be
  subject to cancellation and lose the element of spontaneity
- Extreme care must be taken to avoid simulation equipment and
  consumables entering patient care areas and workstreams (e.g.
  simulated drugs, mislabelled fluids, or non-active equipment being used
  on live patients)

In-situ Simulation checklist

A process of organizing and carrying out in-situ simulations can enable it to
become a routine part of your practice and an invaluable tool for learning,
both for your trainees, but also your organization as a whole.

Prior to an exercise:
- Confirm the learning objectives with commissioners
- Identify all key stakeholders in the location and establish contact, to
  check permission and encourage engagement

- Scope out the location yourself, considering the ease of setting up equipment and identify a location where debrief may occur
- Will you use video or other approaches to recording? You will need to consider consenting all individuals in the clinical area
- Ensure all equipment, especially manikins, are fully charged and in working order! Ensuring a technician is available in-situ is valuable
- Consult your organization's risk officer and planning staff to ensure that you are complying with all processes
- Carefully plan the use of any equipment or consumables in patient care areas, including checking in and out any simulated drugs, therapies, or equipment, even if they are clearly labelled as simulation only

Scenario writing:
- Agree key elements of the scenario with stakeholders
- Ensure all possible adjuncts to your scenario (CXRs, blood results) are available at the highest possible fidelity (i.e. on a computer screen as with PACS)
- Be aware that scenarios in-situ often proceed at a more realistic (i.e. slower) pace than scenarios in-centre. Concentrate on the backstory and responses to likely initial management strategies Be wary of rushing the scenario along to a desired endpoint, as you may lose the opportunity to discuss significant issues that may arise and obstruct the perceived progress of the scenario.

The exercise:
- Recheck the clinical location and permission to continue
- Take all equipment and consumables (clinical and training kit) with you. Make sure you have planned carefully to check out and return any materials, consumables, drugs, or equipment you use
- Be aware of health and safety, cables from manikins running along the floor of a busy clinical area are hazardous
- Perform a pre-brief and familiarization session with your learners, to ensure any training kit is known to them
- Establish protocols for any delays, drop-outs, or cessation of the exercise due to clinical requirements

Afterwards:
- Clean up after yourselves! Thank all those involved
- Identify and arrange restocking of all consumables used, carefully checking your inventory to ensure that no simulated equipment, drugs, or other consumables have entered the patient care workstream
- Circulating learning points to the whole department can help to disseminate that learning and encourage greater engagement with future exercises
- If latent threats have been identified, ensure to highlight these to individuals who have responsibility for running the affected department and offer to reassess those latent threats in future with further simulations

In-situ debriefing model

Debriefing an in-situ exercise carries certain specific challenges:
- Shorter time to debrief. Participants are often keen or under pressure to return to their clinical work
- Psychological safety. Debriefing participants in their actual clinical environment, potentially feeding back on errors made or observed, carries some risk of being perceived as negative criticism
- Separating individual performance from system effects
- Identification and addressing of latent errors. The surest way to engage stakeholders in the value of in-situ simulation is to demonstrate the impact it can have on improving process and patient care

The debrief model we use is based on the DAA structure, with Plus/Delta or advocacy/inquiry (A/I) questioning techniques utilized during the analysis phase (see Debriefing section). The total time for this type of debrief is 20 minutes maximum. We suggest the following 'script':

Description:
- Allow an emotional vent: 'How did that feel?'
- Description of events—involve observers or those on the sidelines if possible.
  - 'Could someone describe what happened?'
  - 'Did anyone see it differently, or see anything else occur?'

Transition:
- Faculty-led description of the clinical aspects of the scenario, highlighting the intended learning to ensure these points are covered

Analysis
- If dealing with systems/latent threats we recommend a
- Plus/Delta approach:
  - 'What went well in this scenario?'
  - 'What could be improved in the team/department/systems in relation to this scenario?'
- If dealing with individual performance, we recommend an A/I approach:
  - 'I noticed that.. [identify behaviour]'
  - 'I know that/I think that… [link behaviour to observed or hypothesized outcome]'
  - 'I wondered what you thought about that?'

Transition
- Sum up the learning points from the analysis phase

Application:
Establish how these learning points, at the individual and departmental/systems level, will be taken forward to create positive changes and how those changes can be sustained

Evaluating practical skills and simulation training

Planning effective evaluation of any training intervention should start at the same time as creating the training programme itself. Establishing appropriate learning objectives for your programme is a vital step, because your evaluation should be measuring the achievement of these objectives. A basic learning objective should contain three things: the behaviour or performance you want the learner to be able exhibit, any conditions under which they perform it, and the standard to which they are required to perform it. Using the language of Bloom's taxonomy can also be helpful in writing learning objectives which can then be effectively evaluated, or in the case of using simulation for assessment, easily assessed.

Technical knowledge and skills learning

Evaluating a programme for its effectiveness in teaching technical skills is relatively straightforward, as you can use the skill itself as a measure of learning, and you can evaluate participants' change in performance as a result of training. However, follow-up evaluations often show that any benefits of a single episode of training attenuate significantly over time.[24] Objective measures of skill performance can include time to completion of the skill, alongside a measure of error rates in skill delivery.

'Non-technical' knowledge and skills learning

❶ It is harder to evaluate impact on behaviours and attitudes towards the so-called 'non-technical skills'. Many observational tools exist, often limited to a particular specialty (Anaesthetists' Non-technical Skills—ANTS, Non-Technical Skills for Surgeons—NOTSS or scenario, Rescue—deteriorating medical patient) and these can have some value in evaluating impacts of training. However, non-technical skills are more complex and contextual in their performance than technical skills. Some evidence points to the potential for self-efficacy—the beliefs that individuals hold about their ability to achieve good performance in a challenging environment—as a valid proxy measure for learning non-technical skills.[25] Though it is not always the first approach considered, the learning that takes place in a scenario-debrief-based simulation training programme, particularly with more complex debriefing models, may benefit from a qualitative approach to evaluation, utilizing interviews and focus groups to explore impacts. For more information on developing evaluation strategies appropriate to your project you may enjoy The Evaluation Toolkit,[26] produced by the authors of this chapter.

Evaluating debriefing

Tools exist for the evaluation of debrief quality, such as the Debriefing Assessment for Simulation in Healthcare (DASH) or the Observational Structured Assessment for Debriefing (OSAD). These are helpful in directing attention to multiple aspects of the debrief and providing guidance to both parties in an evaluation of debrief quality.

Operating and managing a simulation training centre

There are many important elements to consider when running your simulation centre. From day-to-day running of courses, to keeping an eye on the bigger picture and working strategically within your organization, there are proactive steps you can take to ensure that your centre is successful.

At an international level, there is a set of standards and an associated accreditation process for simulation centres offered by the Society for simulation in healthcare. Similarly, some national and regional societies are developing their own standards for simulation education, e.g. the Association for Simulated Practice in Healthcare (ASPiH) in the UK. Ensuring that the work you do matches these standards can be challenging, especially if you are operating as a stand-alone centre. However, they provide valuable guidelines, based on effective practice and emerging research evidence, about how simulation education can be most effective—so refer to them when possible. Increasingly, centres are collaborating across regions to establish networks for sharing resources and expertise. Making links with other centres can also be a source of peer review, with an external quality assurance process. Well-designed quality assurance frameworks can be a useful way to support this process, particularly when starting out, as they give specific targets for the improvement of both individual courses and centres as a whole.

Working interprofessionally is an important element in contemporary simulation training, and it is worth identifying key members of other professions who can support you in establishing your centre and ensuring you have buy-in from all staff. Identifying staff with relevant experience in simulation and debriefing is also important. Opportunities to develop these experiences are increasingly widespread, and you may discover you have experienced debriefers available to you already.

➲ The two elements of running a simulation centre you will probably struggle with the most as a clinician are administration and technical support. These are best run by people with the relevant experience, and retaining these staff is important in maintaining a thriving centre. Career progression for simulation technicians is now starting to be a focus within the field, and in many centres technicians may emerge from other backgrounds (resus officers, administration staff, clinicians).

➲ Sustaining a simulation centre requires good relationships with commissioners and funders of training—lead providers of education for professional groups as well as local health education boards. Importantly, as your centre grows, you will also need to plan for the development of your faculty's interests and skills.

Future of healthcare simulation

Simulation technology is evolving rapidly, as is healthcare. As with any complex and dynamic field, many questions emerge. What is going to happen with different modalities of simulation technology? For example, high-fidelity simulators are currently very expensive. Will prices stay high with the advancement of simulation technology? Many simulators currently are housed at expensive simulation labs and centres. Will the trend of in-situ simulation eventually make these obsolete? Is it possible for individual students to own a toolkit of simulation technologies, which they can use to practice on their own, in their own time?

For simulators, especially task trainers, in general, one task trainer offers limited training opportunities. Due to the high cost, one question for institutions to consider is how many different simulators need to be bought? With technology advancing rapidly, we believe that one or two high-fidelity simulators should be able to demonstrate most of the functions that medical students and junior trainees might need to learn. It is certainly possible that, in time, individual students would be able to afford a simulator for their personal study.

The game industry is also booming. Successful virtual simulations have been developed to improve teaching and training in medicine. Virtual simulation is a potential alternative to task trainers as well as high-fidelity simulators, because they can provide an immersive learning experience. Of course, another attractive aspect of virtual simulations are that they can be fun, and therefore motivating to trainees and valuable for long-term retention (both proven conclusively with learning technology innovations among school children). We believe that future virtual simulations will be developed to make medical learning more interesting and engaging for trainees.

Also, the ubiquitous nature of mobile technologies in other aspects of life will, we believe, make them an attractive platform for simulation learning in medical education. Mobile devices can be compatible with virtual game and high-fidelity simulators, and thus have the potential to make medical education accessible to trainees at any time or place.

Virtual reality in medical education

Virtual reality (VR) refers to an environment in which trainees are immersed in a multimedia, three-dimensional, simulated environment that simulates reality and allows trainees to interact, practice skills, and learn teamwork and collaboration skills, and manipulate medical equipment as well as make diagnostic decisions. The VR environment includes sensory stimulation and is designed to prevent trainees from perceiving influences from the real world outside the simulation. VR has already been applied to a variety of scenarios for training purposes including simple task practice, complex patient interactions, and wholescale clinical scenarios.

A virtual patient is a variation of VR that provides a limited immersive experience where trainees interact with a computer-based simulation of a patient case scenario. Trainees assume the role of the healthcare professional as an avatar, such as a nurse or doctor, and make judgements and clinical decisions based on their assessment of the virtual patient. Trainees learn the role of the professional they represent with regard to assessment, clinical diagnosis, treatment, and care of the patient, just as they would if interacting with a real-life patient.

Serious games are another variant of VR, defined by Zydia[27] as 'mental contests, played with a computer in accordance with specific rules, that use entertainment to further training'. Serious games allow for experiential learning, problem-based learning, and a more learner-centred approach, as the student is immersed in the virtual environment and becomes engaged in the learning process.[28]

VR can allow learners an opportunity to immerse themselves into a constructed, realistic, and most importantly, safe environment where they can practise skills, interact, and collaborate with peers or other professionals, make decisions related to care and interventions, and manipulate equipment without fear of harming a patient. VR simulations can be used in any area of clinical practice, but are especially useful in environments where limited access to the experience is available, such as disaster or perioperative nursing.

With advances in technology including augmented reality and haptics, which generate real sensations of touching and manipulating equipment in virtual procedures, it is likely that VR is here to stay.

References

1. Rodriguez-Paz J, Kennedy M, Salas E, Wu AW, Sexton JB, Hunt EA, Pronovost PJ. Beyond 'see one, do one, teach one': toward a different training paradigm. *BMJ Qual Saf* 2009;18(1):63–68.
2. Huang GC, Smith CC, Gordon CE, Feller-Kopman DJ, Davis RB, Phillips RS, Weingart SN. Beyond the comfort zone: residents assess their comfort performing inpatient medical procedures. *Am J Med* 2006;119(1):e17–24.
3. Wulf G, Shea C, Lewthwaite R. Motor skill learning and performance: a review of influential factors. *Med Educ* 2010;44(1):75–84.
4. Peyton JWR. Teaching in theatre. In: Peyton JWR (Ed.), *Teaching and learning in medical practice* (pp. 171–180). New York, NY: Manticore, 1998.
5. Nikendei C, Huber J, Stiepak J, Huhn D, Lauter J, Herzog W, Jünger J, Krautter M. Modification of Peyton's four-step approach for small group teaching—a descriptive study. *BMC Med Educ* 2014;14(1):68.
6. Orde S, Celenza A, Pinder M. A randomised trial comparing a 4-stage to 2-stage teaching technique for laryngeal mask insertion. *Resuscitation* 2010;81(12):1687–1691.
7. Gaba DM. The future vision of simulation in health care. *BMJ Qual Saf* 2004;13(suppl 1):i2–i10.

8. Lavoie P, Deschênes MF, Nolin R, Bélisle M, Garneau AB, Boyer L, Lapierre A, Fernandez N. Beyond technology: a scoping review of features that promote fidelity and authenticity in simulation-based health professional education. *Clin Sim Nursing* 2020;42:22–41.

9. Kneebone R, Arora S, King D, Bello F, Sevdalis N, Kassab E, Aggarwal R, Darzi A, Nestel D. Distributed simulation–accessible immersive training. *Med Teach* 2010;32(1):65–70.

10. Nestel D, Bearman M. *Simulated patient methodology: theory, evidence and practice*. Oxford: John Wiley & Sons, 2014.

11. Collins JP, Harden RM. *The use of real patients, simulated patients and simulators in clinical examinations 2004*. Copenhagen: Association for Medical Education in Europe (AMEE) Guide, (13), 2004.

12. ten Cate O. Nuts and bolts of entrustable professional activities. *J Grad Med Educ* 2013;5(1):157–158.

13. Issenberg BS, McGaghie WC, Petrusa ER, Lee Gordon D, Scalese RJ. Features and uses of high-fidelity medical simulations that lead to effective learning: a BEME systematic review. *Med Teach* 2005;27(1):10–28.

14. https://harvardmedsim.org/debriefing-assessment-for-simulation-in-healthcare-dash/

15. Steinwachs B. How to facilitate a debriefing. *S&G* 1992;23(2):186–195.

16. Rudolf JW, Simon R, Dufresne RL, Raemer D. There's no such thing as 'non-judgemental' debriefing: a theory and method for debriefing with good judgement. *Simul Healthc* 2006;1(1):49–55.

17. Crichton M, O'Connor P, Flin R. *Safety at the sharp end: a guide to non-technical skills*. Farnham: Ashgate Publishing, 2013.

18. Kahneman D. *Thinking, fast and slow*. London: Macmillan, 2011.

19. Storey J, Holti R. *Towards a new model of leadership for the NHS*. London: NHS Leadership Academy, 2013.

20. Barcan M. Leadership approaches in health organizations. *JoDRM* 2019;10(2):180–187.

21. Willson S, Jaye P. Arts-based learning for a circle of care. *Lancet* 2017;390(10095):642–643.

22. Willers J, Colucci G, Roberts A, Barnes L. 0031 Adamgel: an economical, easily prepared, versatile, selfrepairing and recyclable tissue analogue for procedural simulation training. *BMJ STEL* 2015;1(Suppl 2):A27.

23. Patterson MD, Blike GT, Nadkarni VM. In situ simulation: challenges and results. In: Henriksen K, Battles JB, Keyes MA, Grady ML (eds.), *Advances in patient safety: new directions and alternative approaches (vol. 3: performance and tools)*. 2008. Rockville, MD: Agency for Healthcare Research and Quality (US), 2008.

24. Kneebone R. Evaluating clinical simulations for learning procedural skills: a theory-based approach. *Acad Med* 2005;80(6):549–553.

25. Reedy GB, Lavelle M, Simpson T, Anderson JE. Development of the HUMAN FACTORS SKILLS for Healthcare Instrument: a valid and reliable tool for assessing interprofessional learning across healthcare practice settings. *BMJ STEL* 2017;3(4):135–141.

26. Simpson, T., Kitchen, S., Lavelle, M., Anderson, J.E., Reedy, G., 2017. The Evaluation Practice Toolkit. [online] King's College London. Available at: https://kclpure.kcl.ac.uk/portal/en/publications/evaluation-practice-toolkit [Accessed 11th June 2018]

27. Zyda, M., 2005. From visual simulation to virtual reality to games. *Computer*, 38(9), pp.25–32.

28. Graafland, M., Schraagen, J.M. and Schijven, M.P., 2012. Systematic review of serious games for medical education and surgical skills training. *British journal of surgery*, 99(10), pp.1322–1330.

Assessment principles

David Sales and Bryony Sales

The purpose of assessment and integration within curricula

'Assessment is a good servant and a bad master' French Proverb (paraphrased). The purpose of assessment is to gather sufficient evidence from multiple sources to confirm a standard of learning, or the acquisition of learning outcomes, which subsequently enables decisions to be made about a learner's current abilities. The word assessment comes from the Latin verb 'assidere', meaning 'to sit with'. The origin of the word implies that assessment is something teachers do with and for students, rather than to students.

One of the most common distinctions made between types of assessment within medical education are the differences outlined between formative and summative assessments (Box 6.1).

As the *Tiger* cartoon (Figure 6.1) neatly summarizes, teaching does not always result in learning. The two approaches of assessment for learning and assessment of learning play complementary roles in promoting meaningful, lasting learning.

Box 6.1 Formative and summative assessment

▶ Assessment can be for the sole benefit of the learner when it is described as 'formative', in being an **assessment for learning** or 'summative' for the benefit of external agencies when it is considered an **assessment of learning**. Where students act as their own assessors to monitor their own learning and work towards learning goals, we can consider assessment as operating as **assessment as learning**.

Formative assessments:
• operate as an instructional technique during learning
• are usually not graded, as the focus is on providing rich, descriptive qualitative feedback
• purpose is to evaluate progress, i.e. focused on the process of learning
• assessment for learning
• high impact on learning
• continuous
• typically low stakes

Summative assessments:
• determine, usually at a fixed moment in time after learning, students' knowledge and abilities
• are usually graded, often to a specific mark scheme or set of grade descriptors (may provide evaluative feedback)
• purpose is to assess mastery, i.e. focused on the outcomes of learning
• assessment of learning
• periodic
• limited positive impact on learning
• typically high stakes

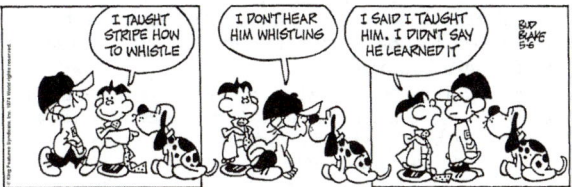

Fig. 6.1 Assessment of learning © King Features Syndicate (reproduced with permission).

Some institutions may have assessment departments that exist separately from those with responsibility for curriculum—in terms of governance arrangements, process, and content. This threatens the full integration of programmes of assessment within postgraduate curricula.

Consequences of this divide include:

- tests that were unrelated to the taught curriculum
- test methods that were intuitively familiar to examiners based on their clinical work (such as the viva) but not students
- off-the-shelf tests that were not appropriately designed for the intended purpose and/or were poorly constructed and that tested what was easy to test, rather than what was important.

The problem is that assessment in medical education addresses complex competencies which require both quantitative and qualitative information gathered from multiple sources and, crucially, involves making professional judgements. There has been an emerging recognition that the content of assessment plays a far more important role than its format. The solution has been a shift in recent years from individual test methods to assessments intertwined within entire education programmes that are more closely aligned to the learning process.[1] ▶ Programmes of assessments should be designed as an integral part of the curriculum—serving and supporting its purposes. Assessments should never be an unrelated, standalone hurdle for other purposes, such as informing decisions about career progression. The challenge for test designers is to ensure that the stated objectives of each assessment within a programme are met—in other words, that it is valid or that it appropriately samples and assesses the stated learning outcomes of a programme.

Having identified the important learning outcomes from a curriculum that need to be acquired by learners, a test designer will set about developing the instruments that will ensure these are robustly assessed throughout the entire programme. The first step in test design is to explicitly define the *purpose* of each assessment (see the MRCGP case example below for further detail, Box 6.2) and then to ensure that important learning outcomes are adequately sampled, guided by a blueprint that explicitly maps the curriculum to the assessments. Typically, such an assessment programme might include a test to assess application of knowledge, a skills test to confirm clinical and practical skills, and a series of authentic observations made in the workplace. In other words, programmes of assessment should, in effect, take multiple [painless] biopsies from the learner using multiple judges,

> **Box 6.2 Case example of an integrated assessment programme for the Membership of the Royal College of GPs (permission obtained)**
>
> The Membership of the Royal College of General Practitioners (MRCGP)[2] examination defines its purpose as an integrated assessment programme that is mapped by a blueprint to an overarching curriculum.
>
> MRCGP is an integrated assessment system, success in which confirms that a doctor has satisfactorily completed specialty training for general practice and is competent to enter independent practice in the United Kingdom without further supervision. Satisfactory completion of the MRCGP is a prerequisite for the issue of a certificate of completion of training and full Membership of the RCGP.
>
> 'MRCGP comprises three separate components: an Applied Knowledge Test, a test of clinical skills (previously known as the Clinical Skills Assessment) which has evolved following the COVID-19 pandemic to the recorded consultation assessment (and has now evolved further to the simulated consultation assessment or SCA) and workplace-based assessment, each of which tests different competencies using validated assessment methods and which together cover the spectrum of knowledge, skills, behaviours, and attitudes as defined by the GP Specialty Training curriculum.
>
> 'MRCGP complies with the General Medical Council (GMC) standards on validity, reliability, feasibility, cost-effectiveness, opportunities for feedback and impact on learning. It also follows good practice in assessment, quality assurance and standard setting.

instruments, and contexts to ensure that the learner has acquired full mastery of the defined learning outcomes and to enable a decision to be made about how competent a trainee is.

A plea for the trainee

The trainee (student or learner) is the central player in any programme of assessments, and test designers should consider the implications of their tests for the trainee. There needs to be explicit transparency about what is to be expected of trainees, such as resident doctors. This can be enhanced by their involvement at every stage from policy making to the implementation of assessments. In addition to the curricular learning outcomes (including syllabic content) and assessment processes, the steps taken to ensure fairness (including validity, reliability, and standard setting) all need to be clearly communicated.

Steps should be taken to ensure that trainees appreciate that each assessment should add value to the overall programme—which, itself, has an acceptable assessment 'load'. Definitions of assessment 'load' vary but typically encompass the volume of assessments (both formative and summative) within a programme of assessment, the proportion of examinations to coursework, and the number of different types of assessment. The assessment 'load' of a programme should be carefully considered and justified. Further, to support trainees' willing and active engagement in the process, apart from ensuring fairness, they should be treated respectfully and with due consideration for their well-being.

It is important to consider the perception of the assessment experience from the users' perspective. It is critical to ensure that assessments feel authentic, and that their content accurately represents the day-to-day work of trainees (which should also inform the content of the curriculum). A written test item that assesses only the application of a trainees' knowledge is, in effect, a poor mimic of actual practice, whereas Objective Structured Clinical Examinations (OSCE) stations as far as possible should mirror clinical experiences. Where approaches to assessment are employed that are perceived as inauthentic to clinical practice, their use needs to be carefully justified, and likely alongside more authentic modalities.

▶ Fundamentally, tests must be fair and robust to ensure that we, as those responsible for training the medical workforce, pass (and progress) competent trainees. Likewise, failing trainees who do not meet the necessary standard is critical in terms of ensuring safe, competent patient care.

Assessment of learning and assessment for learning

Assessment supports learning

Conventional wisdom is that assessment has the collateral benefit of 'driving learning' or more properly 'what is learned'.[3] In reality, there is a symbiotic relationship between the two—with assessment supporting learning through feedback, reflection, and planned further learning.[4]

It therefore benefits curricula and test designers to maximize the positive effects of assessment, such as maintaining the **connection between deeper learning and assessment**; and to mitigate the potential for any negative influences of assessment, such as delivering an undue assessment load and avoiding use of formats that encourage trainees to 'study the test' with only superficial learning (for example, many true/false or multiple choice questions as these assess at the lowest level of Miller's Pyramid, 'knows' see ➲ Chapter 2, and Figure 6.2 below).

Assessment for learning is intuitively attractive, enabling integration of the assessment within the educational process. The use of specific and timely feedback serves to stimulate personal learning which can be tailored to the trainee's needs and pace of curricular coverage.[5] An effective assessment for learning is one that offers supportive but challenging feedback; the learner should be left feeling good about what they have done but also be prompted to develop specific ideas of how they might develop further.

Workplace-Based Assessments (WBAs) have had two important but significantly different purposes: namely the formative need to support trainees to learn and develop (assessment *for* learning); and the summative need to provide evidence for judgements on their progression (assessment *of* learning)—and these must be understood by all parties. At the interface of formative and summative assessments there is scope for the potential blurring of the precise purpose of a formative learning opportunity which might be perceived as having a 'summative spinoff'.

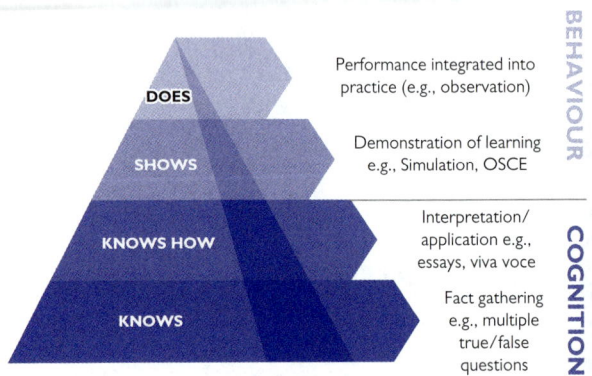

Fig. 6.2 Miller's pyramid. Adapted from Mehay and Burns.[6]

The GMC now distinguishes between two purposes of assessment in the workplace: formative assessment for learning through supervised learning events, and summative assessment used to determine progress, referred to as assessment of progress (similar to assessment of learning, as discussed above).

▶ The precise purpose of any assessment must be explicitly clear to all, especially the learner but also the teacher, examiner, and any other external participants, contributors, or interested parties.

Supervised learning events

Supervised learning events are educational encounters in which assessors observe, and feedback on, aspects of a trainee doctor's clinical practice. Like workplace-based assessments, supervised learning events consist of structured forms which direct the assessor's attention towards particular aspects of clinical practice, such as communication skills or clinical judgement. Supervised learning events are trainee-led formative tools for learning, which show evidence of engagement with the curriculum.[7]

The key elements of the supervised learning events are that:

- it is trainee-focused and encourages reflection, including some degree of self-assessment, based on structured trainer/supervisor feedback
- it is explained to trainees that the process is an opportunity to improve performance, rather than a threat to progression through informed and constructive feedback
- immediate feedback is given, including a specific and mutually agreed educational action plan to guide further supported learning, recorded in the trainee's portfolio
- individual supervised learning events are not scored and will not determine decisions for training progression although the portfolio as a whole will be relevant
- trainee engagement is optimized, the level of which is recorded within the educational supervisor's report
- all supervisors need sufficient scheduled time with the trainee to adequately and appropriately complete extended supervised learning events

Assessment of performance

The key elements of the assessment of performance are that:

- they are 'summative' assessments conducted in the workplace, which make judgements on trainees' level of development and performance at a given time
- they should be planned as a series of events based on a few key clinical activities in which a trainee must be safe and competent at each level of their training
- both trainee and trainer should be clear about what is being assessed at each assessment, and its associated standards
- they must be based on observable performance and assessed against predetermined level descriptors for training progression (which span the entirety of training), with clear links to the Annual Review of Competence Progression (ARCP) process
- multiple assessments should be completed by a range of appropriately trained clinicians across a range of workplace environments covering

a range of specified competences and intended learning outcomes
mapped to the curriculum
- the trainee must be supported in constructing a structured learning plan
prior to assessments of performance and interpreting the evaluation
outcome

The Joint Royal Colleges of Physicians Training Board concluded from
their evaluation that assessments of performance did not function well
as standalone summative assessments and so are not part of their assessment strategy.[6] However, while formative supervised learning events, such
as direct observation of practical skills can be carried out as many times
as trainees wish during training to demonstrate competence in performing
a procedure, trainees are required to gain a summative sign-off. In other
words, Direct Observation of Practical Skills are defined as either formative
(assessment for learning) or summative (assessment of learning).[8]

Formal examinations

Assessments that are designed to measure learning can be used for a variety of purposes, listed in Box 6.3. Formal summative exams are a type of
assessment of learning but, unlike a workplace-based assessment, are conducted in a controlled environment rather than in clinical practice.

Traditional examinations in medical education tended to be mostly assessments of factual knowledge but it is now widely accepted that factual
knowledge alone does not represent good clinical practice.[9] It is difficult to
assess important skills and behaviours with traditional assessments.

Just as assessments of performance in clinical practice have advanced
over time through the evolution of workplace-based assessments, there
have been parallel developments in formal examination tools (and their
quality) used to assess the application of knowledge, practical skills, and
behaviours.

Box 6.3 Assessment of learning (summative assessment)

There are multiple intended uses of assessment of learning (summative
assessment) including to:
- demonstrate career progression within the same training programme,
e.g. exams set by medical royal colleges to confirm progression from
core to higher-level training within certain specialty
- confirm competencies have been achieved to allow progression to
the next stage of training. e.g. that a medical student is sufficiently
competent to begin working as a doctor
- provide evidence to confirm the satisfactory completion of a training
programme and subsequent eligibility for entry onto the specialist or
GP register, following which they can practise independently, without
clinical supervision
- gain membership/fellowship to a medical royal college, specialist
association, or society

Principles of robust and fair assessment design: Blueprinting

Blueprinting is a key step in assessment design. A curriculum identifies the learning outcomes/objectives (LOs) to be learned. The associated programme of assessment is designed to confirm the acquisition of those learning outcomes. Good practice is that the curriculum and programme of assessments are aligned using a blueprint.[10]

Blueprinting can be considered at different levels—the first focuses on the curriculum-assessment interface, and specifies which method is used to assess each intended LO across the entire curriculum. Selecting the most appropriate assessment to evaluate each intended LO is referred to as 'mapping' and ensures comprehensive and systematic assessment of the curriculum. At an 'assessment-learning outcome' level, each tool is mapped to all of the individual LOs that it assesses, or more specifically, cases of importance and smaller domains within the LO.

In programmes of assessment with multiple components, blueprints can be 'stacked' (like *Russian nesting dolls*) to track a candidate's assessment journey. In other words—*Which tools are being used, and when?* This is important when individual exam boards define assessment content in isolation and will assist an educator's overarching view.

What do blueprints look like?

Blueprints are:
- typically a table/grid/template/matrix or spreadsheet, which is usually two-dimensional with two axes
- the top horizontal (x-axis) usually comprises domains, skills or contexts which form the column headings such as 'communicate with patient'
- the vertical (y-axis) comprises content (systems, topics, conditions, or presentations) which form the row headings such as 'chest pain'

An example of an assessment blueprint is shown in Table 6.1. This is a two-dimensional table, but additional information can readily be incorporated, either as hyperlinks or attached explanatory documents. This allows the titles to remain succinct, yet the blueprint is still able to convey additional information that may be relevant to the assessment, e.g. stages in the candidates' training at which the item might be tested.

Blueprints can vary in complexity depending on their intended utility but lend themselves to electronic formats such as a spreadsheet. Using this format, it is straightforward to correctly place test material in the blueprint using the spreadsheet's numerical and alphabetical coordinates.

How to construct a blueprint

In order to produce a comprehensive blueprint that is easy to use, several key steps need to be completed:
1. **Decide on what you want to test:** It is vital to familiarize yourself with the purpose of the test, the LOs defined by your curriculum, and relevant local/national guidelines. Include any other relevant information to ensure the content accurately reflects the breadth of actual practice of the successful candidates, although this should not be at variance with the content of the curriculum.

2. **Agree its format:** Typically, this would be a spreadsheet, grid, matrix, or table with two axes. Ideally it should be 'overarching' that includes all learning outcomes, and all assessment methods used in the overall programme of assessments. However, it's also useful to generate standalone blueprints for individual tests such as Single Best Answers (SBAs) or OSCEs. Whichever format is chosen, make it easily readable and user-friendly for all. Agree on its functionality and intended uses such as linkage to item bank.

3. **'Populate' (complete) the axes:** The x-axis (column headings) comprise skills or domains such as history taking, diagnosis, and management. The y-axis (row headings) are the subject/content areas, which can be system based or 'presentations' derived from the curriculum such as chest pain, shortness of breath, or collapse. Both the content and skills must be mapped to the curricular learning outcomes.

4. **Select the right tools and or design/choose tools that will sample all Los:** Be guided by Miller's Pyramid (Figure 6.2 ➔) and use test instruments appropriately to maximize the efficiency of the programme of assessments. For example, a skills test that is designed to assess clinical and communication skills is less effective at assessing knowledge than a machine markable Single Best Answer test. Each testing format may be used to corroborate different facets of a topic such as the management of anaphylaxis (see Table 6.2) in which the knowledge test might test the correct dose of epinephrine, a skills test might simulate how to administer the drug but only observation in the workplace integrates all these skills in authentic patient management.

5. **'Populate' (complete) the blueprint:** Commission test items that sample all content and skills (see section on item and case construction)

6. **Agree how many test items/cases:** Typically, this will equate to: 100–200 Single Best Answer items over 3 hours; 14–18 OSCE stations over 3 hours

A note on sampling

In an ideal world, one might wish to confirm the acquisition of all learning outcomes. In practice, feasibility dictates a finite approach to the breadth of testing, so sampling is inevitable. The blueprint enables the generation of a coherent and stable sampling strategy of common and important problems, avoids undue duplication or gaps, and ensures the content is consistent over time. The broader the sampling the better the ability to generate a true picture of a candidate's ability.

Individual test blueprint ('Test specification')

Each assessment event should **systematically** sample from the overarching blueprint using a **test specification** or **sampling grid** (Table 6.2). This is a pre-established table of content and processes which is **weighted** to reflect the relative importance of the items encountered in any given test. It provides the link between an overarching blueprint and individual test content. It ensures that each test content and context is stable over time, and therefore will deliver a reproducible standard across multiple cohorts who sit the same examination (but inevitably must be asked different questions).

Table 6.1 Example of an assessment blueprint showing how each intended learning outcome is assessed. Bear in mind that this is a succinct example, and there are many other domains that can be used

Intended learning outcome	Portfolios	Essays	Group project	Exams	Oral exams/ presentations	Practical assessment	Work placement assessment	Computer based assignment	Global assessment of practice
Critically appraise different approaches to teaching anatomy, e.g. virtual, pro-section, and dissection		x	x					x	x
Evaluate art-based teaching methods in anatomy teaching and learning		x	x					x	x
Evaluate different tissue preservation techniques for teaching and learning anatomy		x						x	x
Critically appraise different assessment techniques in anatomy education		x	x					x	x
Develop an understanding of critical appraisal of academic sources		x						x	x
Critically appraise alignment of teaching technique, learning outcome, and assessment technique		x	x					x	x
Demonstrate use of different IT skills in your teaching and research		x	x					x	x

Principles of robust and fair assessment design: Validity including reliability

This section describes fair and robust assessment principles. Descriptions of assessment utility can be found in Chapter 7 ➜.

Validity

Assessment validity refers to the extent that a test measures what it is supposed to measure. Schuwirth and van der Vleuten (2010) proposed validity as the extent to which the competence that the assessment claims to measure is actually being measured.[11]

There are many types of validity:

- **Face validity**: whether a test appears to be valid or not. It is very much a quick look from external appearance as to whether the items appear to measure the desired content or not.
- **Content validity:** how well an instrument covers all relevant aspects of the construct it aims to measure.
- **Construct validity:** the extent to which the test may be said to measure a construct (e.g. a theoretical construct or psychological variable).

Validity can be demonstrated from different sources of evidence. All assessments are required to have demonstrable validity, with appropriate evidence to support the decisions and consequences of the examination outcomes. This ensures defensibility of the assessment.

Reliability

▶ In the context of assessment, reliability is taken to mean the internal consistency, reproducibility, or dependability of test results. Reliability is an estimate of the extent to which the same test used on separate occasions would give approximately the same result.

Evidencing the reliability of an assessment gives sufficient confidence in high-stakes assessments to make **robust** inferences that the candidates' scores accurately reflect their true ability. A totally reliable test would have a reliability coefficient (alpha/G) of 1 and a totally unreliable one would have a reliability of 0. An acceptable reliability is generally taken to be alpha/G >0.7 for an OSCE and >0.8 for multiple choice questions (MCQ). Reliability of a test generally increases the longer the test is, and the more items it contains. However, a balance needs to be struck to avoid the impracticality of, for example, a 10-hour MCQ or a 30-station OSCE.

A candidate's 'observed score' (i.e. actual score) in a test might differ from their 'true score' that reflects actual ability. Error can arise from a number of factors such as:

- **sampling errors** caused by the subset of selected test material not accurately reflecting the true breadth and depth of the curriculum. Test items vary in their degree of challenge and, as competence is context-specific, candidates vary in their mastery of topics, which is reflected by how easy or difficult they find test material. The practical implication is that tests have to be sufficiently long to address these differences (see below).
- **candidate factors**—e.g. misreading a question or instruction.

Table 6.2 An example of Single Best Answer Sampling grid test specification

Item selection derived from blueprint	Domain/skill						
	Disease factors	Diagnosis	Investigation	Peri-operative	Palliative/terminal care	Treatment	Emergencies (including acute care)
Blood and lymph	1	2	2	0	1	1	1
Musculoskeletal	0	2	1	0	0	1	1
Infectious disease	0	4	4	1	1	2	1
Skin	0	2	0	0	0	1	0
Homeostatic	1	1	2	0	0	2	1
Neurological	1	2	1	0	1	1	1
Respiratory	1	5	1	0	1	4	1
Renal	1	2	2	0	0	1	0
Cardiovascular	3	7	2	1	0	3	2
ENT	0	4	1	0	0	1	0
Eye	0	2	0	0	0	1	1
Digestive	1	4	5	1	1	2	2
Women's health	1	2	1	1	1	3	1
Miscellaneous	1	3	0	1	1	1	0

- **exam factors**—such as posing ambiguous questions or instructions.
- **assessor factors**—such as different assessors giving variable scores for similar candidate performances, (inter-rater reliability), or single assessors being inconsistent in awarding marks for almost identical performance, or being inconsistent if re-marking a test item (intra-rater reliability).

Reliability can be estimated mathematically using:
- **Classical test theory**—which is best suited to tests in which the candidates all answer identical questions, such as Single Best Answer, through the estimation of reliability coefficients such as Cronbach Alpha, the Kuder-Richardson Formula 20
- **Generalizability theory**—that is better suited for use in skills tests in which there may be more variability such as caused by candidates not all being examined by the same examiners or facing different cases. Generalizability theory can estimate the likelihood of candidates having a similar result if they had different cases and/or examiners
- **Rasch modelling and item response theory**—which is best suited to high volume knowledge testing but can be used to model test item difficulty, item discrimination, and can estimate reliability

Details of each of these are beyond the scope of this book but see ➲ Cronbach and Shavelson (2004) for further information.[12]

As suggested above, in the past, reliability was considered to be discretely separate from validity and much emphasis was placed on its demonstration in medical exams using a range of precise numerical estimates—notably Cronbach's alpha and the Kuder-Richardson Formula 20. As it could be relatively easily calculated it was often used as the sole metric for demonstrating the effectiveness of assessments at the expense of the rather more conceptual validity. However, within contemporary validity frameworks, reliability is now considered to be just one important part of the evidence supporting the use of any test.

Nevertheless, if a test is unreliable, it may be measuring something other than that which was intended, which would compromise its validity. In order to deliver acceptable reliability, test developers must take steps to reduce these intrinsic sources of error.

These include:
- rigorous assessor selection, training, and through ongoing calibration, and use of multiple assessors to optimize inter- and intra-rater reliability.
- ensuring the quality control of individual cases and items and clarity of associated marking schemes, such as using explicit descriptions of competence 'a passing candidate should be able to … '.
- ensuring that simulated patients, role players, or patients have clear and comprehensive instructions that cover all eventualities about how to portray a case, especially thresholds for revealing information.
- diligent overall test construction informed by a blueprint.
- using long enough testing time and broad sampling—in other words, a sufficient number of items or cases for the specific test/tool, guided by current assessment evidence. The more items or cases included will increase the reliability, even of 'bad' tests.

- allowing candidates sufficient time to complete the test, as any omissions will effectively shorten the test, compromising its reliability.
- ensuring candidates are familiar with the test format and what is required of them.

After the assessment

Following delivery of any assessment, checks should be undertaken to ensure that it's doing what it is intended to be doing. Appropriate psychometric analyses can confirm acceptable overall reliability and/or identify problems within a whole test. However, it's also important to include a review of the characteristics of individual items.

For a Single Best Answer principally this will include:

- **Key validation**—checking that the right correct response has been designated by the assessor
- **Facility**—how easy or difficult an item is. If an item is too difficult candidates might be tempted to guess and it may not discriminate
- **Item discrimination**—such as a correlation between candidates' performance on an individual item with their performance in the test overall, and/or
- **Point biserial correlation**—which is a correlation between right/wrong scores on an individual item and an individual's total scores across the whole exam (expressed typically from –1 [bad] to +1 [perfect]). A low correlation may mean that a question is too easy or ambiguous.

For an OSCE, reliability can be reviewed using item response theory, which may include reviewing the:

- added value of individual stations to the overall **reliability** by omitting a case and recalculating it. The reliability should be lower with fewer cases and, if not, it suggests a problem with the station which merits further investigation
- **correlation** of the global grades and checklist marks within stations (**coefficient of determination,** R^2) which ideally would be good (>0.5)
- **inter-grade discrimination** (average increase in checklist mark difference between global grades) which can identify problems such as variability amongst assessors in their application of marking schedule
- **spread of scores** awarded on each case, such as whether all are deemed 'excellent' or the majority fail
- **between-group variation** (including assessor effects). Unlike MCQs where candidates sit an identical test, OSCEs are not identical as they are examined in groups, which may occur at different times or locations. The total variance for one group on the same circuit can be estimated and then compared to other groups. Good between-group congruence (<30%) would confirm uniformity of the processes whereas values over 40% indicate potential problems at the station level due to inconsistent assessor behaviour and/or other circuit specific characteristics, rather than student performance
- other sources of variance should also be monitored, e.g. any effects related to gender or other candidate characteristics, if there may be non-random allocations of either assessors or candidates, such as by day of the week, candidates taking resits, for example

- between-circuit **error variance** at a station level to identify potential inconsistency by assessors when the same station is marked by different examiners over time
- finally, the spread of scores awarded by each assessor should be monitored especially to check that there are none who are idiosyncratic and/or to establish their degree of hawkish (mark harshly) or dovishness (mark leniently) and can be fed back for their ongoing calibration and training.

For a more detailed review of appropriate OSCE metrics see Fuller et al. (2010).[13]

However, many preventive steps are taken to mitigate sources of error, some degree of error is still inevitable, and this can be quantified using the standard error of measurement (SEM) or confidence intervals (CI). Measurement error is the difference between observed and true scores. The SEM [or confidence interval] estimates the likely range of actual scores that candidates might achieve because of the unreliability of the assessment. Adjustment for measurement error in high-stakes exams is important to ensure that there are no false fails (**fairness** to candidates) and no false passes (to ensure patient safety)—this is especially important for the fair treatment of borderline candidates. As measurement error is decreased, reliability is increased, and the better the assessment.

In addition to the post hoc analysis of individual tests it is also wise to review the whole programme such as by cross correlation of candidates' performance in various components and monitoring candidate characteristics. **Differential item functioning** can be used to determine whether items are measuring different abilities of members of discrete subgroups.

These statistics and an associated narrative can demonstrate the quality and consistency of assessments, enhancing their validity which in turn supports confidence in the **fairness** of test outcomes. Additionally, this review also feeds into the continual quality improvement and refining of each assessment. Only after all these checks have been made can the clear interpretation of results and judgements be communicated to the candidates. Finally, organizations should monitor trends in their examination pass rates longitudinally to ensure that any variations relate to actual changes in the ability of candidates taking a test rather than any flaws in their test design.

Approaches to standard setting

What's the score?

In most written exams the score is based on the number of correct responses. In OSCE cases there is often a scale, which may involve an informed interpretation of the candidate's responses depending on the 'degree of correctness' e.g. a grade of A, B, C, D or E for each domain (A = excellent, B = good, C = satisfactory, D = fail, E = severe fail or not attempted).

What is a standard?

A standard or cut-point is a statement about whether an examination performance is good enough for a particular purpose. A standard is used to define a boundary between those who score well enough and those who do not. Typically, there is a numerical answer to this question. Candidates often ask: 'How much is enough?'…. and the answer is: the pass mark!

Scores vs. standard?

It is a simple exercise to measure and report a score by counting the number of correct responses. However, it is a complex exercise to judge a standard, a conceptual boundary of what constitutes an acceptable performance. It is important to decide which score is 'good enough'.

Measurements and judgements

Measurements are often more objective in nature, whereas judgements tend to be more subjective. For example, measuring how much history candidates obtain from patients or how many physical findings they elicit can be done by simple observation and comparison against a detailed standard. Alternatively, assessing clinical competence involves a complex mix of attributes requiring both measurement and judgements to be made. For example, it would be very difficult to measure how well a candidate responds to patient cues, their approach and professionalism, and their clarity of communication, and therefore these are a matter of judgement.

Standard setting—why bother?

Standard setting is important in a high-stakes assessment to quality assure the product, which is the doctor. It also satisfies the multiple stakeholders throughout a medical career:
• assessors to distinguish between the competent and the incompetent (public interest)
• university to confirm students meet their standards
• regulatory body to certify that graduates are suitable for registration
• employer to be reassured that doctors are fit to work
• specialty societies/colleges to confirm award of postgraduate diplomas

The Gold Standard setting method should be:
• reliable and stable over time
• feasible
• defensible and fair
• supported by evidence in the literature
• acceptable to all stakeholders

The standard setting problem

In an ideal world there would be a bimodal distribution of candidates' scores, that is, there would be clear failures and clear passes with clear water between the two groups. However, competence is a continuous variable and so the distribution of scores tends to be a highly kurtotic normal distribution with numerous 'average' performances peaking around the mean. The pass mark is a conceptual boundary set at the point of maximum uncertainty.

Who should decide on the standards?

Standards are based on making informed judgements about performance against social or educational normative constructs, e.g. standards would be different for a first-year medical student and a first-year doctor. Agreement must be achieved as to what scores or standards need to be reached and across what domains to be acceptable for any given assessment, bearing in mind whether its intended purpose is to confirm competence or define excellence.

Who is best placed to set the 'right' standard?

There are a number of potentially legitimate stakeholders including: examiners, teachers, scientists, academics, jobbing clinicians, workforce planners, recently successful candidates, lay people, and students. Whatever their provenance they must:
- be familiar with the curriculum
- be familiar with breadth of candidate ability
- understand the purpose and level of examination
- understand what is good enough for that particular test
- be a representative and a diverse sample—by experience, age, etc. to minimize bias and maximize information on topics covered

The key points for successful standard setting (any method) are:
- the selection, training, and calibration of judges or 'subject matter experts'
- the process is facilitated by an expert who ensures that judges are familiar with all of the above
- judges need continual reminding to ensure they can reliably conceptualize the just passing candidate

The borderline candidate

In absolute or criterion-referenced methods, the key step involves the definition and recognition of a just passing or borderline candidate, which depends on the precise purpose of the assessment.

▶ It's important that the judges can conceptualize this borderline (or, just passing) candidate who possesses basic knowledge and skills which might be patchy but is fundamentally safe. In an OSCE, the examiner gets to see a real-time breadth of candidate performance, whereas for a knowledge test they need to be already familiar with the breadth of ability of the just passing candidates for whom they then effectively act as proxy. The judges need constant reminding that the borderline is different from both a poor, clearly failing candidate and someone who is performing well.

❗ For standard setting in knowledge tests there are likely to be as many opinions as there are judges and the truth is the mean score. Effectively it's applying the wisdom of a well-informed crowd. Differences of opinion are inevitable, and judges will vary in their hawkishness (mark harshly) or dovishness (mark leniently) which is acceptable—provided they are consistent and balanced in number. Occasionally there is a judge who is idiosyncratic and inconsistent or an outlier despite best efforts of remediation whose score might have to be suppressed from the calculation.

Types of standard setting

There are three main sorts of standards, each will be expanded in turn:
- relative or norm referenced
- absolute or criterion-referenced which can be: test centred such as Angoff or Ebel; or candidate-centred such as borderline regression
- compromise such as Hofstee

Relative 'norm-referenced' standards

Relative standards are based on a comparison of the performance of the group taking the test. Individual success depends on how well a candidate performs relative to other examinees who sit the test, e.g. the bottom 20% will fail regardless of how well they perform... depending on the company they keep.

Strengths of relative 'norm-referenced' standards
- simple method
- does not require dedicated standard setting sessions or employment of subject matter experts or judges
- can identify a predetermined number of candidates such as for selection

Weaknesses of relative 'norm-referenced' standards
- standard is not related to exam content
- some candidates will always fail, no matter how good they are . . . so it's unfair
- pass mark may change depending on the performance of the group in that particular cohort, and will be influenced by overall performance
- the standard required is not known in advance

Absolute or 'criterion-referenced' standards

Success is not dependent on the ability of others. Candidates will pass or fail based on how well they perform. All candidates may pass or all may fail. Absolute standards are preferable!

Strengths of absolute or 'criterion-referenced' standards:
- attention is focused on how well the candidates do . . . their actual competence
- pass/fail decisions based on meeting specified criteria
- takes account of the difficulty of test content
- sound evidence base so defensible, fair and suitable in high-stakes testing
- (relatively!) easy to use

Weaknesses of absolute or 'criterion-referenced' standards
- even with training, risk of variable standards reached with different judges, different methods, or different exam content
- the concept of a 'borderline group' is sometimes difficult to agree and internalize
- more costly and time-consuming than relative (norm-referenced) methods

Relative-absolute compromise standards—Hofstee

Relative-absolute compromise standards combine features of both the above standard settings.[14]

Strengths of Relative-absolute compromise standards

- easy to implement
- educators are 'comfortable' with the decisions
- reassures stakeholders that results seem reasonable
- there is an evidence base

Weaknesses of Relative-absolute compromise standards

- not considered defensible for high-stakes assessments
- the cut score may not be in the area defined by the judges' estimates (if they do not have access to actual exam data)
- perceived to be less credible because judgements are global rather than based on individual items
- some of the disadvantages of relative standard setting like not taking account of variability in test difficulty over time

Examples of the absolute or 'criterion-referenced' standards and the Hofstee standard

Absolute or criterion-referenced standard setting

The most popular contemporary test-centred methods are Angoff and Ebel, and the most commonly used candidate-centred test is borderline regression.

Angoff method

A representative reference group of typically 6–10 judges (or subject matter experts)[15] chosen to fulfil the criteria enumerated above is convened. Following a tutorial to ensure they are familiar with the task and especially agreeing on the characteristics of the borderline candidate who is 'only just good enough to pass'. Working individually the judges are tasked with deciding on the percentage probability that this just passing candidate would get each test item correct. In the Single Best Answer format, there is a 1:5 chance of guessing correctly so usually the advice would be to score each item 20–100, where 20 is the chance of guessing an item correct and 100 would be the probability of all borderline candidates getting an item correct.

The individual scores are collated and if there is a large range within the predicted scores, such questions are discussed and in particular the outliers are asked to briefly explain the rationale for their contrasting judgements. Following this discussion any judge may change their scores, but this is not obligatory. The cut or pass/fail standard is the average of percentages for all the items from all the judges. Practical tips are shown in Box 6.4.

It is worth noting that many people describe using a modified Angoff method, without specifying the nature of the modification. Modified Angoff is the most popular method. The distinction is that the Angoff method is a predetermined criterion-referenced method and test-centred method. Whereas modified Angoff method enables the panellists to be given information such as test result and other panellists' rating result to discuss the cut score.

Ebel's method

Ebel's method starts similarly to Angoff in that the judges initially agree on the definition of the just passing or borderline candidate.[16] The method differs in that the judges are also asked to make 'difficulty-relevance' decisions and so the judges also need to reach a common understanding about each of these categories. Subsequently they are instructed to make two judgements about each item, firstly the difficulty of a question which is categorized as easy, medium, or difficult, and secondly their relevance whether the knowledge is deemed essential, important, or acceptable ('nice to know').

The next step is to request that the judges estimate the percentage of items in each of the nine categories that the just passing candidate would answer correctly, e.g. in the example in Table 6.3, 90% of the essential/easy questions but only 20% of the harder 'nice-to-know' items. The next step is to add the weighting by multiplying this percentage by the actual number

Box 6.4 Practical tips for running an Angoff standard setting session

- Select judges carefully—they should be representative and familiar with the breadth of ability of those on whom they are setting the standard
- The judges must have good communication and group skills. They should be able to offer an informed opinion but also willing to listen to those of others and modify their own ideas if need be!
- Discuss the characteristics of a borderline 'only just good enough to pass' candidate and give a brief tutorial to ensure they are familiar with the task
- Remind them that each judge has to decide on the percentage probability that the just passing candidate **would** not, **should** or **ought** to get each item correct. They may need reminding that if they personally do not know the answer to an item it does not necessarily make it difficult! They also need reminding not to regress to the mean with their scoring
- Do have a dry run and give judges a chance to practice a few questions before going live
- Instruct them that they are standard setting and not proofreading or critiquing your paper (you can give them permission to give such feedback separately)
- Think about how you will collect and project the data—our experience is that a projected spreadsheet that automatically highlights significant differences operated by an administrative colleague who is able to input a large amount of data faithfully works best. Apart from the questions that are being standard set, provide simple tables for the standard setters to record their scores and include their name!

Table 6.3 Grid used when applying Ebel's method

	Easy	Medium	Hard
Essential	90% n = 10	80%	70%
Important	60%	50%	40%
Acceptable	40%	30%	20% n=5

of test items in each category. The passing score is set by averaging the category scores.[16]

So just for illustration if there were 10 items in easy-essential it would be $10 \times 90 = 9.0$ and 5 items in acceptable-hard it would be $5 \times 20 = 1.0$, so if there were only these 15 items on the basis of this very small sample the passing score would be calculated by the sum of the scores divided by the number of items and multiplied by 100 or $10/15 \times 100 = 66.6\%$.

Borderline regression method

Successful standard setting for OSCEs depends on the similar understanding of what constitutes a borderline candidate performance as knowledge testing which must be understood by all of the examiners.

However, unlike the number correct scoring (candidates score is their number of correct responses) used in machine markable tests OSCE marking relies on the professional judgement of assessors. The assessors are effectively setting the standard on any station, so they need to be carefully selected, trained, calibrated, and provided with explicitly clear guidance about what is required to ensure that they make judgements that are consistent between examiners and across sites or time. Borderline regression is the currently preferred candidate-centred absolute or criterion-referenced standard setting method for OSCEs.

This method calls for the assessor to give a candidate's performance of individual scores across various domains in any station, e.g. communication skills, clinical management, practical skills, etc. The individual scores will be guided by the mark sheet and a summation of these scores will give a total mark for that station. In addition to the domain scores the candidate is awarded a separate overall or 'global' score typically using five grades for each station (such as clear fail, borderline fail, borderline, borderline pass, clear pass).

For each station, each candidates' score is plotted on a graph against the global score they were awarded for that station. Where the line of best fit (line of regression) intersects with the 'borderline' global score indicates the 'cut-off' mark for the station (see Figure 6.3). This potentially allows for low scores, for example due to a problem with the OSCE task or timings but still allows good candidates to pass.

Borderline regression has a number of advantages over other methods of standard setting that can be used in skills assessments, notably the production of quality metrics that support its fairness and defensibility.

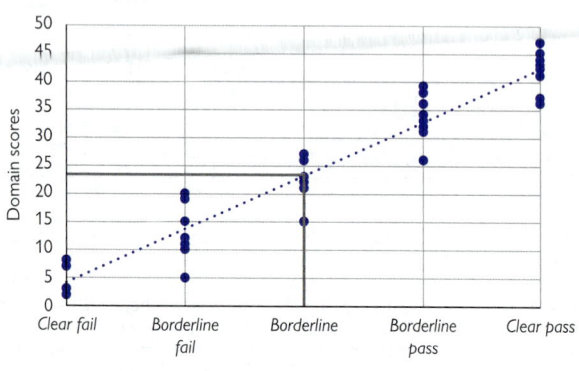

Fig. 6.3 Graph highlighting borderline regression method

Other methods that are used include the borderline group and contrasting groups, which typically use only three grades: fail, borderline, and pass. The assessors discuss the attributes of the borderline candidate before the test takes place and once this group of candidates has been identified, their median score becomes the pass/fail cut-point.[17]

Relative-absolute

Hofstee described presenting actual exam performance data but if this isn't available other exam data such as historical or similar tests are used.[14] Judges are asked to define the minimum and maximum acceptable passing scores and failure rates (see Figure 6.4).

A note on standard setting

▶ Deciding who should pass and who should fail is a question of policy rather than arithmetic, there is no single method that is appropriate for every assessment, and it must be conducted according to best practice and with due diligence to ensure fairness.

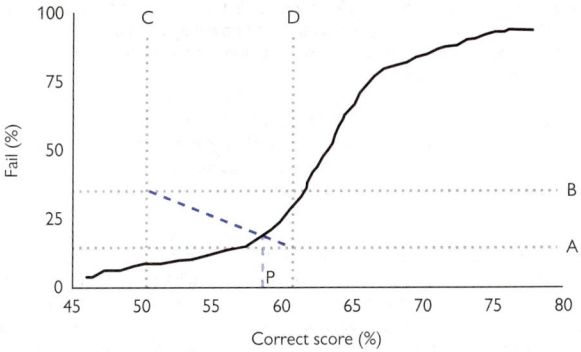

Fig. 6.4 A Hofstee plot—reference group of judges agree: lowest acceptable fail rate (A); highest acceptable fail rate (B); lowest permissible passing score (C); highest required passing score (D). The passing standard P is determined by the midpoint of the 'box'.

Overview of assessment instruments (written)

The wide range of assessment tools in healthcare professions education reflects the broad spectrum of skills required to ensure competency and readiness to deliver optimum patient care; skills range from listening and talking to patients, to intricate and physically demanding interventions. When deciding which assessment method to use, it is important to consider the validity, reliability, educational impact, feasibility, and cost of the proposed assessment tool.

The next section will outline several different types of assessments that are currently used, including written exams, OSCEs, and workplace-based assessments. This chapter focuses on the assessment tools from the perspective of why they are used and includes the pros and cons of their use.

Traditional essay questions

Essays enable the candidates to demonstrate their knowledge, generally about one topic, in depth. The candidate is usually marked on their analytical skills, critical thinking, application of knowledge, and problem-solving abilities, for example within the examinations required by the Faculty of Public Health in the UK.[18]

Essays can be used both for formative and summative assessment. Essays can demonstrate a range of learning, from the understanding of the concepts being taught, to the ability to write clearly and concisely.

Essays can be of benefit to enable the candidate to draw together a number of themes or knowledge from across the delivered course. An essay could allow the candidate to explore issues in depth and/or demonstrate an understanding of more conceptual issues such as ethics and law.

When constructing essay questions, marking criteria need to be clearly drawn up. The marking schedule should include indications of where marks can be gained or lost. Examiners are required to use their experience and judgement when marking essays as candidates have more scope to stray away from anticipated answers and for some topics there are no right or wrong answers. Essays are susceptible to marker and subjectivity bias and are therefore considered less reliable than other methods.

One of the main issues with using a few long essays as the only form of summative assessment is that it only allows a limited sampling of the syllabus. To overcome this, Modified Essay Questions or Structured (or Short) Answer Questions can be used to cover more of a curriculum (often with 10–15 questions which take 10–15 minutes each to answer).

Modified Essay Questions or Structured Answer Questions can provide a highly structured case vignette, followed by questions on any aspect. Extended short answers/short answers usually require a paragraph or two, which may address different aspects.

Strengths of Structured (Short) Answer/Modified Essay Questions:
- good for assessment of higher-order cognitive functions (able to examine at a deeper level than MCQs (improved validity))
- promotes critical thinking and problem-solving
- potential for constructive feedback

Weaknesses of Structured (Short) Answer/Modified Essay Questions:

- lack of reliability and consistency
- intra-rater and inter-rater variability in scoring—examiners require training and quality assurance programmes to ensure reliability
- potential limited content coverage and validity—need to ensure sampling is wide enough to cover the curriculum
- time-consuming process to formulate the marking scheme and to mark
- the criteria are potentially not transparent to candidates

Overview of assessment instruments: MCQ/Single Best Answers/Extended Matching Questions

Technology is assisting in the development of assessments. The next few assessment methods can all be undertaken on the computer (or on paper and marked on computer).

Multiple choice questions

MCQs have become a significant feature of assessment of knowledge in medicine and other professions over the last 60 years.

Traditional Multiple True False questions usually offer 4–6 answers from which the correct one(s) must be chosen. The title is referred to as the stem; each question is called an item, with each item being marked as true or false. While Multiple True False questions assess factual recall of essential knowledge, they do not test the application of knowledge or problem-solving—which are essential in clinical practice. Previously 'negative marking' was used commonly within MCQs, where a wrong answer would incur a mark being deducted. However, this risk-taking behaviour was apparently more prevalent in male candidates, creating a gender bias, therefore negative marking is no longer commonplace.

Strengths of MCQs/Multiple True False Questions
- MCQs take less time to complete so more questions can be answered, thus giving wider curriculum coverage
- MCQs can be administered as online assessments, therefore reducing examiner marking
- handwriting/clarity of presentation is not assessed in responses

Weaknesses of MCQs/Multiple True False Questions
- can be gender biased (towards men) if negatively marked
- do not reflect how adults, learn, retain, and recall knowledge
- typically assesses knowledge only (often superficially)
- MCQs test recognition (choosing an answer) rather than recall (constructing an answer)
- application of knowledge is difficult to assess
- answers can be guessed

The negative aspects of Multiple True False questions make them now a less common and less desirable format. The National Board of Medical Examiners guide suggests the use of true/false questions restricts the choice of questions to a subset that can be classified as completely true all of the time or completely false all of the time.[19]

Single Best Answers

Single Best Answers are used widely in medical education and allow the candidate to demonstrate declarative knowledge. Educationalists are now preferring the use of Single Best Answer questions to assess application of knowledge, integration, synthesis, and judgement. Single Best Answers consist of a stem, lead-in question and usually five options. The options consist of a key (the correct response) and four distractors (wrong answers). Most clinical Single Best Answer questions present a scenario, with plausible options or 'items' from which the candidate must choose the most appropriate. It can be challenging to produce high-quality, discriminating Single Best Answer questions that ensure fair, valid, and reliable assessments.

Single Best Answers are mapped (as should all test tools) to a blueprint, to ensure the full curriculum is assessed during an assessment, ensuring efficient sampling of knowledge. Single Best Answer questions and papers can be prepared in advance. Often a few questions are used repeatedly over time as anchor questions for linear test equating purposes to corroborate the standard over time. Most Single Best Answers are scored optically or directly by computer, reducing examiner time postpreparation and each item can then be analysed for its discrimination and facility.

Strengths of Single Best Answer questions
- easy to administer, machine markable
- tests a predefined broad range of topics/scenarios according to a test blueprint in a short time
- tests application of knowledge with multidimensional professional competencies including knowledge, technical, clinical, decision making skills in addition to safety skills

Weaknesses of Single Best Answer questions
- takes practice to write well
- can be difficult to test higher-order skills such as team working skills
- can cue the right answer and have redundant distractors

Extended Matching Questions

Extended Matching Questions are in effect a cluster of Single Best Answers around a common theme. Single Best Answers have a number of advantages over Extended Matching Questions notably the increased breadth of sampling. If a candidate knows one of the causes of say chest pain in a set of five, they are likely to know them all so it's preferable to ask four additional single items in other testing areas. Single Best Answers also generally have better psychometric properties including spread of scores, discrimination, and internal consistency.

Very Short Answers

In order to overcome some of the obvious flaws of SBA questions notably cueing, guessing, and redundant distractors, Very Short Answer questions are a valuable addition in particular for numerical questions such as calculation of drug dose or statistics. Essentially these are identical in construction to the SBA but without the option list. These are especially good for single word or number answers and typically improves item performance (point biserial) and tend to be marginally harder.

However, their marking can be problematic in that automatic marking currently is restricted to a few key words and typically requires scrutiny by human markers. A policy must be agreed on all possible versions of even numerical answers such as 1,1.0, and one, etc.; partially correct responses and spelling errors such as 'cirosis' (*sic*) when the intended correct response is primary biliary cirrhosis. Equality impact provision must be made for those with specific learning difficulty. Standard setting can be challenging when the standard setters are required to rapidly recalibrate from SBAs. Very short answer questions are also referred to as 'Fill in the Blanks' or 'Constructed Response' questions.

Overview of assessment instruments: OSCEs

The next section will outline assessments that have been designed for the simulated setting as well as those for clinical settings.

Objective Structured Clinical Examinations

Traditionally assessment in medicine has involved oral activities—ranging from formative discussion at the bedside or on the ward round, to workplace-based case-based discussions. In recent years, there has been a drive to provide a standardized approach to allow the candidate to demonstrate skills in assessments. The OSCE was first developed in 1975 by Harden and colleagues in an attempt to find a fair and practical way to assess clinical skills in undergraduate medical students in Dundee University, UK.[20] This approach was further developed by Harden and Gleason (1979), where students were described as moving around a structured set of tasks, many involving simulated patients, and were observed by examiners using a checklist.[21]

OSCEs comprise a series of stations (often 10–15). Candidates are asked to perform specific tasks and/or address specific structured cases. The candidate enters a series of stations in sequence and is given a fixed amount of time before moving onto the next station. Each station contains a task with instructions, assessment 'material' (e.g. a mannequin, a simulated or real patient, a laboratory test result) and an examiner. During the candidate's performance, the examiner observes and then scores their performance against a predetermined marking scheme. A wide range of competencies can be measured e.g. history taking, physical examination, communication skills, counselling skills, data interpretation, and practical procedures appropriate for the stage of assessment. Norcini (2002) suggests OSCEs provide a good test of the candidate's actual performance.[22]

OSCEs were developed in response to unstructured cases to provide higher reliability. Reliability was improved by providing structure to the observation, creating short cases, allowing an increase in different observations, and allowing the candidate to move between cases, to allow assessments by different examiners. OSCEs are often used as a summative assessment. A minimum average of two hours of testing per candidate is required to achieve an acceptable reliability for summative decisions. Most undergraduate OSCEs are held in the medical school environment and can provide an excellent opportunity for learning. Using an OSCE to explore general knowledge is not an efficient use of the format, although it is reasonable to include assessment of the application of knowledge that has a direct relationship to the case.

More recently the OSCE-style assessment has been used in other areas of medical education, for example as 'Mini Multiple Interviews' (MMIs) which replace traditional interviews in recruitment processes throughout medical training.

Strengths of OSCEs

- standardization of scenarios for all candidates
- psychometrically reliable when done well: candidate marked by multiple assessors against a standardized marking schedule
- block of candidates can be examined at the same time
- potential for constructive feedback to candidate (albeit often in practice candidates are only given a grade)
- feedback from actors/simulators
- a wide sampling of curriculum can be achieved
- allows demonstration of emergency skills
- stations can be tailored to level of skills being assessed

Weaknesses of OSCEs

- can be expensive to run
- requires a lot of resources and organization (e.g. closure of an outpatient clinic for a day)
- many examiners needed
- simulated patients need to be trained and be consistent between candidates
- scenarios often don't mimic real-life situations—it can be difficult to holistically examine complex tasks

The assessment instruments described above all provide an assessment of learning. The following assessment instruments provide assessment for learning.

Overview of assessment instruments: Workplace-based assessments

Formal workplace-based assessments were introduced over the last decade across postgraduate medical curricula. Workplace-based assessments evaluate clinical performance throughout a healthcare professional's training in the authentic context of the workplace. Workplace-based assessments are designed to distinguish between the 'can do' (competence) and the 'does do' (performance) of medical professionals.[23] Miller's pyramid can be used to conceptualize assessment (see Figure 6.2),[24] whereby as one ascends up the pyramid, professional authenticity increases (pertaining to knowledge, skills, and attitudes).

Workplace-based assessments are encouraged to be learner-led, with the trainee identifying areas for observations and feedback. It must be noted that workplace-based assessments can also be trainer-driven, depending on the circumstances. Workplace-based assessments provide feedback to trainees about their progress, enable trainers/supervisors to share their experience and support Annual Review Competency Progression panels in making recommendations for progress through training.

Evidence of competence is usually recorded in a web-based portfolio (ePortfolio). A portfolio comprises evidence collected over time. The portfolio collates and organizes workplace-based assessments in addition to captured reflective practice. Workplace-based assessments provide focused and timely feedback to trainees and provide evidence to support longitudinal judgements about a trainee's progression. The Academy of Medical Royal Colleges suggests the main purpose of workplace-based assessments is 'to help trainees identify areas for improvement and is thus formative not summative'.[25]

While it's inevitable that a range of workplace-based assessment instruments are deployed across variable contexts and settings to observe the required attributes, their broad conceptual structure and rating systems should be as similar as possible across specialties.[23] There are many different types of workplace-based assessments, examples that may be of interest for further reading are shown in Table 6.4.

Strengths of WBAs

- Assesses skills in a real-world setting
- Allows for direct observation of performance and real-time feedback
- Led by the trainee
- Can be used to sample practice widely within a workplace
- Can engage multiple assessors to triangulate judgement and assessment

Weaknesses of WBAs

- Negative feedback or marks may be avoided due to close working relationships
- Given the need for training, can be time-consuming for both the assessor, and the trainee
- Can be opportunistic, rather than needs-driven. This can be addressed by also providing scope for WBAs to be instigated by trainers
- Does not assess knowledge directly, and there can be issues in terms of reliability. Should be used alongside other forms of assessment that meet 'shows' and 'knows how'
- If there are issues with the supervisory relationship, it can make seeking out WBAs and engaging with this process challenging

Table 6.4 Example and descriptions of WPBAs

Workplace-Based Assessment Instrument	Description	Assessor(s)/ Evaluator(s)	Remit: Discrete Task or Multiple Competencies Assessed
Mini-clinical evaluation exercise: e.g. 'mini-Cex'	Evaluates elements of good clinical care (history, examination, or clinical reasoning)	More senior clinician in same/similar specialty	Discrete: e.g. taking history
Case-based discussions: e.g. 'CBD'	Allows discussion of a case and demonstration of wider knowledge and reading around the topic	More senior clinician in same/similar specialty	Multiple: i.e. initial consultation skills plus wider reading and interpretation of evidence
Direct observation of procedural skills: e.g. 'DOPs'	Assessed specific practical procedure	More senior clinician in same/similar specialty	Discrete: e.g. intravenous cannulation
Patient satisfaction questionnaires: e.g. patient surveys or feedback	Gathers feedback from multiple patients within a stipulated timeframe	Patients/ clients who have had interaction with the doctor	Multiple: will gather evidence on clinical care, communication, professionalism, etc.
Multisource feedback—e.g. 'MSF', 360 degree feedback, team assessment of behaviour	Gathers feedback from multiple colleagues (clinical and non-clinical) within a stipulated timeframe	Colleagues (clinical and non-clinical)	Multiple: will gather evidence on competence, teamworking, leadership, etc.
Teaching observation	Assesses teaching skills, e.g. delivery of didactic teaching session, or bedside teaching	More senior clinician in same/similar specialty	Single/ Multiple: depending on the teaching session, could be very limited (to specific skills) or include communication, organization, and evidence synthesis
Evaluation of Clinical/ Management Events: e.g. 'Supervised learning event'	More longitudinal assessment of patient management and/or service provision: e.g. conducting a ward round	More senior clinician in same/similar specialty	Multiple: i.e. initial consultation skills plus wider reading and interpretation of evidence

(Continued)

Table 6.4 (Contd.)

Workplace-Based Assessment Instrument	Description	Assessor(s)/ Evaluator(s)	Remit: Discrete Task or Multiple Competencies Assessed
Quality Improvement Project Assessment Tool: e.g. 'QIP', Audit	Assessment of the undertaking of quality improvement project: e.g. audit, research project	Usually a clinical or educational supervisor	Discrete: assesses qualityimprovement domain on portfolio
Clinical/ educator supervisor's report: e.g. 'CSR'/'ESR', end of placement/ year report		Clinical or Educational Supervisor	Multiple: will gather evidence from all above assessments (and other information, e.g. exam success, CPD, etc.) to summarize outcome of placement/year

Assessments in undergraduate and postgraduate medicine

It should be noted that medical assessments are continually under review and development. Traditionally undergraduate assessments have been made through essay coursework and Single Best Answers in the initial years. However, as medical students nearing the end of their training have had clinical exposure, workplace-based assessments, as a formative tool, and the OSCE, as a summative tool, are introduced. Medical finals generally comprise a combination of OSCEs and Single Best Answer/Extended Matching Questions. After qualification, trainees can apply for specialty-specific examinations. These follow a similar pattern assessing both the clinical and knowledge skills: Single Best Answer/Extended Matching Questions and OSCE/simulated surgery.

Future developments of assessments

Over the past 40 years, there has been a considerable change in the approaches to assessment for the UK medical profession; from medical school entry to postgraduate training as well as established clinical practice; regular assessment is now the norm. The days of utilizing exit exams, which were often considered by the candidate as being poorly constructed and unrelated to the taught curriculum are gone. The assessments now in place must be robust—supporting the doctor and protecting the patient, as well as providing accountability. Assessments drive learning; assessment also facilitates learning—through feedback, reflection, and planned further learning.

Entrustable professional activities

Entrustable professional activities aim to bridge the gap between the theoretical aspects of competency-based education and authentic clinical practice. Competency-based education initially appeared valuable to formally observe what a trainee actually did in the workplace as opposed to what they were able to show they could do in an exam. However, supervisors can find this competency-based approach difficult to implement in a consistent way (the calibration and consistency of completion of workplace-based assessments, especially if supervisors are assessing trainees from several different specialties). Furthermore, confusion has arisen over the formative nature of workplace-based assessments, i.e. an 'assessment for learning'. Trainees have considered workplace-based assessments as summative and high-stakes 'assessments of learning', which they were not intended to be.

A new approach to assessment in medical education, which focuses on the outcome of training and is defined in terms of the work that a trainee is trusted to do, is increasingly common. By the end of training the doctor is 'trusted' to undertake all work tasks independently and without supervision.

Ten Cate and Young (2012) defined entrustable professional activities as 'units of professional practice, defined as tasks or responsibilities to be entrusted to a trainee once sufficient specific competence is reached to allow for unsupervised practice. They are independently executable within a time frame and observable and measurable in the process and outcome'.[26]

The mastery of most entrustable professional activities does not exclusively happen at the end of training. Trainees should be trusted to work unsupervised once they have met an appropriate threshold of ability. In clinical practice, ad hoc entrustment decisions are taken by those supervising trainees every day and rely on the judgement of many variables: the trainee, the supervisor, the activity type, the context, and the trainee-supervisor relationship.

There are several important trainee factors for enabling trust: competence, truthfulness/honesty, conscientiousness/reliability and discernment of one's own limitations. It is envisaged that entrustable professional activities, being triangulated, can contribute directly and more meaningfully to ARCP decisions.

An alternative wording used for the entrustable tasks are 'competencies in practice'. A competency in practice is defined as 'a critical part of professional work that can be identified as a unit to be entrusted to a trainee once efficient competence has been reached'.[27] Competencies in practice highlight the importance of the supervisor's role in observation and judgement, and replication of real-life practice.

Currently UK medical colleges, faculties, and the *Foundation Programme* are developing their curricula and assessments from being outcome driven to competency-based. The new curricula will incorporate all of the GMC's generic professional capabilities.

Other likely future developments

The COVID-19 pandemic significantly impacted not only on the content and delivery of clinical practice, but also the assessment landscape, notably onsite clinical testing. Nevertheless, it behoves educationalists to ensure that assessments are adapted both in their content to reflect changes in clinical practice and also format such as being deliverable remotely.

Finally, it is crucial to be mindful of the multi-determined nature of assessment, and the reality that any new system aims for pragmatic improvement rather than achievement of perfection.

Quality assurance of programmes of assessments

Organizations quality manage their programmes of assessments to check how well they are working, by gathering and monitoring evidence to ensure acceptable validity and reliability. Typically, this information is reported as a blend of psychometric and narrative analyses throughout programmatic assessments both on a whole test level but underpinned by item-level quality data. Such reviews may be performed internally and regularly by assigned educational experts such as the royal colleges and/or by sporadic external review.[28]

In the UK the General Medical Council (GMC) is the statutory regulator for all medical doctors, with responsibility for protecting, promoting, and maintaining the health of the public by ensuring proper standards in the practice of medicine. Alongside setting the standards for professional practice in *Good Medical Practice*, the GMC also has a legal duty for quality assuring undergraduate and postgraduate medical education and training, including curricula and assessments.

In order to achieve this, the GMC has defined an integrated standards framework to guide the development, approval, and provision of undergraduate and postgraduate medical education and training in the UK, accessible on their website. The same is true for regulators globally.

The GMC has issued supplementary guidance that describes the current best approaches to assessment and sets out the steps and principles to be followed when planning and designing a programme of assessment and maintaining its quality and validity in practice.[29] Such guidance can be of useful for those designing and delivering assessments within medical education.

References

1. van der Vleuten CPM, Schuwirth LWT. Assessing professional competence: from methods to programmes. *Med Educ* 2005;39(3):309–317.
2. Royal College of General Practitioners. The RCGP curriculum. 2019. https://www.gmc.uk.org/-/media/documents/gp-curriculum-2019-101-10611_pdf-79017777.pdf
3. Van Der Vleuten CPM. The assessment of professional competence: developments, research and practical implications. *Adv Health Sci Educ* 1996;1(1):41–67.
4. Jolly B. National licensing exam or no national licensing exam? That is the question. *Med Educ* 2016;50(1):12–14.
5. Schuwirth LWT, Van der Vleuten CPM. Programmatic assessment: from assessment of learning to assessment for learning. *Med Teach* 2011;33(6):478–485.
6. Mehay R. *The essential handbook for GP training and education*. London, UK: Radcliffe Publishing, 2009.
7. Joint Royal Colleges of Physicians Training Board. Recommendations for specialty trainee assessment and review. 2014. https://www.jrcptb.org.uk/sites/default/files/April%202014%20Recommendations%20for%20specialty%20trainee%20assessment%20and%20review.pdf
8. Joint Royal Colleges of Physicians Training Board. DOPS and potentially life threatening procedure. 2014. https://www.jrcptb.org.uk/sites/default/files/October%202014%20DOPS%20and%20potentially%20life%20threatening%20procedures.pdf
9. Academy of Medical Royal Colleges. Improving assessment: further guidance and recommendations. 2016. https://aomrc.org.uk/wp-content/uploads/2016/06/Improving_assessment_Further_GR_0616-1.pdf

10. Coderre S, Woloschuk W, McLaughlin K. Twelve tips for blueprinting. *Med Teach* 2009;31(4):322–324.

11. Schuwirth L, van der Vleuten C. How to design a useful test: the principles of assessment. In: Swanwick T, Forrest K, O'Brien BC (Eds.), *Understanding medical education* (pp. 275–289). Hoboken, NJ: Wiley-Blackwell, 2018.

12. Cronbach LJ, Shavelson RJ. My current thoughts on coefficient alpha and successor procedures. https://journals.sagepub.com/doi/10.1177/0013164404266386

13. Pell G, Fuller R, Homer M, Roberts T, International Association for Medical Education. How to measure the quality of the OSCE: a review of metrics—AMEE guide no. 49. *Med Teach* 2010;32(10):802–811.

14. Hofstee WKB. The case for compromise in educational selection and grading. In: SB Anderson, Helmick JS (Eds), *On educational testing* (pp. 109–127). San Francisco, CA: Jossey-Bass Publishers, 1983.

15. Angoff WH. *Scales, norms, and equivalent scores* (p. 156). Princeton, NJ: Educational Testing Service, 1984.

16. Ebel RL. *Essentials of educational measurement*, 2nd edn. Englewood Cliffs, NJ: Prentice Hall, 1972.

17. Downing SM, Tekian A, Yudkowsky R. Procedures for establishing defensible absolute passing scores on performance examinations in health professions education. *Teach Learn Med* 2006;18(1):50–57.

18. Faculty of Public Health. Structure of the diplomate examination (DFPH). https://www.fph.org.uk/training-careers/the-diplomate-dfph-and-final-membership-examination-mfph/the-diplomate-examination-dfph/structure-of-the-diplomate-examination-dfph/

19. Case S, Swanton D. *Item writing manual*, 3rd edn. Philadelphia, PA: National Board of Medical Examiners, 1998.

20. Harden RM, Stevenson M, Downie WW, Wilson GM. Assessment of clinical competence using objective structured examination. *Br Med J* 1975;1(5955):447–451.

21. Harden RM, Gleeson FA. Assessment of clinical competence using an objective structured clinical examination (OSCE). *Med Educ* 1979;13(1):41–54.

22. Norcini JJ. The death of the long case? *BMJ* 2002;324(7334):408–409.

23. Postgraduate Medical Education and Training Board. Standards for curricula and assessment systems. 2008. https://www.gmc-uk.org/-/media/documents/Standards_for_curricula_and_assessment_systems_1114_superseded_0517.pdf_48904896.pdf

24. Miller GE. The assessment of clinical skills/competence/performance. *Acad Med* 1990;65(9 Suppl):S63–67.

25. Academy of Medical Royal Colleges. Improving assessment. 2009. https://www.aomrc.org.uk/wp-content/uploads/2016/05/Improving_Asessment_0709.pdf

26. ten Cate O, Young JQ. The patient handover as an entrustable professional activity: adding meaning in teaching and practice. *BMJ Qual Saf* 2012;21 Suppl 1:i9-12.

27. ten Cate O. Entrustability of professional activities and competency-based training. *Med Educ* 2005;39(12):1176–1177.

28. Royal College of General Practitioners. Preface to the HPAC 10-year review and the RCGP response to the recommendations. 2018. https://www.rcgp.org.uk/getmedia/70ab45db-1eec-4cc6-b550-f9b8c26e340d/RCGP-HPAC-10-year-review-of-MRCGP-response-oct-2018-(1).pdf

29. General Medical Council. Designing and maintaining postgraduate assessment programmes. 2017. https://www.gmc-uk.org/-/media/documents/designing-and-maintaining-postgraduate-assessment-programmes-2109_pdf-70434370.pdf

Assessment techniques

Chris Valerio and Luci Etheridge

Introduction

Assessment invokes images of final clinical examinations with real patients and anxious students. Every doctor has been there and will have some idea of what an assessment looks like. However, there is variation between universities and furthermore between postgraduate institutions in how they assess, so everyone's experience of being assessed is likely to be a little different. When writing assessments these memories and experiences can be invaluable but preconceived ideas of assessment may also be a hindrance. There are many different forms of educational assessment. Not all assessment tools are appropriate within the sphere of medicine and some of the tools used in medical education do not work outside of it.

Before creating examinations, it may be worthwhile taking some time to reflect on your own experience and consider the purpose of assessments that you underwent. They should have allowed you to demonstrate that you have achieved the aims and objectives of the curriculum. In order to achieve this there is usually a process called blueprinting involved in selecting exam 'items'.

When constructing an assessment strategy, understanding the nuances of different assessment techniques will enable a coherent approach. Bear in mind that the ideal assessment strategy will be reliable, valid, feasible, and transparent. This process is usually undertaken by an assessment committee of experienced educationalists. Usually, one's first involvement in assessment will be writing an item or a question for an exam to fit in with this strategy. Creating assessments is a skill in itself, and this chapter aims to provide a guide through the process of writing and delivering assessments (in case you have been thrown in at the deep end).

If writing one assessment is easy, writing several is less so and writing a lot is difficult. Creating the ideal, overarching assessment strategy for doctors' training can seem Sisyphean (from Greek mythology, the eternal punishment of Sisyphus was to roll a boulder up to the top of a hill at which point it would roll down the hill so he would have to start all over again).

Principles

Assessments are a balancing act, and any assessment is a compromise between the principles that form an ideal assessment. No one assessment can comprehensively cover all of these principles, and you will likely need several assessments to ensure that the below principles have been met.

The utility (how useful or beneficial an assessment is) of an assessment can be considered using the utility equation,[1] shown in Box 7.1. It is important to note that this is not an equation in the true mathematical sense, but rather should be used to consider the relationship between the principles of an ideal assessment. If any items in the equation equal zero, then the utility of an assessment is also zero. The equation includes the following variables:

- Reliability—the degree to which an examination could be reproduced and elicit the same results
- Validity—the measure what is intended
- Educational impact—encouraging students to engage in deep learning, and have timely formative benefit
- Acceptability—considers human resource, physical resources, impact on other partners, e.g. patients, consider assessment load
- Cost effectiveness—includes cost of staff, resources, incentives, as well as opportunity cost.

Box 7.1 The principles of an ideal assessment can be thought of using the 'utility equation'

- $U = R \times V \times E \times A \times C$
- U= Utility; R= Reliability; V=Validity; E=Educational impact;
- A=Acceptability; C=Cost effectiveness

Adapted from van der Vleuten[1]

Assessment strategy

Selecting and using an assessment is no different to anything else in education; preparation and planning is key. This applies to the students, examiners, and those setting assessments.

It is important to remember that assessments can have different purposes depending on the context. An assessment may be used to encourage learning (it can be a strong driver) or to obtain feedback about how effective teaching has been or to determine if a learner has achieved an adequate level of skill or competence.

Summative and formative assessment

Though summative and formative assessments have different purposes they can be written and constructed using the same format. Contrastingly, delivery of feedback may be very different; in a summative objective structured clinical examination (OSCE) the station assessor provides no feedback to the candidate before they leave (it may be documented and provided at a later date), yet in a formative OSCE station feedback can be given before moving on to the next station.

Simple formative assessments can be used from the start of any course or programme. They can be used to gauge the baseline abilities of the cohort—which may result in tailoring of lesson plans to address weaker areas. This can be an ongoing process. As students progress, the feedback generated from formative assessments can be a valuable guide to what areas they need to focus on or develop.

Undergraduate assessment

Very broadly the medical undergraduate curriculum allows time to guide students up through the levels of Miller's pyramid[2] (see ➔ Chapters 2 and 5) with the aim that when have completed their undergraduate training, they can 'do'. The way students are assessed therefore changes as they progress through medical school.

Miller's model is a pyramid and as such the knowledge base is important. While curricula have become more integrated and progressive it is difficult to 'know how' to do anything in a knowledge vacuum. In the early stages of any curriculum, testing foundations of knowledge is vital, however, over the 4–6 years of medical school the relative amount of knowledge testing is likely to diminish and that of clinical skills ('shows how') will increase (see Table 7.1).

Table 7.1 Example of an undergraduate assessment scheme covering one year of clinical medicine. (MCQ= Multiple Choice Question, OSCE = objective structured clinical examination)

Module	Formative	Summative
Module A	written report supervisor feedback Formative MCQ	MCQ
Module B	written reportsupervisor feedback	MCQ
Module C	written reportsupervisor feedback	MCQ
End of year		OSCE covering all modules and themes for the year

Postgraduate assessment

In the postgraduate world, workplace-based assessments are used to 'show how'. This is because doctors are now in training and practising at the same time. Postgraduate exams typically exhibit a progression towards the higher levels of Miller's pyramid[2] with extensive clinical knowledge tests being followed by clinical exams. An example of a postgraduate examination format is detailed in Table 7.2.

Table 7.2 An example of postgraduate assessment: the MRCPsych examination within the UK (Psychiatry)

Exam paper	Focus of assessment	Format
Paper A	The scientific and theoretical basis of psychiatry	Three hours, 200 marks Two-thirds of the paper = MCQs, one-third = EMIs (Extended Matching Items)
Paper B	Critical review and clinical topics in psychiatry	Three hours, 200 marks. Two-thirds of the paper = MCQs, one-third = EMIs (Extended Matching Items)
CASC	Clinical assessment of skills and competencies	Based on the OSCE format with 16 stations: The first circuit includes 4 pairs of linked stations, each lasting 10 minutes with an additional 90 seconds of preparation time. The second circuit consists of 8 stations, each lasting 7 minutes with 90 second preparation time

Creating assessments

The more people involved in generating and setting the assessments, the less likely they are to reflect one person's view of a subject. Trying questions and scenarios out on colleagues or discussing them in meetings will help to ensure constructive alignment with the curriculum.

A mental checklist of things to consider when writing assessments

Not all the qualities on the below checklist may apply to every question being created, but it aims to provide a sense of what the assessment is for, or why the assessment is required, which may in turn help direct the selection and content of the optimal type of assessment.

What are we assessing?

- Product (an outcome), a process (how it was reached), or both?
- Knowledge > reciting information
- Application of knowledge > stating facts
- Learning > teaching
- Formative or summative
- Convergent, i.e. taking multiple measures of the same construct (divergent less often in undergraduate assessment)
- Cumulative or end point
- Deep/strategic/surface learning
- Holistic > serialism
- Ipsative (compares performance to own student's past performance) > time or context-specific using external benchmarks
- Norm (compares student to their peers) or criterion (compares student to predetermined standard, e.g. pass mark).

(> implies the former option is generally preferable if not impractical)

General top tips

- Pick the right assessment tool for the planned assessment
- Get to know the software used to manage the institution's questions or the person who manages it
- Spread the load with colleagues
- Use your knowledge and experience
- Remember the context.

Assessing clinical knowledge: Written tests

Written tests can be valid, reliable, reproducible, and relatively cheap. Every medical student is familiar with them in some form and most postgraduate assessments have a written component. Computer systems have enabled easier storage, blueprinting, compilation, and marking of items.

Questions can be either open-ended, where candidates spontaneously generate answers, or closed, where they are selected from a list.

General question writing tips

- The better the quality of each individual item, the better the overall quality of the test will be
- While it is simple to write a question it is harder to write several good-quality items and even harder to write an entire test's worth
- Practice helps—but prolific writers are rare as writing questions can become tedious
- Remember authors tend to stick to their area of expertise, so the greater the number and variety of a writer's interests the better
- Latest guidelines (e.g. NICE guidelines) are a good source of ideas
- Check if there is a 'house style' for the institution. If not, develop one to allow consistency and improve item quality
- There is a place in most tests for both difficult and easy questions
- Writing workshops can be productive in increasing the number and quality of items written
- The proof of the pudding is in the eating—collect item data on how new questions perform and use this in your quality assurance processes and for author feedback.

Computerized tests

Computerized testing can also enhance the delivery and security of exam questions. There are a variety of software programs available for the secure electronic storage and compilation of tests. It may be worth becoming familiar with the institution's system if one are likely to spend a significant amount of time compiling examinations. Examination papers can be printed out or many systems now allow for the creation of a computer-based test.

Since the onset of the COVID-19 pandemic, a number of issues have been raised with respect to online testing:

- The security of online testing has been questioned where assessments have been taken at home
- Remote proctoring has raised issues with equality, diversity, and inclusion, e.g. racial profiling with identity checks, as well as its efficacy, and cost
- Artificial intelligence has raised concerns over the reliability of tests.

A writing template for SBA/MCQs

The use of a standardized template allows easier transfer to a computer system with all necessary fields completed. This helps when compiling papers.

AUTHORS:	DATE WRITTEN:
QUESTION TITLE:	BLUEPRINT:
INTENDED ASSESSMENT:	ALTERNATIVE EXAMS:

Options:
Vignette:
Stem (lead-in):
Which is the single ... ?

A	
B	
C	
D	
E	

Correct Answer (key)=
Additional comments or explanation.

Single Best Answer (SBA) 1

SBAs may only assess knowledge, and this may be appropriate for the early years of medical school. For clinical exams they should, and can, address application of knowledge ('knows how'). They should focus on a single clinical issue, usually something clinically important, but this depends on the purpose of the exam (e.g. difficult items about less common conditions may discriminate students who deserve a distinction). Within a test, an SBA is known as an 'item'. Its construction is as follows:

Vignette/scenario
- A brief scenario that provides all the information required for the candidate to reach their decision.
- Presented in a standard order: demographic info, presenting complaint, associated history, examination, and clinical observations then investigations.
- The candidate may only have a short time to read, so keep the information clinically relevant.
- Don't include misleading information.
- Don't repeat words from the stem in any of the options.

Stem (lead-in question)
This should read 'Which is the single ... ' for SBAs.
- Avoid using subjective terms (e.g. important, best, dangerous, useful) as candidates will guess the most immediately life-threatening option irrespective of the clinical stem.

- Negative lead-ins, i.e. asking for the **least** likely diagnosis is unhelpful and usually tests irrelevant knowledge. As assessments help promote learning they should align to what is important and common.
- Commonly used lead-ins: 'Which is the single most likely diagnosis?', 'Which is the single most appropriate investigation?', Which is the single most effective therapy?'
- Should suggest the answer without needing to see the options—'the cover test'—which replicates clinical reasoning and decision-making.

Correct answer and distractors (options)

- A selection of alphabetically or chronologically listed potential answers
- One answer is indisputably correct ('the single most likely', known as the 'key')
- Incorrect options (distractors) should be credible and plausible and not completely wrong, i.e. part of a reasonable differential. Every obviously wrong distractor increases the odds of a correct 'guess'
- Homogeneous, that is, all options should be on the same axis, for example, investigations or all infectious organisms etc. This is because a mix means some options are easily rejected or the candidate struggles comparing apples and oranges
- Concise and similar in length; the longest option is usually correct as it takes more words to define the correct option than a wrong one
- Correctly written—erroneous spellings are more likely to be distractors
- Values are listed in numerical order and the correct answer should not be obviously different, e.g. the only odd number. It should not always be the middle option
- Avoid absolute terms, e.g. 'always', 'never', as these are rarely correct
- Avoid fillers; nonsense options will be discarded by candidates immediately. It can be difficult for writers to find the final option especially if the number of options is prescribed (e.g. five), but writing in groups can help with this as the group can generate and test out ideas
- Convergence-free; if options contain similar elements, the correct answer can be deduced by a logical process of counting and elimination. This is also referred to as 'test wiseness'

All the items in a paper should contain the same number of options. Having only two options effectively makes it a true-false scenario (where one is false and one true). The use of 'none of the above' or 'all of the above' transforms an SBA into a multiple true-false question. A correct option which indicates no illness or no active management can be discriminating as it tests true understanding rather than superficial knowledge. Tests should be inclusive and avoid stereotypes.

▶ *Question quality check 1: Homogeneity*

Question: A 70-year-old man has shoulder girdle aching, a throbbing headache, and reduced visual acuity in his right eye. What is the single best next step?

a. Computerized tomography (CT) head
b. Erythrocyte sedimentation rate (ESR)
c. Ophthalmology review
d. Prednisolone
e. Temporal artery biopsy (this cues the whole scenario)

Answer: The options include investigations, a referral, and a treatment, and therefore the options are not all equal/comparable in terms of being legitimate options.

Single Best Answer (SBA) 2

▶ *Pitfalls—test-wise candidates*

Candidates will attempt to gain an advantage any way they can. A test-wise candidate uses their knowledge of the subject alongside their knowledge of the test format and technique to increase their chance of picking the correct option. They reject options which don't fit the pattern and favour the one which stands out. While this approach can never be completely removed, it is important to promote learning of clinical knowledge rather than test technique. Keeping the test-wise candidate in mind when writing and reviewing SBAs will reduce the number of questions which are rewarded by these tactics.

How to answer SBAs: 10 tips for students (and writers to be aware of)

- Read the stem and lead-in with the options covered up. Try to come up with the correct answer before looking at the options
- Remember there is only ONE correct answer, others may be plausible but not quite right. Never be tempted to put down two answers (machine read sheets will give you 0 marks)
- Eliminate as many distractors as possible before making an educated guess
- Read the stem to look for cues, word matches, and stereotypes
- Check if the lead-in asks for a specific type of option, i.e. investigation, then rule out any answer that is not concordant
- Look at all the answers and decide if any look out of place or different from the rest. These are usually wrong and can be ignored
- Don't overcomplicate the question. The obvious answer is often correct. It's harder to generate plausible distractors than implausible ones
- If there are a set of ranked values, the middle value is often correct (writers pick the correct value and then two above and two below to make up five options)
- If you really don't know the answer, then guess the option that is longest
- Even if the answer is not clear, guess. If there is no negative marking a guess between all five answers still has a 20% chance of being correct

▶ *Question quality check 2: Convergence*

Question: A 48-year-old man with cirrhosis and portal hypertension presents with haematemesis. The patient has good intravenous access. What is the single best management?

a. antibiotics, beta-blocker, and blood products
b. antibiotics, beta-blocker, and terlipressin
c. antibiotics, blood products, and PPI
d. antibiotics, blood products, and terlipressin
e. blood products, PPI, and terlipressin

Answer: D

Four of the answers contain antibiotics and four contain blood products so it is likely they are correct. Three of the options contain terlipressin so again the likelihood is that this is correct. Logical deduction should lead the candidate to answer D, which is correct. Therefore, you cannot tell if the candidate knows what to do in this clinical situation or can simply apply logical deduction.

▶ *Question quality check 3: Cover test*

A 34-year-old woman has had dysphagia for four weeks. She has a history of Raynaud's phenomenon. She has shiny tight skin affecting her fingers and multiple telangiectasia. What is the single most likely diagnosis?

a. Chagas disease
b. Iron deficiency anaemia
c. Limited cutaneous systemic sclerosis
d. Mitral stenosis
e. Pseudo-bulbar palsy

Answer: C limited cutaneous systemic sclerosis (scleroderma), formerly known as CREST (calcinosis, Raynaud's, oesophageal dysmotility, sclerosis, telangiectasia) syndrome.

In the scenario she has four of the five features and no history to suggest the other diagnoses, e.g. history of rheumatic fever to cause mitral stenosis. Note also the longest answer is correct.

True-False Questions

True-False questions use a stem that is correct to supply correct information to the candidate followed by a series of options linked to the stem. Multiple true-false formats include those where the candidate is asked to tick all the correct options (without the number being specified). Using the same stem for multiple items (e.g. five) is common practice and mitigates the issue of candidates only demonstrating that they know something to be untrue. For educational and practical purposes, it is more important to know what is true.

Construction

Include all clinical information that is **not** part of the question. Avoid mentioning any of the answers in the stem. Well-defined or quantifiable terms, e.g. 'twenty per cent' are much easier to use than those like 'seldom' and 'often'. Absolute terms direct the exam savvy student to the correct (usually FALSE) answer and very open questions tend to be TRUE. Double negatives should be avoided; remember that a 'false' answer is seen as a negative. Providing an obverse, positively worded question, means that phrasing can become tortuous in order to satisfy the binary nature of the question.

Example Multiple True-False Question

Question: A 31-year-old man with a cough has mycobacteria on sputum culture. The reference laboratory has not been able to identify the organism yet.

Which of these *Mycobacterium* species are NOT associated with pulmonary disease? (Please select all correct answers)

a. avium complex
b. kansasii

c. leprae
d. malmoense
e. tuberculosis

Answer: There is only one TRUE answer here (option C). It might be better as a best of five Single Best Answer (SBA). It is also an unnecessary negatively-posed question, as the four options that are FALSE are associated with pulmonary disease—thus the question could read which species ARE associated with pulmonary disease, in which case it would not work as an SBA.

Extended Matching Questions (EMQs)

EMQs focus more on decision-making. They work within a theme, e.g. diagnosis, and supply up to 26 options. The lead-in asks the question to be applied to the vignettes that follow, e.g. the most likely diagnosis. The vignettes that follow will each have a correct option contained within the list. Its construction is as follows:

Theme:
Determine this first as it will focus all the options.

Options:
- Short and clear (less likely to give away hints)
- All options should be theoretically possible for all vignettes
- Avoid verbs
- Should all be on the same axis (homogenous), e.g. not a mix of five cranial nerves and five arteries

Stem:
It should be clear and well-defined: 'For each of the following vignettes, please select the most likely diagnosis from the list of options.'

Vignettes:
Need to be kept related to the options. More than one vignette can have the same correct option!

Example EMQ
Theme: Causes of liver disease
A. Alpha-1 anti-trypsin
B. Autoimmune hepatitis
C. Budd-Chiari syndrome
D. Drug-induced liver injury
E. Ethanol-induced liver disease
F. Haemochromatosis
G. Hepatitis B virus
H. Hepatitis C virus
I. Ischaemic liver injury
J. Non-alcoholic fatty liver disease
K. Primary biliary cholangitis
L. Primary sclerosing cholangitis
M. Wilson's disease

For each of the following vignettes, please select the most likely diagnosis from the list of options.
1. A 24-year-old man who recently started treatment for tuberculosis.
2. A 68-year-old man with multiple inpatient stays for alcohol-related issues.

Short Answer Questions (SAQ)

These require the candidate to generate a short written answer; they should be open-ended.

Construction

- As these questions take longer to answer than MCQ formats, it is prudent to make the questions brief and clear.
- Short sentences will help to avoid reading errors but if needed for the purpose of clarity then more words are warranted.
- Double negatives should be avoided.
- The ideal answer and alternative acceptable answers need to be pre-defined for markers.
- Ideally the answer key (i.e. the mark scheme or example answer) should be clear enough that more than one person and non-experts can mark the paper.
- Candidates can be unclear what kind of answer is expected of them from SAQs.
- Stating the length of answer or number of responses expected (e.g. the three main causes) and the marks attached to the question may help.
- However, the level of detail may still be unclear. For instance, if small cell lung cancer is needed to obtain the marks and lung cancer isn't enough, the question needs to convey this to the candidate.
- Candidates may take a visual cue from the size of the space for writing or typing into—so this should be standardized.
- Candidates may try to fill the available space to ensure that the right answer can be found somewhere in the word salad that their mind has produced.

For reasons of reliability, when marking, it is better for each question to be assigned to a marker for correction than dividing the answer scripts. In this way, each marker is familiar with one question and is able to benchmark and sense check their marking; and each student has their overall test marked by multiple assessors, offering multiple viewpoints on their performance.

General writing tip

Extraneous or redundant information is a waste of a candidate's time and adds nothing to the assessment. Especially when reviewing other questions, it is worth considering if there are statements that can be cut, e.g. a history of recent travel should include locations if it is possibly a tropical disease, however if the cause is thromboembolism, a long-haul travel is all that is needed—it does not matter if they flew from Colombia.

Example SAQ (1)

Question: The origin of which bronchus has a straighter course at the carina?

Answer: Right main bronchus

There is no clinical correlation and only two possible answers left or right, so a T/F format might be better (and certainly quicker).

- A child has inhaled a small toy. Which bronchus is it most likely to be lodged in?

Although now clinically relevant the question does not clearly state what generation of bronchus or the size of the toy. If first generation bronchus then the options are still only left or right, but the author's intended answer may be the second-generation right lower lobe bronchus. To assess understanding, it would also be better to ask why.

- Example SAQ (2)

A 20-year-old student has been unwell since returning from Southeast Asia. His temperature is 39.1°C. What investigations should be sent?

This is a more appropriate SAQ. It also reflects what a practising doctor does: they order investigations. This would not work in an SBA format, although a T/F list could be given. However, without an indication of how many marks are available students may just write the first two or three answers that occur to them OR they may write every test they can think of. Changing the question to ask which two investigations should be sent first will be more challenging but will focus the candidates and remain relevant to clinical practice.

Structured essay questions

These are also open-ended but require a longer answer. This will allow the candidate to demonstrate application, reasoning, or evaluation in a novel scenario related to a core learning outcome. This does mean they need to be marked by hand. Also, the writing style of the candidates can influence scores. Its construction is as follows:

The question needs to be phrased clearly and should indicate what level of detail the candidate needs to provide. They can contain more information than SAQs. Candidate information should include the maximum length for an answer (or they will adopt a blunderbuss approach) and number of marks for each answer to allow proportionate division of testing time.

To offer some standardization guidance to examiners, an answer key must exist and include the correct answer, acceptable alternatives and incorrect but conceivable answers.

Choices

If candidates are to be offered choices of essay questions care needs to be taken to ensure they are likely to produce a similar distribution of marks—a seemingly easy question may have a high 'pass' rate but may disadvantage those trying to achieve a top grade compared with an alternative which may 'fail' more candidates.

Special type: Modified essay question

Typically, this involves a case history followed by a sequence of questions. This is prone to interdependency as if a candidate answers incorrectly initially they may not be able to answer subsequent questions correctly. This can only be overcome if the candidates have to submit answers before they can proceed to the next question—this can be achieved with computer-based approaches.

Example structured essay question

A 57-year-old woman presents with an episode of syncope. When she arrives in the emergency department, she has a temperature of 37.2°C, heart rate of 110 bpm, BP 106/62, respiratory rate of 24, and oxygen saturations of 96 on air. She is found to have a pulmonary embolus on CTPA (CT pulmonary angiogram). Define syncope and explain how this episode may have occurred in relation to where in the pulmonary vasculature the clot is seen on the CT images.

New question and test types

Key-feature approach questions

In this type of assessment, problem-solving is assessed by presenting a case (or cases) and asking for decisions to be made. The response format can vary. ALL the important information must be included in the case, including context. The questions must ask for essential clinical decisions. The answers can be presented either as a short written answer or selection of options from a menu. Care needs to be given to the scoring key, with selection of correct key features scoring one, but over or under selection, or selection of 'killer' options (which would represent dangerous practice) scoring 0. Care also needs to be taken to test different key features, e.g. history-taking, investigations, rather than making correct answering of one part of the item dependent on correctly having answered previous parts.

Script concordance tests

These tests use ill-defined problems and an aggregate scoring system. The clinical scenario does NOT contain all the data and the candidate scores the likelihood of a menu of options in relation to the solution from +2 to –2. The original developers suggest expert teams are needed to construct items and the scoring key.

Prescribing safety assessment (PSA)

The PSA has been designed to test all UK final-year medical students on their knowledge, skills, and judgement in relation to prescribing. The content has been designed to be directly relevant to the prescribing tasks a Foundation Year 1 doctor is expected to perform. It is an open book exam—students have access to the BNF (British National Formulary) throughout. It is set as a pass/fail assessment with the benchmark being safe, competent prescribing practice.

Situational judgement test

Situational judgement questions use hypothetical scenarios to assess real-world understanding, behaviours, and professional attributes. They were created to look at psychometrics as much as knowledge.

Table 7.3 Blueprint for OSCE stations organized by skill to be examined and body system and list of stations below

Skill/System	Breathing	Circulation	Digestion	Locomotion
History-taking		7 Chest pain		
Physical exam			1 Ascites	6 Shoulder
Diagnostic procedure		8 Venepuncture		
Data interpretation	2 ABG			10 Hip X-ray
Patient education			9 Endoscopy	4 Gout
Patient management	11 Prescribing			
Communication	3 Cancer		12 Drug error	
Critical appraisal		5 Paper		
Problem-solving			12 Drug error	10 Hip X-ray

Station key/List

1. Real patient examination—ascites
2. Arterial blood gas—interpret and explain
3. Cancer—discussion of complications
4. Gout—dietary education
5. Paper—interpret for a student
6. Shoulder exam—normal simulated patient
7. Chest pain—history of acute coronary syndrome
8. Venepuncture—with manikin
9. Endoscopy—explanation
10. Hip X-ray—diagnosis and management planning
11. Prescribing—drugs for acute asthma
12. Drug error—explanation and management planning

Assessing clinical competence

Objective structured clinical examination (OSCE)

The OSCE is a competence-based examination in which candidates are observed and scored as they progress through a circuit of stations laid out according to a blueprinted plan. Each OSCE station should focus on an element of clinical competence and the candidate will interact with a real or simulated patient, interpret investigations, or perform a clinical task while being assessed.

Planning

When planning and designing an OSCE many of the factors that will influence the format are already predetermined, but you should take note of:

- The number of candidates to be assessed, e.g. the entire fourth-year cohort of 200
- The purpose of the OSCE, e.g. summative assessment of progression
- Breadth or focus of assessment, e.g. finals or psychiatry only
- Venue(s) and capacity, e.g. clinical skills centres on two different sites
- Resources attainable, especially real and simulated patients
- Stage of training of candidates, e.g. finals students

The variables that can be set for an OSCE are:

- Number of stations (generally 10–30)
- Length of time for each station (commonly 5–15 min)
- Number of circuits (one or more)
- Use of 'procedure' and 'question' stations
- Use of 'double' and 'linked' stations
- Order of the stations in a circuit
- Provisions for feedback to the candidates

These need to be agreed and consistent across multiple sites to ensure a fair exam for all candidates. This can involve a fair degree of negotiation and flexibility in planning.

Blueprinting for OSCEs

One of the key elements in planning any OSCE is the development of a blueprint. This is a road map of what your OSCE will look like and contains details of the stations and how they map to the curriculum or learning objectives. It is usually constructed as a simple grid or table, with topic areas plotted against skill areas. Blueprinting allows you to ensure that your OSCE samples widely from across your curriculum—it prevents duplication.

Example of OSCE blueprint

Table 7.3 illustrates a simple blueprint for an undergraduate 12-station OSCE. Every skill is covered, and the four modules are equally represented by the stations selected.

OSCE terminology

There are many terms used by experts when talking about OSCEs that are easily confused.

Split circuit

Where an OSCE is broken up into two equal circuits, e.g. a 14-station OSCE becomes A and B each with seven stations. This is usually for logistic reasons, e.g. lack of space for students. Circuit A can be taken on day one by all students and circuit B on day two of the assessment.

Rest station

At a rest station the candidate has a rest in between stations. They are used when there is a need to accommodate more students than there are stations.

Gaps

When there are fewer candidates than stations the examiners will experience a 'gap' in the flow of candidates.

Double station

A station that is twice the normal length of the standard for the OSCE circuit. This requires two stations (a and b) to be set up and run with alternating candidates entering a and b as they finish the preceding station. It also requires either an early start for one of the candidates, who will consequently finish a station early, or a rest start with a late finish.

Linked stations

Where the activity of a station is then taken further forward at the next station, e.g. an examination station followed by a station where the candidate must explain a management plan. A candidate cannot start on the second linked station. Caution needs to be applied to prevent candidate deficiencies in the first station from being penalized again in the second station.

OSCE station writing: Preparation

Writing an OSCE station or scenario requires a deep understanding of the problem and the possible approaches to it. Within an OSCE station there are three variables: the candidate, the assessor, and the patient. Candidates, simulated patients or role players, patients, and examiners can be unpredictable, and it is the clarity of instructions and the forethought of what might happen that makes a scenario work consistently. Depending on your learning and working style you may develop the scenario in different ways. Stations can be written single-handedly but a second author makes it more likely that problems will be corrected in the writing phase.

The first step is to come up with a scenario and sketch out what the task is. This may have been determined by a need to round out the OSCE, e.g. an exam lacking an ethics and law station and with few orthopaedic patients might necessitate an orthopaedic-related ethical scenario. OSCEs should typically place the volunteer in a role they would or could be expected to perform (on passing the assessment). If defining a role, then it should reflect the candidate's expected context, e.g. asking a trainee paediatric doctor sitting a membership OSCE to fulfil the role of a surgical registrar in theatre would be invalid. It is imperative that the information is consistent for all parties and if changes are made to the station that this is reflected in all the different instructions.

Candidate instructions

Upon reading the instructions the candidate should have a clear idea of what the station will involve. Keep the scenario information brief as the candidates have limited time to read it and will probably forget any detail once they start the station anyway. Give them a clear instruction as to what they are expected to do and, if necessary, state what part of the tasks they are not expected to do.

Equipment list

Better to overdo this as it needs to include everything. The bare minimum is three chairs, a table, tissues, alcohol hand rub, pencil and paper, plus the assessor's marking equipment. Some 'props' may need to be specifically designed, e.g. drug charts—many institutions have templates for these. Again, where possible, it is best to have things as they are in practice, so radiology on computer screens but electrocardiograms (ECGs) printed out. If information sheets are not meant to be written on by the candidates, then laminate them.

Example OSCE station: 'Finals' examination—10-minute station
candidate instructions

You are a Foundation Year 1 doctor in medicine.

Mrs Foster has come to speak with you about her mother, Betty, one of the patients on the ward. Betty is recovering from pneumonia. The team have identified memory problems and suspect she has dementia.

Mrs Foster is concerned that her mother has not been eating well and has lost weight. She has asked to speak to a doctor to discuss feeding options to help her mother recover from her recent illness.

Please discuss feeding options for Mrs Foster's mother and answer her questions.

This is a 10-minute station.

Equipment list
• Table
• 3 chairs
• Tissues
• Hand gel
• Pen
• Paper

OSCE station writing: Simulated patient

Simulated patient instructions

In contrast to the candidate information, the more detail given to the simulated patients the better they are able to inhabit the role. Age, size, gender, and ethnicity can all be cast according to the station. Clear guidance about clothing helps actors get into the role. There are several examples of institutions successfully using child-simulated patients in OSCEs. UK laws govern the work of child actors, and good practice guidance covers the use of child patients or healthy children. Generally, children cannot comfortably role-play for too many candidates in succession as they tire easily. Therefore, two or more children may be recruited for each role. Stations that are written to allow flexibility on age, gender, ethnicity, and appearance will work better.

Give a full life background—consider what questions would be asked by a candidate taking a full history—as the simulated patient will have to answer them. Remember that candidates could ask almost anything. They won't always stick to a concise history.

The salient points of the presenting complaint or reason for attending come next. It is good practice to give simulated patients an opening line: 'my chest hurts and I feel like I'm dying'. They will need to be able to give a believable and consistent response to any probing questions asked by the candidate relating to the problem.

Some medical terms may have to be explained and providing background leaflets may help but write instructions so they are understandable. Remember if the simulated patient doesn't understand a candidate's question, then it is unlikely a real patient would either.

There is a limit to how much script actors can retain, but 'standard' details like past medical history, allergies, drugs, and family history can be listed for ease. Conversely, listing a lot of negative responses is not helpful. Experienced role players know that the default answer is a neutral or negative response.

A simulated patient's genuine reaction to a leftfield question usually prompts candidates to consider their line of questioning. The script should contain all the information they need about symptoms, signs, timing, associated features, and treatment that a good candidate might ask to exclude other diagnoses and identify related problems. Again, having a second person think through how the scenario will play out is helpful, and practising a run through of the station with a simulated patient and a mock candidate can be invaluable.

Actors like instructions that tell them how to act, e.g. become angry if you do not get what you want. They can be incredibly effective at portraying difficult roles. They may need to have specific questions to ask, e.g. 'won't chemotherapy make my hair fall out?' or prompts 'do you want to call for help?' to make sure that the candidate moves on and covers all the competencies being assessed. They may need to be provided with particular beliefs or concerns that the candidate needs to elucidate to understand the problem.

Simulated patients may be asked to assign a mark to candidates based on their feelings about the interaction with the candidate. If this is done, then the simulated patient should be asked to score the candidate on a specific question, e.g. did the candidate understand my concerns and seek my opinion?

Example OSCE station: Finals 10-minute station

Simulated Patient information

Mrs Foster: middle aged woman, any ethnicity, smartly dressed

Background and context

You are a 59-year-old accountant. You live with your husband (Dave) and have two grown up children. Your mother (Betty) is 87 years old. She lives nearby and has lived alone since your father died four years ago. Your father died of cancer. He seemed to 'waste away' as he wasn't eating anything due to his throat cancer. You recall your mother talking to him about how important it was that he continued to eat. There was some talk at the time about him possibly having a feeding tube put in to help. Betty was admitted to hospital with pneumonia a week ago—her first serious illness.

Opening statement

You are speaking to a junior doctor who works on the ward. You asked to speak to them today when you were visiting. After they introduce themselves say: 'Thank you for speaking to me. I'm very worried that my mother isn't eating and wanted to discuss what to do.'

Your worries

Your mother has needed help at home for the last two years; carers currently come once a day. When possible, you try to prepare her meals, but she also has a neighbour who pops by a couple of times a week. It's a friendly neighbourhood and she has lived there for a long time, so everyone knows her. While in hospital your mother has not eaten well. She says she does not like hospital food, and it is often cold. When she is given a meal, she starts eating then seems to stop and do something else. You have seen some of the staff try to help make sure she eats but it doesn't always happen. Your mother looks thin and gaunt and seems down. If allowed to freely speak about your worries, talk about your father's demise and ask if your mother could have a feeding tube. The doctor may ask you about the feeding tube. Say you cannot remember much about it but that it was mentioned as something that might help your father to keep his strength up.

Questions you should ask at an appropriate point:
• What are the options to ensure my mum gets nourishment?
• What is the safest option?
• How does tube-feeding work?
• Are there any complications?

Your feelings

You feel helpless as you don't know how to get your mother to eat, and you are worried this might be the beginning of the end. You think the consultant should be speaking to you to update you and if the doctor does not take time to listen to you and explain things in a clear way then you can become argumentative and say, 'I want to speak with the consultant in charge'.

OSCE station writing: Assessment

Once the scenario has been mapped out, thought needs to be given as to how it will be scored. Institutions will have policy and guidance as to how stations should be scored (see ➌ Chapter 6, Assessment principles). However, the specifics for each station will need to be completed and guidance drawn up for assessors on how to score candidates in a standardized way across circuits and venues.

Assessor instructions

Examiners should be given copies of **all** the information for the station. They should also be given a brief overview of what the candidate is expected to do. Sometimes it can be helpful to provide a model answer. Assessors in OSCEs often need reminding that they are supposed to be passive observers of candidate behaviour rather than interlocutors as in clinical viva exams. Ideally there should be no prompts for the assessor to give (they should come from the simulated patient), but if assessors are expected to ask questions, these should be clearly written in advance and instructions given as to when to ask them. Assessors should not indicate from their communication, verbal or non-verbal, as to how the candidate is doing. An

Table 7.4 Example of global ratings marksheet

Skill to be assessed	Rating				
	A—Excellent	B—Clear pass	C—Pass	D—Borderline	E—Fail
Initial approach to the patient	A	B	C	D	E
Information giving: clinical content	A	B	C	D	E
Information giving: Communication	A	B	C	D	E

advantage of this is that assessors do not need expertise in the station they are assessing; in fact, this is often best avoided for undergraduates.

Marksheets

Marksheets are the dark art of OSCEs. Students and doctors have little idea of what may be on them, and they can make a difficult and stressful station yield high marks and an apparently easy station difficult to pass. Early undergraduate OSCEs often utilize checklists whereas later undergraduate or postgraduate scoring may be based more on global scoring (see Table 7.4) and broader competencies.

Example: global ratings marksheet (for example station)

The marking categories can depend on the institution and may be just straightforward pass/fail or numeric or graded marks.

The style may depend on the method used for standard setting (see ➲ Chapter 6, Assessment principles).

▶ *Testing/piloting*

Even experienced OSCE writers can be unsure as to how long a station will take or if some aspect has been forgotten. It is recommended that where possible the station is piloted, even if this is a run through with some colleagues (one of whom is naïve to the scenario). This helps to pick up problems and check that the time allowed is reasonable and to amend stations before going live.

OSCE station types

OSCEs have the advantage that they can test a range of clinical skills. However, due to time constraints, whole 'consultations' are generally not advised as the extra station time needed would reduce the overall number of stations that can be tested, thereby reducing reliability. For this reason, many institutions have a number of templates for testing skills in different areas.

History

The candidate instructions should normally give the presenting complaint to guide the candidate along the right path. Candidates should generally be instructed to conclude the consultation by using the final minute to explain to the patient what they think the problem is. The simulated patient script is obviously important here and may need to be simplified or honed down to be manageable in the time available. It is reasonable to instruct actors to hold back key information, e.g. sexual history, unless specifically asked.

Examination

The candidate instructions should state exactly what they are expected to examine, and this should be achievable in the time available (e.g. not a full neurological examination). Time should be allowed for presentation of findings to the assessor. This can be with a simulated patient/volunteer, in which case the method of examination can be assessed rather than the ability to detect abnormalities. The simulated patient can be instructed to portray some abnormalities, e.g. tenderness, or to have picture props or make-up showing signs, but these are less realistic. Real patients can be used but can be difficult to standardize. They are selected because they have good signs. It is wise to check on their medical details before each sitting and the assessor(s) should always examine them to check they agree with the clinical signs. An assessor guide sheet and grid to fill in is helpful here.

Certain clinical assessments create a lot of difficulty, e.g. the Glasgow Coma Scale (GCS). There are a limited number of GCS scores that an actor can be asked to simulate because the motor score must always be 6/6 and eye 3 or 4 (for ethical reasons). An alternative is to use a video recording of a GCS assessment. Similarly, child development is, of course, progressive, but a video may capture a snapshot that illustrates certain points that a candidate can watch and report on.

Verbal communication, patient education

There are a large variety of verbal communication stations reflecting scenarios where verbal communication is integral to competence. The station should not require advanced knowledge of medicine so that some candidates may be disadvantaged. Candidate instructions need to explain the scenario and state who the person being addressed is, e.g. a difficult relative or problem colleague or student. Candidates may expect these to be bad news or ethics type stations, but they can be about phone referrals or health promotion. These can be remarkably true to life with a well-simulated patient. Actors will naturally find it easier to perform as lay people than as experts (e.g. colleagues) and so extra information or even coaching may be needed from assessors. There may be specific points for assessors to consider, e.g. Candidates demonstrating they can meet responsibilities under duty of candour guidance, which will need to be built into the actor's brief to ensure they come out in the scenario. Some institutions also include marks given by simulated patients.

Written communication

Much medical practice involves written communication, e.g. writing discharge summaries and safe prescribing is a key skill for all doctors. These stations usually require some mocked-up medical notes. A formulary should be available if prescribing. Marking can be done after the candidate has left the station or at the end of the exam. A note of caution however: if designing a station with a written element, make sure that it could not be tested in another format (e.g. a written test of knowledge) to avoid 'wasting' an OSCE station.

Practical and technical skills

There is a variety of low-fidelity and high-fidelity equipment on the market for teaching and assessing practical and technical skills. Where possible, candidates should be tested using equipment they are familiar with from teaching. The main concern is ensuring all the equipment needed is listed and available with plenty of spares. These stations may require an able volunteer to assist candidates and to ensure equipment changeover between candidates. It is also possible to combine technical skills with clinical communication by using a simulated patient along with equipment.

Simulation stations

With the increasing sophistication of simulation, there are models that can demonstrate changing and adaptive physiology in critical situations for doctors to respond to. This does make the station more complex and an agreed scheme for how the patient responds needs to include responses for conceivable treatments that might be given. Quite a long list of equipment may be needed, assessors need clear and specific instructions and actors may need help in understanding the more technical aspects of the scenario and the simulation system.

Problem-solving/data interpretation

These stations usually require the candidate to do some thinking and work out what to do with some clinical information. The way this is assessed can vary, so you can be creative: recreating a multidisciplinary team meeting or a discussion with a patient or relative. The data is best presented as it would normally be in real life, e.g. CT images rather than the report.

OSCE delivery

Preparation is everything. Your team will thank you if your equipment lists are exhaustive, the instructions are clear, and all the paperwork is prepared and correct. Finalizing the master list of OSCE stations, mapping out the circuit(s), identifying patients, and checking the necessary equipment is working and available can all be done well in advance. By far the best way to ensure all tasks have been assigned and completed in time is to have a standard operating procedure (SOP) document that everyone works to.

Candidates will need to be allocated to a start station and examiners will need to be assigned a station to assess. A schedule for the day should be provided to all involved so they know when they are expected to arrive and when their participation will finish.

Sequestering may be used if OSCE circuits run in the morning and afternoon to stop students leaking information; this needs to be planned and the students need to be informed. Administrative staff can look after this so more clinical staff can be present at the OSCE.

The 'walk through' is traditionally the last check that the exam centre is set up to run the OSCE. This is usually done the afternoon before, once everything is set up, and is a last chance to spot potential problems and make changes. These are vital if the OSCE is running on multiple sites: site representatives can walk through at one lead site and can then disseminate last minute changes to all sites to ensure standardization.

Assessor training

Never forget that clinicians, especially consultants, are independent-minded people and liable to do things their own way, regardless of what they have been told. Assessor training is vital to ensure assessors understand the purpose, scope, and aims of the assessment and are familiar with mark schemes and best practice. Favourite tricks are inadvertently showing candidates the mark scheme and talking to the candidates or asking them viva-like questions. It is always useful to have reserve assessors available at the start as it is much easier to send someone away on the day than to find a last minute available trained assessor who may take time to arrive and delay the start of the exam. There are a number of different ways to run assessor training, but using videos of actual stations and asking assessors to mark and then take part in a facilitated discussion of their scoring allows for a valid and real-life experience.

▶ *Top tips for OSCE day*

- Take some time to get to know the stations—remember there may be different stations and information on different days
- Assign someone to look after any real patients and child actors and make sure they get a rest
- Assign someone to brief the students and lead them in
- If external examiners are expected, have some spare examiner information packs for them
- Check where you work—but marksheets and feedback forms are usually delivered and collected on the day

On the day itself:

- Arrive early and check the venue
- Brief assessors and allocate stations, allowing assessors marking the same station to confer and ensure they will all mark in the same way
- Guide assessors, patients, and simulated patients to stations and allow them time to familiarize themselves with the exam environment
- Students should have a briefing before being brought to the OSCE circuit
- When all candidates and assessors are present signal the start of OSCE (don't forget about early starters if needed)
- Assign a dedicated timekeeper to give time warnings and announce the change of stations
- Written responses can be carried around, posted in a box, or removed after each candidate
- When the OSCE finishes collect the examiner mark sheets and briefly check them for missing marks
- If there is another group of candidates, they should be assembled and held away from the group that is finishing the circuit/examination
- Encourage assessors across different circuits to talk at breaks and ensure standardization
- Supply refreshments during breaks
- Repeat as necessary
- Thank everyone at the end

Long cases

Traditionally in a long case, the candidate would interview a patient and then present them to an assessor. This doesn't actually assess beyond 'knows how' and the objective structured long examination record was developed to include observation of the patient interaction. To make case examinations reliable, several cases need to be included and observed, which logically leads many to decide to use OSCEs.

Viva Voce ('Vivas'—oral examinations)

Vivas are the principal way that expert knowledge can be assessed (by other experts, e.g. in a doctoral, PhD, viva). The benefits they offer in medicine are limited because on the job assessments cover much of the same ground and allow for a broader assessment from a greater number of senior sources. If they are used, they should have a structured mark scheme. However, they remain difficult to standardize. Multiple Mini-Interviews (MMIs), used in medical selection, involve an oral assessment but are significantly briefer than a true viva. In the MMI, there are multiple stations which enable some level of comparison and standardization.

PACES—a recognizable OSCE

At the time of writing, the MRCP(UK) Part 2 Clinical Examination (Practical Assessment of Clinical Examination Skills—PACES) is perhaps one of the most recognized acronyms in UK examinations. Medical students wishing to excel in their finals will often use PACES revision guides because the subject matter is so similar. The PACES format has evolved to encompass five stations and eight patient encounters. Six of these patients are real—this is a much higher proportion than in most undergraduate exams and so it is difficult to standardize. To aid with reliability there are two 'independent' examiners at each station.

Assessing performance: Workplace-based assessments (WPBA)

Because performance describes what an individual actually does, these assessments have to take place in the work environment. Although 'does' is at the pinnacle of Miller's pyramid, these assessments do not have to be summative and in fact are more valuable to trainees as formative learning events.

Currently in the UK a wide range of WPBAs are used by the various Royal Colleges and training boards. Although we discuss the principal tools used, we have highlighted some areas of significant variation. Other institutions may use bespoke tools to suit their trainee's needs.

Assessors

The general rule regarding assessor suitability is that it can be any clinician with experience beyond that of the trainee at completion of their training. Some institutions will have specific requirements that a certain proportion of WPBAs in a programme be completed by consultants. It is important that assessors are well-versed in giving educational feedback. Efforts are being made to train assessors and certify this process. The prescriptive nature of the portfolio system is not understood and or liked by some assessors; it is unlikely that a trainee will derive educational benefit if this is the case.

In brief, trainees should receive constructive feedback outlining their strengths as displayed by their performance, suggestions for development, and an agreed action plan for future progress.

The Joint Royal Colleges of Physicians Training Board (JRCPTB) has piloted a new type of assessment to gauge physician trainee progress; Entrustable Professional Activities (EPAs) or Competencies in Practice (CiP). A CiP is defined as 'a critical part of professional work that can be identified as a unit to be entrusted to a trainee once efficient competence has been reached'. The trainee completes a self-assessment and the educational supervisor completes the CiP using other assessment tools and clinical supervisor information. A meeting between supervisor and trainee allows discussion before a final decision is made.

General WPBA tips (for trainee and trainer—i.e. if both parties do it then it will work)

- Do lots of WPBAs, whether you are a trainee or a trainer
- Review the portfolio to identify learning objectives to link to or focus on
- Start completing them early in any attachment
- Set aside dedicated time for completion and feedback
- Provide feedback in a comfortable, quiet environment
- Keep a look out for suitable opportunities and, where possible, plan the encounter in advance
- Engage in verbal feedback and transcribe this into the form
- Complete the form as soon as possible after the event, ideally immediately after
- Contribute to the action plan

Mini-Clinical Evaluation eXercise (mini-CEX)

This tool evaluates skills essential for good clinical care, e.g. history-taking, examination, and clinical reasoning.

How to do it (best practice)

- Vary the setting and focus of the encounter, e.g. ward rounds for snapshots of management, clinic for first encounter histories
- Reserve time when the trainee, assessor and a patient are available so an entire encounter can be assessed <could be a requirement if SUMMATIVE>
- A whole encounter may not be required; five minutes of observation may provide enough to usefully comment on the trainee
- Ask the trainee to present findings in the presence of the patient—this encourages focus and succinct presentation of information
- Only give feedback about those elements directly observed in the encounter
- Give immediate feedback in a constructive fashion and complete the mini-CEX paperwork

Troubleshooting/problem-solving

- Decide the focus in advance to make the best use of the time
- Use your questioning skills to probe for deeper trainee reflections

Taking notes may help if there is a delay between observation and feedback.

Assessment of clinical expertise (ACE) and mini-ACE

These are used in psychiatry and have been modified from the mini-CEX. For an ACE the entire encounter is observed. The rating addresses a trainee's ability to perform a complete assessment. The mini-ACE focuses on part of the encounter, e.g. history-taking.

Directly observed procedural skills (DOPS)

A DOPS evaluates the performance of a trainee in undertaking a practical procedure.

Troubleshooting

- Remind trainees that WPBAs are principally formative
- A form completed early in training may include several 'development required' selections. This should simply reflect that they need training and in later years it will serve to remind the trainee of how far they have come
- Areas for development that arose from other WPBAs can be addressed with DOPS, e.g. patient interaction
- Forms should not be completed retrospectively
- Assess every time a procedure is carried out rather than the bare minimum suggested
- It is not recommended to assess the same trainee performing the same procedure twice
- A trainee can write up the procedure note while the assessor completes the form (N.B. documentation should be assessed)

Procedure-based assessment (PBA)

A PBA is a surgery-specific tool which assesses the trainee's operative and professional skills. PBAs use two principal components:

- A series of competences within six domains. Most of the competences within the six domains are common to all procedures, but a small number within certain domains are specific to a particular procedure.
- A global assessment that is divided into four levels. The highest rating is the ability to perform the procedure to the standard expected of a specialist in practice within the NHS (the level required for an award of completion of training).

The form is supported by a worksheet consisting of descriptors outlining desirable and undesirable behaviours. An assessor will observe a trainee undertaking agreed sections of the PBA in the normal course of work (usually scrubbed). Trainees carry out the procedure explaining what they intend to do throughout.

Case-based discussion (CBD)

The CBD is a tool for supervised learning events based on a trainee's management of a patient. It focuses on assessing the trainee's clinical reasoning, decision-making, and medical knowledge application in relation to patient care.

How to do it (good practice)

- Negotiate the case to be discussed (e.g. there is little point in the trainee presenting a case where they are the relative expert)
- Use a recent or current case so both parties can recall the relevant details
- More than one case can be discussed at a time
- Trainees can bring the patient's notes: this will help if you do not know the case so well and you can review the trainee's entries
- Try to encourage the trainee to expand on their thoughts and to reflect
- Don't spend too much time on minutiae
- Cases can be followed up and feedback can be amended or updated, or a later case can be used to address the action points
- Discuss wider issues that the case brings up
- Let the trainee do the majority of the talking but provide tailored teaching and advice

Case-based discussion group assessment (CBDGA)

This has been developed by the Royal College of Psychiatry to provide structured feedback on a trainee's attendance and contribution to case discussion groups (also known as Balint-type groups).

Multi-source feedback (MSF)

This is also known as: mini-peer assessment tool (mini-PAT), team assessment of behaviour (TAB), and 360-degree feedback. This type of assessment seeks the views of those who work with the clinician. A valid MSF requires at least six responses, but research indicates that this is the minimum requirement and that a minimum of 8–10 responses is better.

How to do it (good practice)

As a supervisor your first role is to ensure the trainee understands the process and how the feedback will be used. Encourage them to complete their own form as this may identify areas that they want feedback on and in turn suggest the most appropriate people to participate. The list of invitees should be agreed between trainee and supervisor and include as broad a range of clinical staff as possible. Ensure you both know the institutional rules for their portfolio/stage of training; there may be specific requirements, e.g. for nurses or doctors who are their peers. Selecting a few extra participants will assist in reaching the target but as a supervisor you may also encourage those selected to complete their forms, especially to try and overcome bias from only people who like the trainee making the effort to complete these forms.

You do not have control over the quality of the feedback in the individual forms. Take some time to go through the feedback and prepare for the discussion with the trainee. It may be useful to co-ordinate it with writing a supervisor report and it will certainly make more sense in the wider context of the trainee's portfolio. The MSF often reveals something to the trainee that they were not expecting.

The exercise can be repeated.

Multiple consultant report (MCR)

The MCR was introduced by the UK JRCPTB in 2013 to formalize the overall opinion of consultants rather than rely on this being informally fed back to educational supervisors who completed a second-hand single supervisor's report. The MCR requests feedback on clinical performance and must be completed in addition to an MSF if they are both requested. Each MCR form is completed by a single consultant. Therefore, if four MCRs are required, four consultants should complete a form each—resulting in four MCR forms. MCR forms are automatically collated and summarized in the MCR Year Summary Sheet which should inform the educational supervisor report. Educational supervisors should not be asked to complete an MCR for their own trainees as they will complete the educational supervisor report.

Patient surveys

These capture the trainee's performance from the perspective of the patient in areas such as interpersonal skills, communication skills, and professionalism. They should be undertaken as a survey to obtain a range of responses, rather than just the positive or negative ones that typically generate evidence.

Example selection of appropriate respondents

Clive is a Foundation Year 2 doctor. He has sent TAB/MSF requests to a large number of medical staff already. He has sent requests to:
- six fellow FY2s that he has worked with previously
- the two firm FY1s
- the two firm core trainees
- the three registrars in the team
- one consultant (your departmental colleague)

There are two problems with the selections made that require your advice and intervention. Firstly, as Clive's supervisor you should advise him that he needs more consultants to complete the questions and secondly there are no staff from the wider multidisciplinary team (e.g. nursing staff included). A multiple source feedback should try to get responses from as broad a range of healthcare workers as possible.

Acute care assessment tool (ACAT)

The ACAT is used to capture and assess all aspects of a patient's management—from initial assessment, decision-making, team working, time management, record keeping, and handover for the whole time period and multiple patients. It is most commonly employed during an acute medical take (or a ward round or covers a full day's management of admissions and ward work). A minimum of five cases ensures the validity of an ACAT assessment.

The ACAT is an increasingly utilized tool as it specifically deals with the 'acute take' and associated presentations and behaviours. A difficulty with this is that it is based on the presentation of cases on the post-take ward round rather than direct observation of management: that is the assessor only observes the effects rather than performance itself.

Other assessments

There is a large array of assessment tools that have been created by postgraduate training boards to reflect the different skills expected of doctors in training. Some not mentioned above are briefly discussed here. The same principles of assessment and feedback apply to all.

Audit assessment (AA)

This assesses the trainee's competence in completing an audit through oral presentation of their findings and/or a written report.

Discussion of correspondence (DOC)

A SLE (supervised learning event) based on written communication (i.e clinic letters) created by the trainee. The assessor should have the clinical notes available and make an objective assessment of the trainee using a structured approach.

Handover assessment tool (HAT)

A formative, flexible tool used to evaluate the effectiveness of handover. It is not dependent on a single handover model.

Quality improvement project assessment tool (QIPAT)

This assesses the trainee's competence in completing a quality improvement project through oral presentation of their findings and/or a written report. Assessors can be any doctor with suitable experience.

RCPCHStart (specialty trainee assessment of readiness for tenure)

This is primarily an assessment of Clinical Decision Making and of Level 1 competencies not assessed elsewhere in paediatric training.

Teaching observation (TO)

The TO is designed to provide structured, formative feedback to trainees. It can be based on any instance of formalized teaching by the trainee which has been observed by the assessor. The process should be trainee-led, identifying appropriate teaching sessions and assessors.

Portfolio assessment

At undergraduate level, tutors may have to make judgements about their students in addition to providing pastoral care, feedback, and support. Within the undergraduate environment, institutions generally have well benchmarked standards and good longitudinal performance data on students, allowing clear decisions about progression and licensing to be made by faculty that know students well.

Postgraduate training is more complex as the "Peter principle" may apply (● this is the concept that people competent in a particular area are then promoted or selected to positions where they lack competence). The realization that WPBAs are not generally effective as summative assessments led to the reconsideration of how they were implemented, with a move away from using them as a single guide to progression. This change to formative SLEs and summative AoPs has perhaps placed greater importance on the review of the trainee's progress by their supervisor and training panel at annual review. This is because, while a single WPBA is not reliable or valid as an assessment, a portfolio of several WPBAs looking at different curriculum areas and completed by different assessors is.

▶ Portfolios are not just restricted to trainees; maintaining a portfolio of supporting information is necessary for all licensed doctors in the UK to undergo revalidation.

Annual review of competence progression (ARCP)

It is important to consider WPBAs in the wider context that is the portfolio—record of training—which uses WPBA as one tool amongst many to demonstrate competence. While in training, the ARCP is the equivalent of an annual appraisal. The validity and reliability of individual WPBAs is improved by performing multiple assessments of different kinds. The ARCP is a summative assessment of the year's progress culminating in the signing-off of training in the final year—when the portfolio should demonstrate completion of all curriculum components.

▶ There are different requirements for different specialties and stages of training. However, this should not be a box-ticking exercise.

Educational supervisor (ES) report

The ES report serves as a means to interpret the evidence in the portfolio and how it relates to the trainee's engagement with the curriculum. It has become structured to reflect this.

The ES's report is (according to the *Gold* guide) supposed to be a triangulated judgement that should support (the ARCP will affirm) the trainee's progress. It should be difficult for an ARCP panel to overturn a properly considered recommendation from an ES that a trainee progresses.

Penultimate year assessment (PYA)

An external assessor (out-with the training region) appraises the trainee's portfolio making recommendations about what areas need to be addressed.

Sign-off/certificate of completion of training (CCT)

A judgement is made at the final ARCP as to whether the trainee should be recommended for the specialist register.

Name of Trainee		NTN	
Hospital	Specialty	Dates	
Programme Number		Post no. in Programme	
Name of Educational Supervisor			
Comments			
Has the trainee satisfactorily completed this attachment (YES/NO)?			
Recommendations (state where special attention should be given in future attachments)			
Signature of trainee		NTN	
Signature of educational supervisor		Date	
YEAR OF TRAINING (please circle)			
ONE/TWO/THREE/FOUR/FIVE/SIX			

Fig. 7.1 Example supervisor report based on the 2002 Royal College of Physicians format.

Figure 7.1 illustrates an example of an old version of the supervisor report before moving to the online system. It allowed for free text (handwritten) comments, although with no guidance as to what these comments should be about, followed by free text for future recommendations. Some of the additional structure that is required now is to ensure that WPBAs have been reviewed when writing a report.

Appraisal and revalidation

Revalidation

The revalidation process exists in the UK with the aim of ensuring that all licensed doctors continue to meet professional standards set by the General Medical Council (GMC). That is, they are able to provide a good level of care and remain up-to-date and fit to practice in their chosen field. Revalidation will occur every five years but requires participation in an annual appraisal that covers all of a doctor's practice. A responsible officer has to make a recommendation statement to the GMC.

Responsible officer (RO)

You can act as an RO for doctors connected to your designated body, e.g. training programme director for a specialty within a deanery. Three broad recommendations are submissible:

- the doctor is up-to-date and fit to practice
- defer the doctor's revalidation submission date
- non-engagement in revalidation

℘ See GMC website[3] for in-depth guidance.

Appraisal

The GMC has developed a framework for appraisal and revalidation consisting of four domains (with three attributes):

- Knowledge, skills, and performance
- Safety and quality
- Communication, partnership, and teamwork
- Maintaining trust

The GMC's intent is to encourage reflection on practice and approach to medicine using supporting information. This should enable doctors to identify areas for improvement and development. Areas where doctors are up-to-date should be demonstrable according to the framework criteria.

Supporting information falls under four broad headings:

- General Information
  - Personal details
  - Scope of work
  - Record of annual appraisals
  - Personal development plans and their review
  - Probity
  - Health
- Keeping up-to-date
  - Continuing professional development
- Review of your practice
  - Quality improvement activity
  - Significant events
- Feedback on your practice
  - Feedback from colleagues
  - Feedback from patients
  - Review of complaints and compliments

By providing all six types of information over the five-year revalidation cycle you should have demonstrated your practice against all 12 attributes in the Good Medical Practice framework through reflection and discussion at appraisal.

Further reading

➲ *The Gold Guide*. A reference guide for postgraduate specialty training in the UK, which sets out the arrangements agreed by the four UK Health Departments for core and/or specialty training programmes.

🕮 The General Medical Council publishes standards (in effect from 1 January 2016) for education and training http://www.gmc-uk.org/education/standards.asp and also standards expected of doctors (Good Medical Practice)

http://www.gmc-uk.org/guidance/index.asp

Foundation school

https://foundationprogramme.nhs.uk/curriculum/assessments/

🕮 Intercollegiate Surgical Curriculum Programme

https://www.iscp.ac.uk/iscp/surgical-curriculum-from-august-2021/about-the-surgical-curriculum/

🕮 Joint Committee on Intercollegiate Examinations* (for The Royal College of Surgeons of London and Edinburgh and the Royal College of Physicians and Surgeons of Glasgow)

https://www.jcie.org.uk/content/content.aspx?ID=1

🕮 Joint Royal College of Physicians Training Board assessment pages, deal with Core Medical Training, MRCP (UK) and Physician Specialty training including the SCE

https://www.jrcptb.org.uk/assessment

🕮 The Royal College of Anaesthetists

http://www.rcoa.ac.uk

🕮 The Royal College of Emergency Medicine

http://www.rcem.ac.uk

🕮 The Royal College of General Practice

http://www.rcgp.org.uk/training-exams.aspx

🕮 The Royal College of Obstetricians and Gynaecologists

https://www.rcog.org.uk/en/careers-training/

🕮 The Royal College of Paediatrics and Child Health http://www.rcpch.ac.uk/training-examinations

🕮 The Royal College of Pathologists https://www.rcpath.org/trainees.html

🕮 The Royal College of Physicians https://www.mrcpuk.org/mrcpuk-examinations

🕮 The Royal College of Psychiatrists http://www.rcpsych.ac.uk/traininpsychiatry.aspx

🕮 The Royal College of Radiologists https://www.rcr.ac.uk/clinical-radiology/specialty-training

References

1. Van Der Vleuten CPM. The assessment of professional competence: developments, research and practical implications. *Adv Health Sci Educ* 1996;1:41–67. https://doi.org/10.1007/BF00596229
2. Miller GE. The assessment of clinical skills/competence/performance. *Acad Med* 1990;65(9):S63–67.
3. General Medical Council (GMC) website. https://www.gmc-uk.org/doctors/revalidation

Chapter 8

Feedback and evaluation

*Karim Keshwani, Matthew H.V. Byrne,
and Eleana Ntatsaki*

Feedback

What is it?

Feedback is a technique that is used to share information between two individuals. In doing so, the difference between what was expected and what was achieved can be reduced, and areas for supportive development can be identified.[1] ▶ Feedback is 'a dynamic and co-constructive interaction in the context of a safe and mutually respectful relationship for the purpose of challenging a learner's (and educator's) ways of thinking, acting, or being, to support growth'.[2]

What is the theoretical background of feedback?

Feedback has a wide-ranging theoretical basis. For example: feedback is an interaction between individuals within a team to promote learning (Socioculturalism); it can act as a positive or negative stimuli to change a behaviour (Behaviourism); and it can be used to explore why a learner behaved the way they did (Humanism). For more information about these theories please ➔ see Chapter 2 .

Why do we do it?

Feedback is fundamental to an individual's medical education as it helps learners identify how they can develop their knowledge, skills, attitudes, and behaviours.

How should we do it?

By breaking down the definition of feedback, Ajjawi and Regehr help us identify some of the ways in which we can support feedback[2]:

- **'Dynamic'**—feedback is a back-and-forth discussion; it is not a passive process and requires initiative and engagement from both sides.
- **'Co-constructive'**—feedback is a process where a 'shared understanding or solution' to a problem is built by the learner and the educator together.
- **'Safe and mutually respectful'**—if individuals do not feel safe, they may not want to discuss feedback. If there is not mutual respect, feedback may be ignored.
- **'Challenging ways of thinking, acting, or being'**—feedback can be challenging, and be more helpful than banal positive comments. However, it is important to separate an observed action from the individual.
- **'Support growth'**—all the above is fruitless if it does not help support the learner's development.

Types of feedback

Feedback covers a wide range of activities, it may be informal and delivered while working, e.g. noting the angle that a lumbar puncture needle is held during a procedure, or it may be delivered more formally, e.g. an education supervisor meeting, or as a formative assessment.

Feedback can be weak or strong[3]:

- **Weak feedback**—non-specific and too general, not based on direct observations or expertise, indirect, and without support for development or a plan for a repeat review.

- **Strong feedback**—specific, based on first-hand observation and supported by expertise, direct, delivered with the goal of supporting improvement and with a plan for review.

Barriers to feedback in medical education

Feedback can be a challenging process for all individuals involved: learners feel as though they do not have enough feedback; whereas educators feel that learners do not fully recognize the volume or value of the feedback shared.[2] 🛈 Identified barriers to sharing feedback include[1,2]:

- Misalignment of perceptions around what feedback comprises.
- Limited awareness of learner's curriculum and the standard they should achieve.
- Limited training in feedback techniques.
- Avoidance of critical feedback and concerns that feedback may impact the individual's self-confidence and the learner-educator relationship.
- Uneasiness in communicating feedback, especially around patients and other team members.
- Limited time and opportunity for direct observation of learners and to support learners' growth.
- Lack of commitment from learner or educator.

How feedback can help students learn

Ripples on a pond

The 'ripples on a pond' model of feedback describes that components of learning, e.g. wanting, doing, making sense, and feedback can happen at the same time rather than as separate events.[4] Learning can be thought of as a ripple in a pond (see Figure 8.1). An initial stimulus causes a ripple, but if no further stimuli are introduced that ripple will diminish. In the same way, without extra stimuli learning can diminish. Feedback is a process that can cause this 'ripple' of learning to rebound and rather than disappearing it can cause the ripple to strengthen. Using this metaphor Race describes that feedback is a stimulus that can cause learning to continue developing, and it can even be the stimuli that causes the ripple of learning to start in the first place.[4]

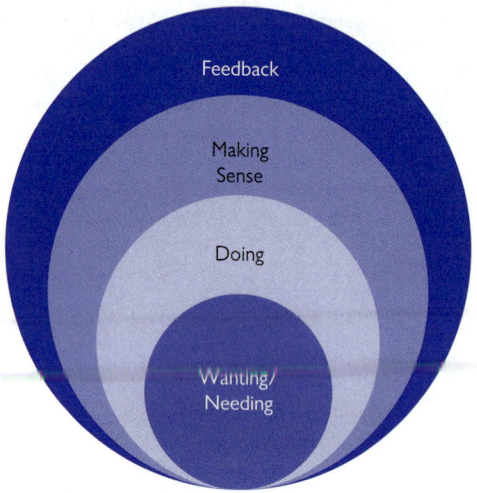

Fig. 8.1 Ripples on a pond, adapted from Race, 2004.[4]

Kolb's experiential learning cycle

Kolb's experiential learning cycle describes how experiential learning, i.e. 'learning by doing' occurs. There are four steps to this cyclical process (see Figure 8.2): a concrete experience—a personal experience that others can relate to; reflective observation—thoughts about the experience; abstract conceptualization—developing ideas to help understand the experience; active experimentation—using these ideas to inform future learning; and then the cycle continues.[5] Feedback can assist students by providing support and insight at each step of Kolb's learning cycle and can even be the concrete experience that can start the learning cycle.

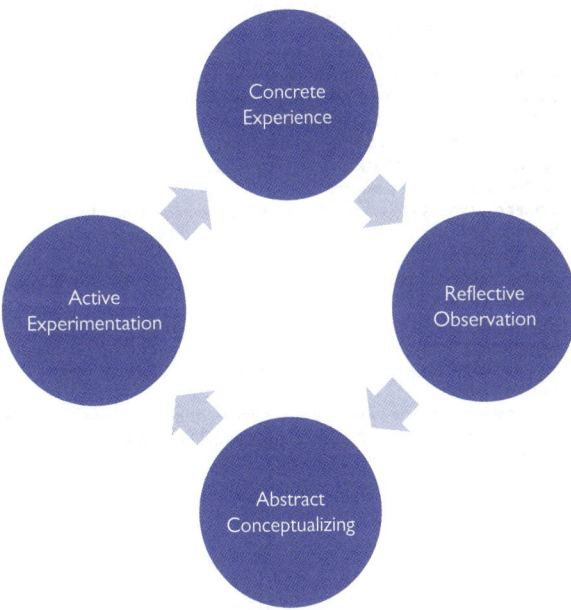

Fig. 8.2 Kolb's Experiential Learning Cycle, adapted from Kolb, 1984.[5]

Considerations before a feedback conversation

Below are some considerations that you may wish to reflect on prior to having a feedback conversation[3]:

- **Content**—what specific information is going to be delivered? Does the feedback relate to an action, a desired standard, the result of that action, providing a conceptual background to an action?
- **Aim**—what do you want to achieve by sharing feedback? Do you want to help the learner identify areas for improvement? Do you want to explore an opportunity for reflection?
- **Recipient**—is the feedback for a single individual or is it to more than one individual? E.g. discussing feedback after a cardiac arrest situation may involve multiple participants who may each have separate specific feedback needs to consider.
- **Form**—how are you going to deliver your feedback? What is the best form to deliver feedback in? Ajjawi and Regehr argue that when information is provided to a learner in a form that does not allow for a back-and-forth discussion it is not feedback.[2] Therefore, you may wish to avoid written feedback and organize a face-to-face meeting with the learner to maximize learning.
- **Source**—who is the source that provides the information for the feedback discussion? Is it a personal reflection of the learner? Is it a direct observation you had? Is it second-hand information from another person? Generally, second-hand information leads to weak feedback.
- **Provider**—who is exploring the information to the learner? Are you the best person to explore this feedback? Do you have the required expertise or training? Did you observe the behaviour? If not, is there someone more appropriate who could support the learner in this situation better?
- **Setting**—where and when are you going to have your discussion? Is it appropriate to have the discussion right away? Does the conversation need to be scheduled and somewhere private?

Considerations during a feedback conversation

There are many sources with recommendations for how to hold a feedback conversation. We discuss some of the common recommendations for feedback discussions below.[4,6]

Feedback should be:

- **A conversation**—feedback is not unilateral. It is a discussion that aims to develop a shared understanding that empowers and supports a learner to grow.
- **Credible**—for effective feedback, learners need to perceive it as credible—e.g. an informed opinion that is supported by direct observations and delivered appropriately by an individual who is trusted and has sufficient expertise.
- **Consensual**—without consent, feedback is less likely to be perceived as credible and could be perceived as an unwanted opinion that negatively affects the learner-educator relationship.
- **Tailored**—feedback should be tailored to each learner's unique feedback needs. This can be supported by establishing a shared learning agenda early in the feedback discussion or by identifying the structure of feedback the learner prefers (see: Methods of sharing feedback).
- **Specific**—the more specific the better. Rather than delivering general comments about the quality of an action, e.g. you were slow taking that history, you need to be quicker; instead, think about the specific things that led to that conclusion. E.g. your history overran because you spent too long discussing the patient's family history in your history. This was because the patient went off topic, next time you could try bringing them back on topic sooner, you could have done this when the patient said.
- **Actionable**—feedback should have practical points that the learner can implement. You can discuss with the learner what support they need, or if they are unsure, you can provide a framework that describes the steps that they need to take to improve.
- **Part of the culture**—regular quality feedback should form part of the workplace culture and allow individuals to integrate into the team. Feedback-seeking behaviours should be cultivated.
- **Timely**—feedback can be discussed during an action, immediately after, or in the future. Feedback after a considerable delay is less credible, but not all feedback needs to be explored immediately. Sometimes a period of reflection by both learner and educator may be beneficial.
- **Manageable**—while it can be tempting to try to discuss everything, too much feedback can overwhelm a learner and make prioritizing learning points difficult. Instead, you can focus on discussing either the most important feedback or the feedback that addresses the shared learning agenda.

Feedback should not be:

- **Isolated**—feedback is most effective when learners are given a chance to demonstrate change and to seek new feedback on this. This results in incremental improvements over time.
- **Careless**—understandably, negative feedback can negatively affect learner's emotions. Care needs to be taken when discussing negative feedback and appropriate support needs to be provided for the learner subsequently.
- **Personal and judgemental**—feedback should be objective and based on facts, rather than on personal attributes that are unchangeable. Feedback should be framed as 'I saw this' rather than 'you did that'.
- **Based on second-hand information**—it is often less credible, specific, and effective.
- **Based on assumptions**—learners may have reasons for their actions that you are not aware of. E.g. the reason they are struggling to meet deadlines is because they are now caring for a sick relative.

Informal feedback and feedback in busy clinical environments

Formal feedback is structured and planned. Whereas informal feedback is shared during an action. For example, if a learner was performing an ultra-sound examination and did not use the optimal settings the educator could discuss this with them at the time.

Informal feedback is particularly useful within busy clinical environments, as there may not be time for a scheduled formal feedback session. While informal feedback is brief and focused, many of the points discuss previously can still be applied to informal feedback.

Generally, learners feel that they do not receive enough feedback and educators feel as though learners do not recognize they are being given feedback. This discrepancy may be due to learners not recognizing informal feedback. Educators can highlight that they are giving feedback to learners by asking them whether they want feedback before the activity begins. This also allows the educator to ask whether there are any areas that the learner wants to focus on. During the action the educator can discuss specific and actionable points with the learner. If a more in-depth discussion is needed, this could occur at a later date when time allows.

In the ➲ 'Methods of sharing feedback' section of this chapter, we discuss the one-minute preceptor model. This is a particularly useful technique for discussing feedback during busy clinical environments where time is limited.

Sharing feedback in a busy clinical environment is challenging and it may not be possible to observe the activity of the learner. It may not be possible to engage in the feedback process at all, if this is the case it should be discussed with the learner early and an alternative plan made.

Common feedback pitfalls

We have discussed how to promote constructive conversations around feedback. Even when a learner is open to feedback, a defensive reaction is natural when they perceive negative feedback. In situations where serious negative feedback is discussed, strong defensive reactions are even more likely. To handle defensive reactions from a learner you can try the techniques in Table 8.1.[7]

These techniques are valuable as they are less confrontational and give agency back to the learner. They allow the learner to give their opinion of the issue, provide opportunities for support, and help the learner take responsibility for their actions and learning going forwards. It is also important to avoid being defensive when discussing feedback (see Table 8.2).[7]

It is easy to fall into these traps, especially when sharing negative feedback. However, they undermine the learner-educator relationship. At best they affect the quality of the feedback, and at worst they negatively affect a learner's growth.

Table 8.1 Techniques to handle defensive reactions from learners

Technique	Example
Articulate and uncover the issue	This seems to have troubled you. So that I can help you, can you tell me why?
Remain positive	Shall we summarize the things that went well so that we can identify if any of your strengths could be used to help improve this issue?
Promote ownership	I noticed that you became angry during the situation, do you accept that it affected our discussion?
Promote responsibility	What are you going to do so that you can learn from this?
Negotiate	We can address this problem but for me to help you I need you to assure me that you will work on …
Pause	We have discussed some difficult things today, shall we take a break so that you can think more about this, and we can meet again later?

Table 8.2 Behaviours to avoid being defensive when discussing feedback

Behaviour	Example
Obligation	As your supervisor, I am obliged to inform you …
Moral authority	You need to do this for your own benefit.
Avoidance	Discussing irrelevant things to avoid the main issue.
Minimizing	This happens to everyone, so you shouldn't worry about it.
Colluding	Actually, I agree with you, and I think that behaviour wasn't that bad.

Written feedback

The practicalities of clinical training programmes mean that tracking verbal feedback from a wide range of sources is seldom feasible. As a consequence, educational programmes around the world incorporate written feedback as a core component of the feedback process. This feedback often consists of anonymous responses submitted by many members of the multiple disciplinary team multiple times each year. Examples of written feedback tools include: 'multiple source feedback', 'team-assessment of behaviour', and '360-degree feedback'.

Format

Written feedback can include open and closed questions. For example, free-text responses about that a healthcare professional has done well or areas for development. Closed questions collect responses such as outstanding, satisfactory, or needs development across different domains including skills, knowledge, behaviour, communication, relationship with colleagues and patients, and overall opinions. Written feedback may be used formatively or summatively as an assessment tool. For example, satisfactory multi-source feedback is required every year for the progression of UK postgraduate doctors in training programmes.

Benefits
- Written feedback is easier and quicker to collate from a wider range of individuals.
- Information can be standardized and mapped to learning objectives. This information can be logged, tracked over time, and used as a tool to monitor progress and growth.
- The identities of those submitting information can be anonymized for the learner, so that individuals can give honest opinions. Some feedback tools allow the individual to select the individuals they want feedback from, whereas others require input from all relevant parties.

Limitations
- The risk of written feedback is that information is delivered to the learner in a unilateral fashion rather than discussed with the learner as a two-way conversation. To avoid this the information may be sent to the learner's supervisor who can subsequently meet with the learner to have this conversation.
- Written information may be brief, and it can be difficult to obtain a deeper understanding of comments.
- Those who are asked to provide feedback might not be aware of the learning needs of the person requesting the information.

We can use the considerations we have already discussed earlier in this chapter regarding feedback conversations to inform how we can write better feedback and how learners can make the most of it.

How to write better feedback

- Be specific about what was positive or what needs to be improved, the reasons why, and the actions the learner should take to develop.
- Include sufficient detail. Feedback that is too brief is rarely useful.
- Be mindful that while feedback might be anonymous to the learner it may not be anonymous to the learner's supervisor. Feedback must be professional and should not be a personal or judgemental. Written feedback may be part of the learner's permanent record.
- Concerns can be raised within written feedback. However, it is our opinion that anonymized written feedback should not be the first time a learner is made aware of any major issues. If there are serious issues these should be discussed with the trainee in advance, as often these issues are complex and benefit from more in-depth discussion.

How to make the most of written feedback as a learner

- What content do you need from the people you approach and what do you want to achieve by asking for this information? Are you using a multi-source feedback tool or are you asking them for specific information pertinent to you? If you do not ask them for the information you want, you might not get it. Similarly, if you are too restrictive in the information you ask for, you might limit your opportunity for growth.
- Who are you asking? If you value someone's opinion you are more likely to act on the feedback you receive, but you may have asked them for verbal feedback and know their opinions already.
- Negative written feedback can be surprising. There can be a delay between when the event occurred and when the written feedback you may have forgotten about it, someone might have a different perception of the situation than you, or you may have simply asked people that you thought would give you purely positive feedback. Negative feedback can be anxiety inducing if the written feedback forms are used as an assessment tool. However, if you have no areas that you can develop, the feedback is going to be less useful.
- To avoid unilateral feedback, you can ask your supervisor to discuss the feedback with you—they can provide an alternative viewpoint, help you understand the written feedback, and can help structure a reflective discussion.
- Reflect on the feedback. There is no point in asking for feedback if you subsequently do not engage with it.

Impact of hierarchy on feedback

Hierarchy is entrenched within medicine. There have been some positive changes towards flattening hierarchies, so that junior team members and those that hold less 'power' do not feel intimidated by more senior team members or those that hold more 'power'. The overall aim of flattening hierarchies is to improve patient care by reducing mistakes—as team members are more likely to raise concerns. Despite these positive initiatives, power dynamics are still prevalent throughout medicine, and feedback is no different.

Credibility of feedback is affected by trust and a sufficient level of expertise. When a learner does not recognize the credibility of feedback or the person exploring the feedback, the feedback may be ignored.[3]

It follows that being more senior might equate with delivering better feedback. Those people have more knowledge or power, and so they may be perceived as more credible. However, this is not always the case. Like our example of raising concerns during clinical care, the hierarchy within medicine can adversely affect delivery of feedback. If learners are intimidated by the power dynamic within a learner-educator relationship, they may be less likely to ask for feedback and negative feedback may affect negative emotions more strongly. Indeed, some of the most insightful feedback might come from peers—they can also be trustworthy and have appropriate expertise. For example, a recent graduate might be able to have a feedback conversation with a final year undergraduate about exam technique within that local context.

When having feedback conversations, it is important to reflect on how your own status within the hierarchy of the clinical environment might affect the learner-educator relationship. ➔ Following our considerations before and during a feedback conversation can help reduce the impact of power dynamics. For senior team members, any steps that promote the agency of the learner, i.e. the feeling of control over the situation that the learner has, will help flatten the hierarchy. For more junior team members, you may feel anxious that you do not have the required expertise to deliver quality feedback. However, expertise is not limited to clinical knowledge alone, and simply taking a learning through the steps that facilitate a feedback discussion can be immensely valuable (see methods of sharing feedback) ➔.

Student peer feedback

Peer feedback can improve learning for the person who requests feedback, but it can also help the student discussing the feedback to reflect on their own learning. It can allow an opportunity for students to think about how they would have acted within a similar situation, to identify gaps in and deepen their own knowledge. Students also appreciate the opportunity to develop their own feedback skills.[8]

Most students feel confident discussing feedback for their peers and feel it is a valuable process to be involved in. However, students do not like exploring negative feedback, especially when considering the impact this may have on their friendships. Students may worry about the accuracy of the feedback they discuss, and that they do not have sufficient knowledge to comment on their peers.[8] These are areas where the educator facilitating student peer feedback can support the feedback discussion.

Feedback from peers in training

Healthcare professionals that have completed their initial qualification and have entered postgraduate training pathways also value peer feedback. Peer feedback can be seen as more authentic and therefore credible as colleagues at a similar stage are more aware of their own needs. As such, feedback can identify areas that more senior educators have not commented upon. The perception is that feedback from peers is less effective for improving knowledge. Rather, it is valuable when discussing teamworking, communication, professionalism, attitudes towards work, and interpersonal skills.[9]

The following steps can improve the quality of peer feedback: providing feedback training; identify feedback aims; having a clear structure; and discussing feedback 1 on 1.[9]

Feedback from junior to senior team members

Hierarchy within medical education can also impact the feedback that junior team members discuss with senior team members, including between those within postgraduate training pathways at different levels. In part because there are concerns of how this will affect working relationships.[9]

Some individuals prefer providing anonymized or written feedback in these situations. Yet, they recognize the limitations of these formats and that developing feedback skills is an important professional skill. Instead, anxiety around discussing feedback can be reduced by creating a culture of feedback within the team.[9]

The role of the learner in feedback

So far, we have primarily discussed the role of the educator in the feedback conversation. As feedback is a discussion, the role of the learner is vital. An educator can follow all the recommendations and try their hardest to improve the quality of feedback, but if the learner is not engaged in the process this effort will be futile. In this section we discuss how the learner can maximize the benefit they can derive from feedback.

Barriers that learners can create during feedback include: defensive behaviours when exploring negative feedback; preconceived opinions of themselves; misattributing feedback as a wholly negative approach. These barriers can cause learners to avoid seeking feedback, to not engage, or to not fully embrace any learning points. These barriers can be compounded by barriers that the educator faces.[10] For example, if it is a busy clinical environment a learner may not want to ask the educator for feedback, or they might feel as though they must rush through the discussion and therefore not gain as much as they could from it.

Because of these challenges, it is important to prepare learners as best as possible for these feedback discussions. Below are some recommendations for how learners can make the most of the feedback discussion.[10]

How learners can make the most of the feedback discussion

Start with self-assessment

Self-assessment is a reflection on your knowledge, abilities, skills, and attributes for a given situation. When we reflect on how an activity went, we tend to look at it generally. E.g. that discussion went badly, I need to do more work next time. As such, it is something that many learners are not particularly good at. To improve your ability to self-assess, instead of thinking about the whole performance, learners can break down the performance into its components.[10] E.g. I find it hard to structure my answers to questions during difficult conversations. In the same way, we have discussed the importance of sharing specific feedback, it is important to be specific in your own self-assessments. Through having a deeper understanding of where your abilities lie, you will be able to seek more specific feedback and provide a more detailed agenda during the feedback discussion.

Use feedback as a tool to identify areas you are not aware of

After self-assessment there will be areas that you know you need to improve. However, there will also be areas that you do not know that you need to improve, but others may be able to see. Feedback is a tool that can provide us with information about these 'unknown' areas (see Figure 8.3).[10]

Build rapport with your teacher

Feedback is influenced by the relationship learners have with their educator. A stronger relationship is likely to be more trusting, which impacts on the credibility of feedback. As it is a learner-educator relationship, the learner also has a responsibility to nurture it.[10]

Take the initiative and seek feedback

It is easy to miss chances for feedback. Previously we have discussed how the busy clinical environment can be a barrier to feedback. While it may not be possible to have feedback conversations during busy shifts, you could ask to organize a feedback discussion with an educator at a later date. Once

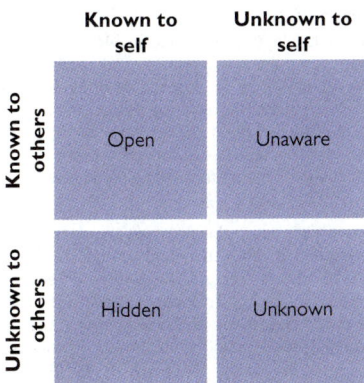

Fig. 8.3 The Johari Window adapted from Algiraigri, 2014.[10] The Johari window describes four states of information divided by whether it is known to yourself and known to others. Open is information that is known by both you and others; the blind spot is information that is unknown to you but is known by others; hidden is information that is known to you, but unknown by others; and unknown is information about you that is unknown to everyone. Unaware is the area that feedback can help develop your learning.

it is established that you want feedback, educators will be more receptive to discussing it.[10] Similarly, if you come to the educator with an agenda or items that you want to discuss this can make the discussion more specific and productive.

Stay calm

Discussing feedback can be stressful, it is natural to experience negative emotions when exploring feedback. Feedback can evoke feelings of hurt, embarrassment, shame, or fear of consequences. These feelings can be exacerbated if feedback is delivered poorly. However, if a learner has a negative reaction to these emotions, it can render feedback ineffective. It is important to remember that mistakes during clinical practice occur, that your feelings towards these mistakes are valid, and the purpose of feedback is to positively modify behaviours for future situations, rather than a personal attack. You do not need to respond straight away to negative feedback. Often the immediate response will be a negative emotion or an excuse. You can take a pause to process the information that has been discussed, which can allow this initial emotion to dissipate.[10] It is okay to take a time out during a feedback conversation if you need to. Similarly, it may be appropriate to say no to discussing feedback, e.g. the morning after a busy night shift, in this situation the feedback discussion may not be productive; however, you should schedule a time when this feedback discussion can occur.

Clarify ambiguous points

Feedback is most valuable when it is specific. Not everyone who discusses feedback has received training in feedback, and just because a person has received training in delivering feedback, this does not guarantee higher quality feedback.[3] Feedback is a dynamic discussion and understanding of the situation is co-constructed.[2] If the educator is not specific, unclear, or not meeting your learning need it is your responsibility as a learner to probe the educator for the information that will help you best.[10]

Make a plan

Feedback should result in actionable points to promote your learning. At the end of your feedback session, you should summarize the pertinent issues you have discussed and co-create a plan with your educator to develop based on these learning points.[10] Once you have a plan you should then schedule a time to for a re-review of the behaviour you discussed. This will allow for incremental feedback and development, as well as accountability.

Feedback-seeking behaviour

Feedback-seeking behaviour is 'the conscious devotion of effort towards determining the correctness and adequacy of one's behaviours for attaining valued goals'.[11] It is not simply an individual asking how they are performing. It is an individual's persistent actions to use feedback to work towards a specific objective.[11]

Why is it important?

Feedback-seeking can improve performance, learning, adaptability, and integration into the team. In particular, it can help[11]:
- Growth through seeking negative feedback
- Identification of development opportunities
- Understanding of team dynamics
- Adaptation to new situations
- Achievement of learning objectives
- Understand actions from alternative points of view
- Improve work satisfaction

Feedback-seeking behaviour has five factors:
- **Method used**—learners can ask another person for feedback or observe the actions of others to inform their own behaviours.
- **Frequency of feedback**—isolated feedback is less likely to influence change, and those who seek more regular feedback are more likely to gain benefit.
- **Timing**—learners wait until an opportune time to ask for feedback. Learners avoid seeking feedback if educators are in a bad mood or may seek feedback after they have achieved a good performance.
- **Target**—learners do not ask everyone for feedback. They tend to ask those who are more approachable and those with more experience.
- **Topic**—learners decide on the topic they wish to seek feedback on.[11]

How to promote feedback-seeking behaviour

Highlight the importance of feedback-seeking behaviours for team members during inductions. Develop a workplace environment that is not intimidating, so that learners feel they can ask for feedback frequently, and to avoid learners waiting for opportune times for feedback. Ask learners what their objectives are, so that you can signpost them to appropriate individuals and topics.[11] An example of feedback-seeking behaviour is in Box 8.1.

> **Box 8.1 An example of feedback-seeking behaviour**
> A surgical postgraduate doctor in training wants to perform an appendicectomy independently. The doctor could seek feedback on the specific parts of the operation they need to develop. They can develop their skills in these areas and seek additional feedback that progresses them towards their goal.

Methods of sharing feedback

Feedback models

There are many well-established models for sharing feedback. These models can provide structure to the way feedback is delivered.

The choice of feedback model is informed by the context of the learning situation and the learner's feedback needs. It is important to remember that while one model may work well for one student, it may not work well universally or as the same learner evolves over time. In this section we will discuss some of the common feedback models used in medical education:

- The Feedback Sandwich
- Pendleton's Rules
- The ALOBA model
- SET-GO approach
- PEARLS model
- Transtheoretical Stages of Change model
- The one-minute preceptor
- BOOST model
- R2C2 model

This is not a comprehensive list, but it provides examples of the options and techniques available. We provide a range of older outdated techniques that are still widely used (e.g. the Feedback Sandwich and Pendleton's Rules), as well as newer more robust techniques (e.g. the R2C2 model). We share their strengths and weakness so that you can make an informed decision about the model you use.

Feedback sandwich

The feedback sandwich is a common feedback technique that consists of a piece of corrective feedback that is 'sandwiched' between two positive pieces of feedback. ❶ We have included this model for context as it is still a commonly used technique; however, due to the limitations discussed below it is considered to be outdated by educators and we recommend considering other models. The feedback sandwich involves the following steps:

1. The educator provides a positive item of feedback
2. The educator then provides areas where the learner can improve
3. The educator closes with another positive item of feedback.

The rationale for the feedback sandwich is to move the learner into a positive mindset and to mitigate negative emotions that might arise from hearing corrective feedback by reiterating the positive aspects at the end. The feedback is biased towards positive feedback so that the learners overall feel the feedback has been positive. Those who advocate this method do so because they feel learners focus more strongly on negative feedback (Figure 8.4).

Strengths and weaknesses

Strengths of the feedback sandwich
- It is quick, as it only comprises three elements.
- It is simple and easy to learn. This is particularly useful for those who are starting as educators, or those who have no formal training in sharing feedback.

Weaknesses of the feedback sandwich
- It is formulaic. Once learners know the structure, they can anticipate the negative feedback and still focus on that.
- It can feel superficial or disingenuous. Learners may realize that the positive feedback is only there to pad the negative feedback.
- It is not always appropriate. Sometimes it may not be appropriate to start with positive feedback. For example, if there has been an especially challenging situation for a learner it may be better to acknowledge that rather than start with a 'this is what went well'.

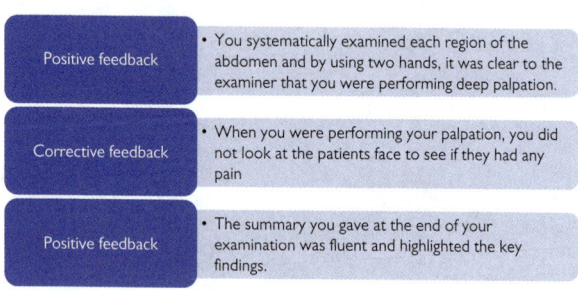

Fig. 8.4 Example of the feedback sandwich adapted from Cantillon and Sergeant, 2008.[1]

- Despite trying to balance negative feedback between two positive pieces, there can be too much negative feedback in the middle of the sandwich.
- Beyond the simple structure there is not much structure for supporting the learner's growth.
- It is unidirectional and does not empower the learner to contribute to the feedback conversation.

Tips for using the feedback sandwich

- Avoid the word 'but' before sharing the negative feedback. This can mean that the learner disregards the initial positive feedback. Instead, you can simply use the word 'and'.
- It is important to achieve balance within this model, but you need to be careful not to spend too long on the positives if there is limited time to discuss how the learner can improve.[1]

Pendleton's rules

Pendleton's rules are another common feedback model and one that is often taught on teaching courses. It is similar to the feedback sandwich as it encourages a balance of positive and constructive feedback. However, unlike the feedback sandwich, Pendleton's rules start to encourage engagement from both the learner and the educator.[12] 🕛 Although this model does encourage interaction, newer feedback models can facilitate more of a feedback discussion, and these are the models we recommend instead.

Pendleton's rules involves the following steps:

1. **The learner says what went well**—this encourages the learner to be proactive and to focus on positives, when it is easy to focus solely on negatives. Often learners will jump straight to what could be improved and need to be brought back to this point.

2. **The educator says what the learner did well**—this helps put the learner at ease and encourages a positive rather than negative initial reaction. It can be used to reiterate positive aspects already identified or to highlight aspects that the learner may not have identified. This step can be particularly useful if the educator has observed the learner performing the same activity multiple times as it can be used to praise positive changes that the learner has made based on previous feedback.

3. **The learner says what could be improved and how they might do this**—more junior learners may list large volumes of things that can be improved, and it may be more useful to ask them to choose a small number of items so that they can develop a focused plan for development.

4. **The trainer says what could be improved and how the learner might do this**—similar to the previous step, it is useful to comment on a small number of specific actions and clearly outline the steps that the learner can take to develop these, rather than commenting on every item that can be improved.

The feedback method may be used one-on-one, or it can be performed as a group—where other individuals also comment on what went well and what could be improved. When performed as a group, it can encourage discussion amongst learners and the other learners in the group can reflect upon their own knowledge, skills, and attitudes.[1] An example of the method is provided in Box 8.2.

Strengths and weaknesses

Strengths of Pendleton's rules

- It is more detailed than the feedback sandwich but is still simple and easy to learn and use
- Learners are encouraged to evaluate their own actions
- Positive points are highlighted at the start of the conversation
- Provides a basic structure for interaction between the learner and the education.

Box 8.2 An example of Pendleton's rules adapted from Brown and Cooke[12]

1. Learner positives	Educator—what did you do well in the history you took?
	Learner—I felt as though my rapport with the patient was good
2. Educator positives	Educator—I agree, you used empathy well to help develop your rapport
3. Leaner areas for improvement	Educator—what do you think could be improved?
	Learner—I asked some questions about the social history at the start and then later as well. I could improve this by using more of a structure next time.
4. Educator areas for improvement	Educator—developing more of a structure in your histories could also help you identify the patient's key symptoms more efficiently, which would help you when you formulate your differential diagnosis. Here is an example of a structure you could use ...

Weaknesses of Pendleton's rules

Formulaic learners can anticipate negative feedback once familiar with the model.

Learners will often skip the first positive steps and discuss what they need to improve. The flow of the discussion is then interrupted by bringing the learner back to the positives. It can seem stilted to clearly separate out the positives from the areas for improvement.[12]

It can be repetitive and time-inefficient, especially in larger groups. By keeping areas for improvement at the end, it can be challenging to have an in-depth discussion if time is limited.[12]

Interaction between the learner and educator can be superficial and the learner is not as involved as other models.

Tips for using Pendleton's rules

It is easy to use the wording: what was correct and what was incorrect? Or what was positive and what was negative? This should be avoided as it can seem judgemental. We suggest the wording: what went well and what could be improved?

Agenda-led, outcome-based analysis (ALOBA)

The ALOBA model is a feedback model that seeks to assist learners in developing their own learning agenda. The ALOBA model was created to mitigate the limitations of Pendleton's rules—which are formulaic and inflexible. The focus of the ALOBA model is to help the learner establish where they need support, and to then facilitate how that goal can be achieved.[13] An example of the ALOBA feedback model is given in Box 8.3.

The ALOBA feedback model:

- **Identify the learner's agenda**—ask the learner where they need help and what they find difficult. This allows the learner to set the agenda, which can reduce defensiveness by recognizing difficulties early and agreeing to work together to create a solution.
- **Explore and identify what tasks or goals need to be achieved**—both the learner and the educator contribute to this.
- **Identify skills to solve the problem**—this is led by the learner and facilitated by the educator. The educator can help the learner explore alternatives ideas and suggestions.
- **Empower the learner**—through positive feedback and highlighting strengths. The educator can discuss new ideas, concepts, and theories to support the learner to solve the problem.
- **Rehearsal of the skills**—this allows the learner to rehearse the skills they will use within a safe environment and allows the learner to discuss further feedback.
- **Summarize**—the educator presents the key learning points from the session.
- **Check the learner's agenda has been addressed**—ask the learner to summarize their learning agenda and whether you have covered it.

Strengths and weaknesses

Strengths of ALOBA

- Learner centred. Encourages self-directed learning behaviours, including generating ideas, solutions, and alternatives.
- Creates a supportive learning environment where solutions can be rehearsed.
- May be used one-to-one or in a group.

Weaknesses of ALOBA

- The model is more complex than others.
- It can be more challenging to achieve balance in the feedback compared to other models.

Tips for using ALOBA

- Similar to feedback it is important that the learning agenda is specific and descriptive with a clear aim.
- The ALOBA model can be used with a video recording of the scenario. The learner can then set the agenda after the scenario has occurred.

Box 8.3 An example of the ALOBA feedback model

Educator: what do you want to focus on improving in the clinical scenario today?

Learner: I want to improve the fluency of the summary I give.

After the clinical encounter the educator can ask the learner's opinion on how it went, ask the learner how they might improve, explore an example structure they can use, give the learner an opportunity the rehearse the new structured summary, summarize the key points, and then check with the learner that the learning agenda was addressed.

SET-GO

SET-GO is a mnemonic to help educators structure feedback. It may be used alongside a video recording of the learner, and provides the educator, learner, or group of learners with a structure to discuss their reflections while rewatching the scenario.[12]

The SET-GO mnemonic[12]:

- S—what did I See?—This is a specific objective description of what the educator observed.
- E—what Else did you see?—Deeper discussion of the events from the perspective of the learner. It can describe what happened because of the initial observed action.
- T—what do you Think?—Reflection on the events and the way in which they progressed.
- G—what is your Goal?—What was the initial aim of the scenario?
- O— Offer ideas for how to progress towards this goal—How can the observations and reflections be used to progress the learner towards this goal?

While in a scenario there may be cues that the patient gives, or actions that the learner performs, that the learner is not aware of. This can be because all the learner's attention is directed towards the verbal information they are receiving, the questions they are going to ask, or pre-emptively forming differential diagnoses or management plans. By using the SET-GO technique with a video recording it allows the learner to step back and for their concentration to be directed towards other aspects of the scenario. The technique can also allow the learner to verbalize the thinking behind their actions to the educator. An example of the SET-GO model is shown in Box 8.4.

Box 8.4 Example of the SET-GO model adapted from Brown and Cooke, 2009[12]

S—I noticed that the patient was distressed when you said they had a relapse of their Crohn's disease.

E—I paused to give the patient time and tried to be empathetic before I continued discussing the diagnosis with them.

T—I didn't appreciate that the last time the patient had a relapse they had to have an emergency surgery. I tried to chunk the information into smaller bits so that it would be easier to remember but the patient still became distressed.

G—The goal of this scenario was to explain the patient's diagnosis had worsened.

O—When discussing a diagnosis with a patient in the future you could establish what the patient's understanding of the situation is, and any potential worries they have beforehand.

Strengths and weaknesses

Strengths of SET-GO

- Highlights areas of weakness to learners (see Johari window in the role of the learner in feedback).
- Prompts learners and educators to reflect on behaviours that they have observed which improves credibility of feedback.
- Links the feedback to an agreed learning objective and encourages discussion around developing a plan to achieve this.
- Can be used in a group as well as one-on-one.

Weaknesses of SET-GO

- Video recording may not always be appropriate, takes longer to set up, and requires a discussion with and consent from the patient beforehand. Learners may be self-conscious about being recorded.
- It can be more challenging to balance positive and negative feedback, as it does not have the same distinction between positive and negative feedback that the feedback sandwich or Pendleton's rules have.

Tips for using SET-GO

- This model is useful when used with an accompanying video recording. Make sure you have tested all your recording equipment before setting up the scenario to avoid last-minute technical issues.

PEARLS of feedback wisdom

The PEARLS model was initially designed for difficult communication scenarios with patients; however, it can be used for sharing feedback to learners. It can be used to build rapport with a learner and develop a more trusting learner-educator relationship. It seeks to engage the learner throughout the feedback process and can be useful in more challenging feedback situations, such as learners who are struggling. These situations may be more emotionally charged and defensive reactions are more likely [14].

The PEARLS model[14]:

- **P**artnership for joint problem solving—The educator should work together with the learner to develop a shared understand of the issue and co-construct the solution to the problem.
- **E**mpathic understanding—During difficult situations it is important to build an understanding from the learner's perspective.
- **A**cknowledgement of barriers to the learner's success—There will be barriers that a learner encounters that may influence their actions, some of these will be modifiable and others less so.
- **R**espect for learner's values and choices—Through developing an understanding of the issue from the learner's point of view you can learn how their choices and values influenced the situation.
- **L**egitimation of feelings and intentions—It is important to validate the learner's emotions to build trust, yet it is easy to unintentionally dismiss them with phrases such as, don't worry about it, or it gets easier.
- **S**upport for efforts at correction—What is the best way that you can support the learner? Does the learner need support from anyone else?

You can use the model in a linear fashion. However, unlike some of the other models in this chapter which are more rigid, you may wish to come back to some of the points as the conversation evolves. An example is shown in Box 8.5.

**Box 8.5 An example of the PEARLS model
when discussing a learner who has received a complaint
from a patient who thought they were rude**

P—I am here to support you. I want to work with you to help understand how this happened, and to develop a solution to help you avoid this in the future.

E—It is difficult to receive a complaint, especially when it is your first. Can you tell me more about the events so I can understand things from your point of view?

A—I agree that having a busy shift makes patient communication more challenging.

R—I understand why you chose to prioritize seeing as many patients as you could over having a more detailed conversation with this patient.

L—It is natural to feel frustrated at this complaint, especially as you were not trying to be rude, you were in a rush. From the patient's point of view, they did not know that and thought you did not want to spend time speaking with them.

S—What are your thoughts on how we can avoid this happening again in the future?

Transtheoretical stages of change model

The Transtheoretical Stages of Change is a theory of behavioural change (see Figure 8.5 and Box 8.6). It is primarily used to promote positive health behaviours. However, educators can also use it as a feedback model. It can allow an educator to identify where the learner is in their willingness to change behaviours. Understanding where the learner is can help tailor the feedback to the learner's needs. The educator can then share feedback that moves the learner through the cycle of behavioural change.[14]

The stages of the model are:

- **Pre-contemplation**—the learner does not intend to change and may resist suggestions that they need to change. They may not have an awareness of the problem.
- **Contemplation**—the learner starts to think about the problem but has not committed to make any changes.

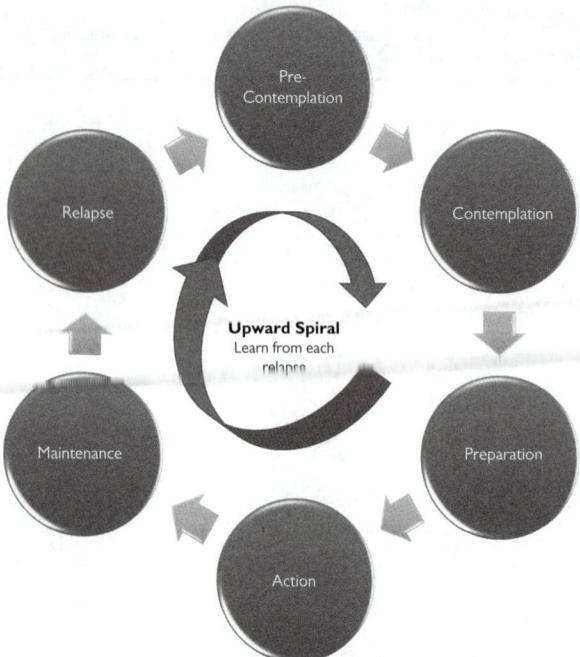

Fig. 8.5 Figure showing Transtheoretical Stages of Change Model, adapted from Milan, Parish and Reichgott, 2006. While displayed as a cycle the learners can move between nodes in a non-sequential manner. For example, a person who has relapsed may more directly to contemplation, and contemplating, preparation, and action can fail to progress to the next step and result in relapse.[14]

- **Preparation**—the learner has decided to change and has started to make plans for these changes.
- **Action**—the learner initiates the change.
- **Maintenance**—the learner consistently continues with these changes.
- **Relapse**—the learner ceases to maintain the changes and reverts to their previous behaviour.

Box 8.6 Examples of the different stages in the Transtheoretical Stages of Change model, adapted from Milan, Parish, and Reichgott, 2006[14]

Those who have not thought about change

'It's the ward clerk's fault that I can't get my work done as they keep booking meetings with relatives all afternoon.'

The PEARLS model can be used to gain an understanding of the underlying issues.

'I understand that it's been very busy, and this makes things more challenging. As speaking to relatives is part of your role how do you think you are doing?'

The educator can encourage the learner to self-assess and develop a deeper understanding of how their own actions may influence the situation and move the learner towards contemplating changing their actions.

Those who are contemplating change

'I always run late but everyone is late to meetings, so it doesn't really matter.'

The PEARLS model can be used to identify barriers to change and to weigh the strengths and weaknesses of changes in relation to those barriers. By encouraging the learner to reflect on these barriers it can help the learner identify any of their own actions that acting as a barrier. This can help move the learner towards making plans for changes.

'What do you think are the barriers that are keeping you from attending meetings on time?'

Those who are prepared to change

'I am always staying late at work after handover. I need to prioritize which urgent jobs need doing overnight that I can handover and which jobs can wait until the next day.'

For these individuals the educator should focus on exploring specific points to help learners in their actions, and to cultivate the learner's belief that they can achieve their objectives.

The one-minute preceptor

The one-minute preceptor (i.e. teacher) model is a time efficient technique for learners to present a patient that they have reviewed to the educator. The benefits of the model are it is quick, simple, and easy to learn. It can improve engagement with learners, effectiveness of clinical learning encounters, and can encourage deeper thinking than simply gathering and presenting information. The model may be used one-on-one or as a group.[15] While the one-minute preceptor was designed for clinical case presentations it can be used in a variety of other teaching scenarios as well. For example: presenting investigation findings such as from X-rays, ECGs, etc.; or communication scenarios.

The model has five steps that the learner and educator use to discuss a clinical case[15]:

1. **Get a commitment**—Ask a question that is relevant to the clinical scenario that starts the discussion. This can be a general question: e.g. what is the next step? Or it can be specific, e.g. what is your management plan in this scenario? This encourages the learner to bring together the information they have received and to form this into a solution.[15]

2. **Probe for evidence**—Ask further questions that aim to uncover why the learner gave the example they did. You can simply ask: how did you make this decision?[16] In our management plan example, you may want to ask why they wanted to order specific investigations or prescribe certain medications, and whether they considered any alternatives.[15]

3. **Teach general rules**—The educator will now understand the learner's knowledge level and gaps in their reasoning and can use this to inform how they can help the learner. This information should use the specific case as an example but be generalizable to other cases. The educator can discuss information in these areas such as key symptoms, communication skills, guidelines, scoring systems.[16]

4. **Reinforce what was done well**—Discuss feedback on positive aspects first. To encourage learner engagement, you can integrate this with other feedback models such as Pendleton's rules asking the learner 'what do you think went well?' before you discuss feedback. You can also ask the learner what their learning agenda is in advance and link your feedback back to that.[16]

5. **Correct mistakes**—This should follow general principles described previously in this chapter (see Considerations during a feedback conversation). Learners can be encouraged to verbalize this themselves, and it can also be integrated with the BOOST model (a model for feedback content described later in this chapter).

Tips for the one-minute preceptor

- The model can highlight areas where there are gaps in understanding or reasoning. These are the areas that the educator should focus on developing. This information does not need to be comprehensive and is best if it is concise.[15]
- For examples of questions, you can ask students to prompt them, please see Bloom's Taxonomy in Teaching in the clinical setting chapter.

- Inexperienced learners may be nervous about sharing a commitment as they may be worried about giving an incorrect answer. Options to assist this include: commenting that you want to hear their reasoning so that you can help them develop; and asking for a commitment before the learner presents the summary of the patient. This way the learner knows what they will be asked to focus on later. By presenting their summary they will be reminded of the salient points and can think about how this relates to the questions in advance.[16]
- Depending on the learner's level of experience you may want to ask some preliminary questions that lay the foundation before you get a commitment. If the learner gave a summary, this might be key information that the learner missed from that summary. E.g. if the patient had a fever in a sepsis scenario.[16]
- For more advanced learners, you should aim to get commitments near the limits of their knowledge to promote growth.[16]

BOOST model for feedback content

Having a structure for feedback is important as it can prepare the learner appropriately, but the content of the feedback is also crucial. The BOOST mnemonic is an easy way to remember valuable components of feedback content. An example is shown in Box 8.7.

The BOOST model:

- **Balanced**—It is important to balance both positive and negative comments within your feedback. Positive comments help to strengthen good actions, and avoid initial defensive responses from the learner, whereas corrective comments can help the learner develop. It is easy to provide too many corrective comments which can overwhelm the learner. This can mean they cannot remember all of them and become demotivated.
- **Observed**—It is best to discuss examples of behaviours you have observed first-hand in your feedback. Firstly, it is easier for you to identify areas that the learner needs to improve, and secondly it allows a deeper discussion with the learner about their actions as the reasons for the feedback are clear to both the learner and the educator. Second-hand information is less credible and therefore learners are less likely to change because of it.
- **Objective**—Feedback should be as objective as possible and based on facts. Feedback should not be personal, as the learner is more likely to be defensive and less likely to act on the feedback.
- **Specific**—Specific feedback is better than general comments as it allows the learner to focus on improving those areas more easily.
- **Timely**—Feedback should be discussed soon after the observed behaviour. This is so it is fresh in both the learner's and educator's minds, which results in a more meaningful feedback discussion.

Box 8.7 An example of using the BOOST mnemonic adapted from Milan, Parish, and Reichgott, 2006[14]

Bad example

James told me you missed three meetings a month ago. You need to make sure that doesn't happen again.

Good example

I noticed that you missed this morning's teaching session as well as the previous two. When James discussed this with you, I saw that you weren't bothered by missing the teaching. Normally you're very punctual, could we discuss this so that I understand this better?

The R2C2 model

The R2C2 model was developed to 'coach' learners, where learners are supported to develop self-directed learning in response to previous feedback or evaluations. It is a model that is more learner-focused by incorporating greater levels of learner reflection. The model can help stretch learners who are doing well as well as those who are struggling by providing them a structure for how they can improve.[17] An example is shown in Box 8.8.

The R2C2 model consists of four steps[17]:

1. **Relationship/rapport building**—The aim of relationship building is to involve the learner and to start developing a good learner-educator relationship where there is trust and mutual respect.
2. **Exploring reactions to the feedback**—What does the learner think about the feedback that was discussed? This can be particularly useful when reviewing assessments or evaluations—when there may have only been a written report. By discussing this with the learner It can validate their feelings and further build the relationship.
3. **Explore the understanding of the feedback content**—Are there any areas in the feedback that the learner should prioritize? How does the feedback relate to their current learning?
4. **Coach for change**—How can you support the learner in the creation of an actionable plan to help them achieve their goals?

Box 8.8 An example of the R2C2 model

1. **Relationship/rapport building**—how is your placement going so far? What do you want to get out of it? What has your experience of feedback been so far?
2. **Exploring reactions to the feedback**—what are your thoughts on the feedback? Was there any feedback that you did not expect or understand?[17]
   Adapted from Sargeant et al., 2018[17]
3. **Explore feedback content**—are there any parts of that feedback that you would like to develop?[17]
4. **Coach for change**—what are your objectives and how are you going to achieve these?

Evaluation

What is evaluation?

While the terms feedback and evaluation are sometimes used interchangeably, they have separate meanings. ▶ Evaluation aims to 'collect, sort and interpret information about the development, implementation and outcomes of programmes'.[18] It can apply to single teaching episodes, and can also extend to components of a programme, the programme or curricula as a whole, and even to educational policies.[18] While evaluation can have a wide range of applications, we will focus on evaluation of single teaching episodes within this chapter. It is important to note that the definition of evaluation in North America is different and is often used to mean assessment ❶.

What is the theoretical background?

One of the most common models for evaluation is Kirkpatrick's model. It is a pragmatic rather than theory-based model that describes four levels that for the effectiveness of an educational intervention[18]:

1. Reaction—did the learner find the teaching useful?
2. Learning—did the learner gain skills, or knowledge?
3. Behaviour—did it alter the learner's behaviour?)
4. Results—was there an impact on clinical outcomes?

⮕ See Chapter 10, 'Researching interventions within medical education' for more information about Kirkpatrick's Model (p. 374).

Why perform evaluation?

Evaluation has a wide range of uses including[18,19]:

- Curriculum—To see whether the educational session has achieved its goals. Understanding the practicalities of new educational methods before they are implemented generally.
- Learning—ensuring learners' needs are met and to measure the impact or effectiveness of the session for learners, to understand how a programme influenced learning.
- Policy—understanding how the service was delivered to inform the allocation of resources and to influence changes.

How should we do it?

There are a wide range of methods that can be used for evaluation[19]: surveys, interviews, focus groups, case studies, diaries, and self-reporting, observation, programme evaluation instruments, cost-analysis, and Delphi studies. The sources can be from learners, peers, supervisors, and external or expert sources.

Common limitations in evaluation in medical education:

- Personal bias—it is important to be aware of your own values and attitudes and how this might influence an evaluation.
- It is sometimes unclear who is responsible for the evaluation—is it your responsibility as an educator, or if you are in a formal educational position is it your supervisor's or funder's responsibility?
- Time limitations—performing a thorough evaluation can be an involved process.
- Limitations related to the method used for the evaluation.[19]

Evaluation methods: Surveys

Why use surveys?

Surveys can be a quick and efficient way to gather a large volume of data from a wide range of participants. They are particularly useful in evaluation as they collect information in a standardized way.[20] A simple example of when surveys could be used is an evaluation form that is handed to learners immediately after a teaching session.

Surveys can be used to collect a wide range of information including both quantitative and qualitative data. The two key aims of surveys are to ensure as many people within the teaching session respond so that we can have a representative sample; and to make sure the information we collect from the learner is as accurate as possible.[20]

One of the most important steps to designing a survey is deciding what you want to ask questions about, and whether there are any existing survey instruments that you could use. As well as asking questions to collect data on what you are interested in, it may also be important to ask questions that could explain those responses, and anything that could confound the data—for example, demographics.[20]

Designing a survey

If you choose to design your own instrument Gehlbach and Artino provide some general principles you can follow[21]:

- **Start with the most important questions**—asking demographics at the start can put learners off and may not be as important for you as the other questions.
- **Ensure questions are clear, unambiguous, and only ask about one item**—for example, if you asked learners whether they enjoyed the session and found it informative, learners who enjoyed the session but did not find it informative might be unsure which option they should select.
- **Ensure response options match the question**—for example, if you wanted to have a Likert Scale for whether learners enjoyed your teaching session rather than asking them whether they agree or disagree, you could use 'enjoy' or 'didn't enjoy'.
- **Avoid negative wording**—these can confuse the learner, e.g. double negatives, not, anti-, un-, etc.
- **Keep formatting and scoring consistent**—if the formatting or the scoring you use for Likert scales changes it can confuse learners. Learners may enter a response accidentally and this can affect the validity of your data.
- **Keep the survey an appropriate length**—surveys that are too short are not going to be informative. However, if they are too long, learners are less likely to complete them accurately, as the learner can rush through it and not pay sufficient attention to each question.

Questions can be closed or open-ended

Surveys can include both closed and open questions. There are both positives and negatives to using either one. Open questions can also be used to supplement lists of closed questions, as an 'other' box, so that participants can write a 'free-text' response if their answer is not present in the list.

Closed questions benefit the educator as the data generated is easier to interpret. They are suitable for evaluation but are not as effective at generating novel information as they limit the learner in the responses and information they can share.

Open-ended questions allow the learner the most freedom over their responses. They can provide new insights that the educator has not antici- pated. The information can be left in its raw form and still be meaningful. However, to gain the most out of open-ended data it often needs to be processed in some way before it can be interpreted—for example, by using

---

Box 8.9 The different question types that can be used in a survey, adapted from Leung, 2001[20]

Single choice
These give learners a set of options, and the learner can only choose one.
    For example: What is your favourite learning method?
    [ ] Lectures
    [ ] Small group
    [ ] One-on-One

Checklist
These give learners a series of options and they can select more than one option. For example: What training have you previously received?
    [ ] Basic life support
    [ ] Advanced life support
    [ ] Advanced trauma life support

Likert scale
These give a range of options in response to a question. For ex- ample: How much did you like the teaching session?
    1 = Strongly disliked; 2 = Disliked; 3 = Neither liked or disliked; 4 = Liked; 5 = Strongly liked.

Semantic differential
This is a numeric scale with two labels on either end of the scale. The learner then selects one of the numbers. For example, how often do you revise outside of class?
    Not often 1 2 3 4 5 6 7 8 9 10 Often

Visual analogue scale
This is a scale with two labels on either. The learner can then mark on the scale where their opinion lies. For example: how confident do you feel for the upcoming test?
    Not confident ≤≥ Confident

Ranking
Learners are asked to rank items in order of preference. For example, please rank your favourite learning method, where 1 = your favourite and 3 = your least favourite:
    [ ] Lectures
    [ ] Small group
    [ ] One-on-One

content or thematic analysis. This helps place the data into common groups that can then inform practice. While open-ended responses can provide detailed descriptions, the responses can also be brief and not particularly informative if the survey is too long, or the learner is disinterested. The box below shows the different question types that can be used in a survey.[20]

Distributing the survey

To maximize the number and quality of responses in your survey it is important to distribute it to the learners as soon as possible. This may be immediately after the session—in the case of paper feedback forms, or shortly after if you need to send a hyperlink to an electronic version. Anonymous feedback is best for honest responses. Both methods can permit anonymity, and anonymous paper feedback can be collected in a pile or box away from the educator. An example of a teaching evaluation is shown in Box 8.10.

Box 8.10 An example of a teaching evaluation questionnaire that uses a mixture of quantitative and qualitative measures

Session Topic . . . .
Session Date . . . .
Instructor Name . . . .
Session Type: [ ] one-to-one [ ] seminar [ ] lecture

Were the learning objectives clear?

Very unclear	Unclear	Neither	Clear	Very clear

Was the content at an appropriate level for your training stage?

Very inappropriate	Inappropriate	Neither	Appropriate	Very appropriate

Was there a clear summary?

Very unclear	Unclear	Neither	Clear	Very clear

Was the session engaging?

Very unengaging	Unengaging	Neither	Engaging	Very engaging

Overall, how was the quality of the session?

Very low quality	Low quality	Neither	High quality	Very high quality

What did you like?
. . . .

What could be improved?
. . . .

What stage are you in your training?
[ ] student [ ] postgraduate doctor in training [ ] consultant other . . . .

Strengths and weaknesses

Strengths of surveys

- Quick and easy to distribute to a wide number of individuals after an education session.
- Can collect data across a broad range of question types.
- Collects standardized data.
- Can analyse the data to show trends or themes.[20]

Weaknesses of surveys

- May have response bias if you do not collect a representative sample.
- If the survey is poorly designed, you may collect low-quality data.
- Learners are asked to complete many surveys and they may refuse to complete yours due to survey fatigue.
- To make the most out of the information you need to analyse it, which can add additional time.
- Qualitative data is not as robust as when collected during an interview, as you cannot ask follow-up questions.[20]

Examples of written evaluations

Always remember to tailor your evaluation method to allow you to gain the most from your written evaluation. There may be overlap with feedback, depending on whether evaluation is used to evaluate a programme as a whole or how an individual teacher has delivered a teaching session. Consider how useful the following statements might be:

'I dislike Dr A's teaching style—it's so ineffective.'

To identify areas of improvement, it is helpful to ask the student about specific aspects of the teaching style they find ineffective, such as the use of questions or teaching pace. Providing feedback in the form of a specific suggestion, such as 'It would be beneficial if you could speak more slowly presentations', is more likely to prompt changes in the teacher's behaviour.

'This seminar was interesting, and Mrs B was incredibly helpful.'

To ensure that subsequent seminars continue to be engaging, it's essential to ask learners to be specific about what made the seminar interesting. Encourage them to provide examples in their responses to gain a deeper understanding of their feedback. Statements such as 'I would give this course 3/5' do not provide sufficient information on areas for improvement. Instead, free-text responses in addition to Likert scale ratings can offer more detailed feedback that is valuable in improving the course quality. Therefore, encouraging learners to provide examples and explanations in the free-text space to provide enriched feedback.

'Mr C is really nice and friendly.'

While the statement may provide an ego boost, it is unclear what it suggests about the teaching. It could be a reflection of the warm and inviting demeanour, which encourages active engagement and fosters an encouraging learning environment. However, it is also possible that the statement is unrelated to the teaching and open to interpretation.

'At times, it felt like there was too much information to process because the session wasn't divided into manageable segments.'

If this statement is supported by feedback from other students or observations from a peer, then it can confidently make changes to your session. It is possible that the tutor was overly optimistic about the amount of time they had or the level of knowledge the learners possessed before the session began.

'It would have been helpful to have a handout for each lecture.'

By asking for specific ways to improve the session in future iterations, you can gather actionable points to consider when teaching this session again.

Evaluation methods: Sticky notes

Sticky notes can be a fun and interactive way of engaging learners and evaluating your teaching. You can use sticky notes to evaluate learners or your teaching.

Evaluate learners

You can distribute sticky notes to learners at the end of the session and use these to evaluate the learners' experience. For example, you might ask learners to 'create one action point from today's teaching session by writing this down on a sticky note'. Digital, online whiteboards designed for learner collaboration usually include the option to create sticky notes, and so are a useful alternative to physical sticky note use in online learning.

Evaluate your teaching

Sticky notes can be used to evaluate a teaching session; for instance:

- 'Write down three things that you have learnt this morning on a pink sticky note.'
- 'What has been the most useful aspect? Please write this on a blue sticky note.'
- 'What can be improved? Please write this on a yellow sticky note.'

You can then collect the sticky notes or ask the learners to place them on a flipchart in their respective groups. The latter will allow the group to review other students' comments and learn by peer learning. The responses can be analysed using qualitative methods.

Strengths and weaknesses

Strengths of sticky notes
- More engaging for learners as it is interactive
- Easier to review than a survey or focus group

Weaknesses of sticky notes
- Answers are often not anonymous
- May take longer to complete the activity compared to distributing a survey

Evaluation methods: Interviews

Interviews are a method that 'involves the gathering of data through direct verbal interaction between individuals'.[22] They are a commonly used method for generating qualitative data. Three commonly used forms of individual interviews are open, semi-structured, or structured interviews[23]:

- **Open interviews**—these start with a question and then progress depending upon the response to that question. These are the most flexible of the three interview types.
- **Semi-structured interviews**—there is a guide for questions, but the interviewer can ask follow-up questions to expand.
- **Structured interviews**—each question asked is the same and follows the same order. These are the least flexible of the three interview types.

Interviews can be performed face-to-face or via telephone, or videoconferencing software.

Why use interviews?

Interviews can be a tool to gain a deep understanding of a person's perspectives, behaviours, and attitudes. They can be used to explain phenomena and can be a tool to support other evaluation methods.[22]

Strengths and weaknesses

Strengths of interviews
- Generates a detailed descriptions of participants' experiences and perspectives
- Can explore the learner's responses and probe for additional information
- Can be more suitable than focus groups to explore sensitive issues[22,23]

Weaknesses of interviews
- Interviewing is a skill that takes time to master
- It is important to reflect on how your own biases can influence the interview and analysis of data
- Interviews take more time to complete than surveys
- Qualitative analysis methods are needed to gain the most out of the data[22,23]

Evaluation methods: Focus groups

What is a focus group?

Focus groups are a form of group interview that can be used to evaluate specific areas in more depth. Kitzinger described focus groups as 'group discussions organized to explore a specific set of issues… The group is focused in the sense that it involves some kind of collective activity… crucially, focus groups are distinguished from the broader category of group interview by the explicit use of the group interaction as research data'.[24]

Why use focus groups?

The key benefit of focus groups is the additional insights created through the interaction between participants. It is a process that favours the agenda of the participants, rather than the agenda of the facilitator.[22] This is unlike a group interview, where the facilitator controls the group dynamic. Group interviews are between the group and the facilitator, which limits additional information generation from interactions between participants.[24]

Focus groups can create[22,24]:
- A diverse set of perspectives
- Understanding of how behaviours, attitudes, and values are informed among individuals from different backgrounds
- Rich data that explores complexities in depth
- Added meaning to other evaluation techniques such as surveys
- Novel ideas that can be used to inform both the teaching session and other evaluation techniques—e.g. a future evaluation survey may be based on the feedback from the focus groups

Strengths and weaknesses

Strengths of focus groups
- Quicker compared to individual interviews
- Allows participants to react and add their own thoughts to others' comments
- Generates rich descriptive qualitative data[24]

Weaknesses of focus group
- While the groups aim to be representative, they can be influenced by more dominant members, and others may not share their thoughts
- The group dynamic can influence the data collected and the facilitator may not be able to collect responses to all the questions they want
- The volume of qualitative data generated can be overwhelming
- Focus groups can be more challenging to organize than individual interviews[24]

References

1. Cantillon P, Sargeant J. Giving feedback in clinical settings. *BMJ* 2008;337:a1961.
2. Ajjawi R, Regehr G. When I say … feedback. *Med Educ* 2019;53(7):652–654.
3. Van De Ridder JMM, Stokking KM, McGaghie WC, Ten Cate OTJ. What is feedback in clinical education? *Med Educ* 2008;42(2):189–197.
4. Race P. Using feedback to help students to learn. The Higher Education Academy; 2004 Nov. https://www.advance-he.ac.uk/knowledge-hub/using-feedback-help-students-learn
5. Kolb DA. *Experiential learning: experience as the source of learning and development.* Englewood Cliffs, NJ: Prentice Hall, 1984.

6. Lefroy J, Watling C, Teunissen PW, Brand P. Guidelines: the do's, don'ts and don't knows of feedback for clinical education. *Perspect Med Educ* 2015;4(6):284–299.
7. King J. Giving feedback. *BMJ* 1999;318(7200):S2.
8. Burgess AW, Roberts C, Black KI, Mellis C. Senior medical student perceived ability and experience in giving peer feedback in formative long case examinations. *BMC Med Educ* 2013;13(1):79.
9. de la Cruz MSD, Kopec MT, Wimsatt LA. Resident perceptions of giving and receiving peer-to-peer feedback. *J Grad Med Educ* 2015;7(2):208–213.
10. Algiraigri AH. Ten tips for receiving feedback effectively in clinical practice. *Med Educ Online* 2014;19:25141.
11. Crommelinck M, Anseel F. Understanding and encouraging feedback-seeking behaviour: a literature review. *Med Educ* 2013;47(3):232–241.
12. Brown N, Cooke L. Giving effective feedback to psychiatric trainees. *Adv Psychiatr Treat* 2009;15(2):123–128.
13. Chowdhury RR, Kalu G. Learning to give feedback in medical education. *Obstet Gynaecol* 2004;6(4):243–247.
14. Milan FB, Parish SJ, Reichgott MJ. A model for educational feedback based on clinical communication skills strategies: beyond the 'feedback sandwich'. *Teach Learn Med* 2006;18(1):42–47.
15. Gatewood E, De Gagne JC. The one-minute preceptor model: a systematic review. *J Am Assoc Nurse Pract* 2019;31(1):46.
16. Neher JO, Stevens NG. The one-minute preceptor: shaping the teaching conversation. *Fam Med* 2003;35(6):391–393.
17. Sargeant J, Lockyer JM, Mann K, Armson H, Warren A, Zetkulic M, et al. The R2C2 model in residency education: how does it foster coaching and promote feedback use? *Acad Med* 2018;93(7):1055.
18. Allen LM, Hay M, Palermo C. Evaluation in health professions education—is measuring outcomes enough? *Med Educ* 2022;56(1):127–136.
19. Goldie J. The formation of professional identity in medical students: considerations for educators. *Med Teach* 2012;34(9):e641–648.
20. Leung WC. How to design a questionnaire. *BMJ* 2001;322(Suppl S6):0106187.
21. Gehlbach H, Artino ARJ. The survey checklist (manifesto). *Acad Med* 2018;93(3):360.
22. Cohen L, Manion L, Morrison K. *Research methods in education*, 6th edn. London; New York: Routledge, 2007: 638 p.
23. de la Croix A, Barrett A, Stenfors T. How to... do research interviews in different ways. *Clin Teach* 2018;15(6):451–456.
24. Stalmeijer RE, McNaughton N, Van Mook WNKA. Using focus groups in medical education research: AMEE Guide No. 91. *Med Teach* 2014;36(11):923–939.

Chapter 9

Technology and medical education

Iain Doherty; Tim Vincent, and Julie Chen

Introduction

The aim of undergraduate medical education is to prepare medical students, referred to as trainees in this chapter, for the next stage of training. Graduates must have a foundational level of expertise in the domains of medical knowledge, medical skills, along with the attitudes or dispositions that will enable them to deliver patient-centred care.

- Knowledge may encompass the basic and clinical sciences, population health, and the ethics of practising as a doctor.
- Skills which must be mastered include problem-solving, clinical examination, and interpersonal communication.
- Dispositions include professional, humanistic, open-minded, and collaborative attitudes and behaviours to enable doctors to work with patients and as a part of a team providing healthcare support to patients.

Beyond the traditional didactic, lecture-based modalities, teaching and learning in medical school are increasingly incorporating approaches underpinned by adult learning theories and using innovative technology-enabled approaches to help students achieve the desired learning outcomes. In this respect, technologies[1] are used across all three domains of learning that we have identified: acquisition of knowledge, development of skills, and cultivation of dispositions (behaviours).

How technology is incorporated to 'enhance' (complement and add value to) learning is dependent on the intended learning outcomes, the characteristics (including the year of study) of the target cohort, the subject matter, and approaches to teaching, learning, and assessment. The educator using technologies must consider the students, the content knowledge, and the pedagogical approaches that need to be used in the different stages of medical education to achieve optimal impact. It is these factors that drive the use of technologies so that the 'tool' is fit for purpose. Importantly, this takes place within the context of the wider resource environment—what digital hardware and software are available to both educator and learner is highly dependent on personal and institutional constraints (e.g. budgets, existing infrastructure, policies, laws).

In the next sections, we will look at two frameworks that can underpin the use of technologies in teaching and learning. These frameworks are commonly used by learning designers to focus on outcomes, content, and assessment ahead of considering the use of technologies to facilitate student learning. In this way we can avoid the fact that technologies are often poorly integrated with other educational activities. The core reason for this is that pedagogical considerations need to precede technology considerations. ∴ the first sections of this chapter focus on pedagogy or on teaching and learning considerations that should drive the use of any technology for learning.

---

1 Acknowledging that 'technologies' is an extremely broad term (a pen is a technology), this chapter is focused on *digital* technologies.

Technology, pedagogy, and content

The Technological, Pedagogical and Content Knowledge (TPACK) framework can be used to effectively implement technologies in medical education because this model is overt in terms of thinking through the inclusion of technology in relation to pedagogical approaches and content knowledge (ℬ www.tpack.org). TPACK, therefore, provides us with a solution to the challenge that we identified above, namely that teaching and learning considerations should precede decisions about the use of technologies in the curriculum.

In this framework, the 'TK' references technological knowledge (appropriate use of technologies to support student learning) to complement and interact with pedagogical knowledge (PK; how people learn), and content knowledge (CK; discipline and subject knowledge). For example, if the CK consists of basic facts, then we can ask about the optimal pedagogical approach to teaching CK and the most appropriate technologies to support students in their learning. ∴ the teaching method for basic facts might be a pre-recorded video lecture and the technology used to support students in their learning might be the quiz function within an organization's learning management system (LMS) to test students' factual recall and to provide them with contextualized feedback on how they are doing.

In terms of the medical curriculum, it should be clear that students are learning different CK at different times during their degree programme. ▶ This requires different pedagogical approaches to teach ever more complex knowledge, skills, and behaviours, and, in turn, these approaches can be supported using diverse technologies to enhance student learning. Diagrammatically, this relationship can be represented as shown in Figure 9.1.

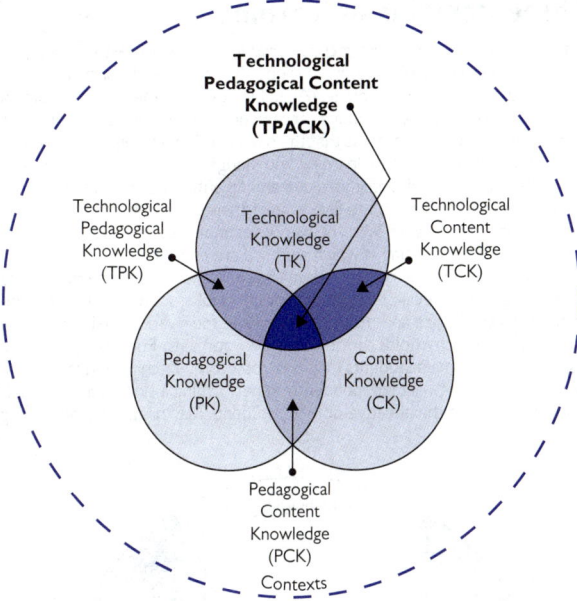

Fig. 9.1 Technological pedagogical content knowledge (TPACK).

Three domains of learning

The three domains of learning considered in this section were developed between 1956 and 1972 and they include the cognitive domain (Benjamin Bloom), the psychomotor domain (Anita Harrow) and the affective domain (David Krathwohl). These domains have undergone revisions over time but the key point for this chapter is that the different domains enable us to conceptualize medical students learning knowledge, skills, and dispositions in terms of a hierarchy of ever more demanding outcomes from the first year of their studies through to the final year of their studies. ▶ These domains are summarized in Figure 9.2. The use of technologies needs to be aligned with the 'level' of learning in which students are engaging.

Broadly speaking, the cognitive domain represents a hierarchy of learning from basic factual recall, through to analysis until students finally have the capacity to synthesize and make evaluations in their various fields of study. This same hierarchy holds in the other two domains. For example, in the psychomotor domain students may progress from watching and imitating a skill to being able to act independently in performing a skill, such as a medical procedure. In the affective domain, students may progress from having

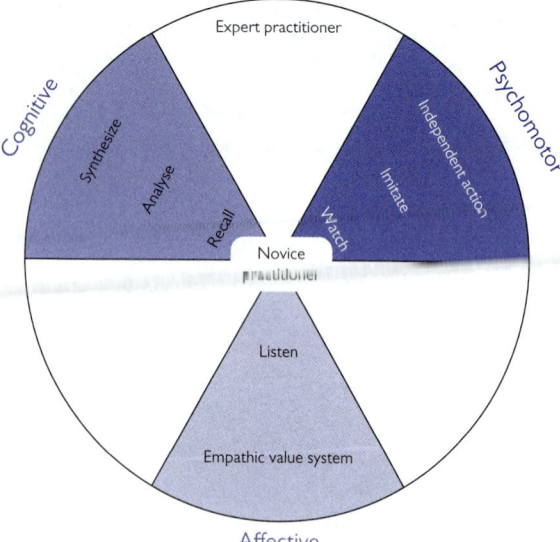

Fig. 9.2 A summary model indicating the progression of the practitioner across three domains of learning, adapted by the authors of this chapter from works by Benjamin Bloom, Anita Harrow, and David Krathwohl.

the capacity to listen to patients to having a developed and empathetic value system that guides them in their interactions with patients and peers and their clinical decision-making.

The medical curriculum needs to be designed to teach students across the cognitive domain, the psychomotor domain, and the affective domain in a way that will see students progressing from the development of basic knowledge and skills to the achievement of the advanced outcomes or competencies required by medical curricula.

∴ the three domains of learning are useful in this respect because they are presented in a hierarchy or in terms of different levels of achievement which can be mapped across the curriculum to scaffold students' learning, building on their basic knowledge, skills, and behaviours to developing more advanced knowledge, skills, and behaviours.

These taxonomies may be new to readers, but Bloom's taxonomy of the cognitive domain has been referenced extensively in the education literature. Davis et al.[1] used the taxonomy when researching student performance in closed-book exams versus open-book exams. In this context, they categorized assessment questions *to determine what domain of cognitive knowledge a question was measuring, or the type of information required to answer it (i.e. factual recall, understanding, application)*. Ahmed and Ishtiaq[2] also used Bloom's taxonomy in the context of reviewing and making recommendations for the use of different assessment types in medical education contingent on the level of 'performance' that is expected from the students.

We can now connect the domains of learning with the TPACK model. The different domains essentially represent the 'content knowledge' that students need to learn if we understand CK in terms of the cognitive, psychomotor, and affective domains. This CK becomes ever more complex as students progress through their medical degree.

▶ This means that different pedagogical approaches need to be employed at different stages in the medical curriculum. Think, for example, of the different approaches required to teach students basic knowledge as opposed to developing students' ability to engage in clinical reasoning. Finally, technologies need to be aligned to support students in the different domains of learning across the life cycle of the medical curriculum.

Technologies in medical education

Digital technologies have come to play a central role in medical education and training, and across all aspects of patient care. In this context, technology-enhanced learning (TEL) approaches can be used to support students in achieving at different levels across all three domains of learning that we have previously outlined with activities aligned to the intended learning outcomes and assessment of those outcomes.

▶ However, technologies need to be used purposefully if they are to be useful in supporting the medical education process. Our aim in the following sections is to provide examples of this purposeful use of technologies in undergraduate medical education.[2] We will be looking at digital technologies provided through educational institutions, such as LMS that offer free access at the point of need and are supported by organizational infrastructure, along with digital technologies available to educators and learners operating outside institutions—a plethora of tools and services provided by commercial organizations or through the valuable global 'open education' community (such as peer-to-peer communities or those labelled as Free Open Access Medical Education (FOAMed)).

While the rest of this chapter is structured into general domains of learning or application, we recognize that there are few hard boundaries in educational tools—digital tools can be used across several domains, at different stages of curriculum, and one tool can have a variety of functions or modes. Further, it is important to recognize that students have agency over the use of digital tools in their learning journey—students may use tools provided in a way different to that which you intended and different to their peers. On top of this, the relative speed of change in the digital world and the need to adopt new tools is well known. ∴ as skilled educators we need to be aware and prepared for this reality by guiding learners in the use of tools but allowing them the freedom to explore; by keeping a loose hold on particular technologies while holding onto the key learning objectives and pedagogic principles; by embracing the need to be continual learners ourselves (Box 9.1).

Digital accessibility and inclusive practice

Before diving into the main discussion, we wish to highlight an important overarching area of practice that is pertinent to us as individuals, as professionals, and as members of organizations: Digital accessibility. ▶ Ensuring that digital information is equally accessible to all users, irrespective of any disability (e.g. visual, or audiological), has always been important but the lack of consideration of this during the rapid rise of digital technologies has led to poor 'digital accessibility'. The sudden reliance on digital communications arising from the COVID-19 pandemic has brought the need to the fore.

The World Wide Web Consortium's Web Accessibility Initiative (W3C WAI) has derived an extensive evidence-based standard called the 'Web Consortium Accessibility Guidelines 2.1 AA' (WCAG) that aims to ensure

---

2 While postgraduate education is outside the scope of this chapter, many of the principles and activities apply but more commonly take place in the practice setting rather than in higher education institutions.

> **Box 9.1 Learning theories and technology**
> ▶▶*What learning theories are technologies based on?*
> An important question! Broadly speaking, the use of digital tools in
> teaching is to facilitate learning. These methods may seek to align with
> several learning theories, although, it can be difficult to identify and iso-
> late specifically. For more detail on learning theory, see Chapter 2:
> - **Active learning**—engage learners in tasks, provide opportunities
>   to participate—digital tools can facilitate active participation and
>   engagement activities.
> - **Constructivist**—Build on existing knowledge to understand and
>   develop new understanding—digital tools can facilitate gathering
>   existing knowledge; provide opportunities for independent learning;
>   to explore new understanding.
> - **Social/Contextual**—learning within the context of other people,
>   communities of practice, and professional contexts—digital tools can
>   facilitate interaction, engagement, and connection across social and
>   professional networks. Relevant to the context of application (e.g.
>   healthcare).
> - **Constructive alignment**—provide learning tasks that align with
>   the learning aims and assessment—digital tools can facilitate providing
>   learning tasks that meet the learning aims; active engagement rather
>   than passive.

that digital content is created with inherent functions to maximize accessibility for all users. Many countries are now voluntarily adopting the WCAG
standard into legislation which places a legal mandate on compliance. In
the UK, for example, the Public Sector Bodies (Websites and Mobile
Applications) Accessibility Regulations 2018[3] means that all publicly funded
organizations must ensure their published digital content complies.

What does this mean (in reality) for medical education?
In the UK, for example, it currently requires publicly funded organiza-
tions to:
- Educate staff on digital accessibility principles and requirements;
- Publish an accessibility statement on their website or mobile app
  (organizations);
- Provide users with an easy means of reporting where content may be
  inaccessible and request it in a more accessible format.

  For medical educators themselves it means:
- Be aware of digital accessibility principles and requirements.
- Create digital resources for all users—learners, patients, colleagues—
  that have key accessibility features (see Box 9.2 below).

3 See https://www.legislation.gov.uk/uksi/2018/852/contents/made

Box 9.2 Digital accessibility

What are digital accessibility features in practice?

These are wide-ranging, depending on the digital resource, and include both 'natural content' (text, images, sound) and encoded content. It includes:

- Sufficiently high contrast between the background and text.
- Effective use of colour (factoring in colour vision impairments such red-green).
- Size and style of the typeface.
- Alternative text ('alt text') and descriptions added to images.
- Closed captions on videos and the ability to download a transcript.
- Logical heading structure and meaningful layout of objects.
  Functions for the user to adjust factors such as contrast and size.

What is digital content?

It can include a wide range of materials including:

- Websites (external and internal, thus including a university virtual learning environment (VLE))
- Mobile apps
- Digital documents such PDFs or Microsoft Word or PowerPoint files
- Videos
- Audio recordings

There are tools available to help you assess and improve digital accessibility:

- The UK Government provide guidance and resources at this page ℘ https://www.gov.uk/guidance/guidance-and-tools-for-digital-accessibility.
- AbilityNet (℘ https://abilitynet.org.uk) and WebAIM (℘ https://webaim.org/) explicitly aim to improve web accessibility and provide helpful resources to improve accessibility of web content.
- Many Microsoft Office® applications also now include a 'Check Accessibility' function which is a helpful tool for highlighting potential improvements in accessibility.

Becoming 'digitally accessible practitioners' does require us all to adopt new practices in our digital content creation to meet legal requirements. However, most legislation allows time to achieve the standards and also for the assessment of 'disproportionate burden' effort versus benefit delivered.

▶ The sooner we can all become 'digitally accessible practitioners', the sooner we achieve the goal of a digital ecosystem that is inherently accessible and inclusive for all and not perpetuating the reverse.

Factual knowledge

Lectures

The lecture modality has a core role in medical education, but the pedagogical value of the didactic lecture has long been questioned and ● its value for teaching students is still contested today both in general and in the medical education literature, with researchers proposing alternative, more engaging approaches.

Further reading

Questioning the value of the lecture has a long history in educational research and those interested
might like to start with these references.

➲ King A. From sage on the stage to guide on the side. *Coll Teach* 1993;41(1):30–35.
➲ Easton G. How medical teachers use narratives in lectures: a qualitative study. *BMC Med Educ*
2016;16(1):3.
➲ Luscombe C, Montgomery J. Exploring medical student learning in the large group teaching
environment: examining current practice to inform curricular development. *BMC Med Educ*
2016;16(1):184.
➲ Tuma F. The use of educational technology for interactive teaching in lectures. *Ann Med Surg*
2021;62:231–235.

In this context, it can be argued that the move away from transmissive lectures (passive learner) to the use of interactivity (active learner) in medical
lectures is solidly grounded in what we know about cognition in learning
and what we know about the requirement for students to construct new
knowledge and robust mental models that will enable them to retain and
apply new information.

Mehta and Bhandari (2016) have proposed a move away from traditional
lectures to a more interactive pedagogical approach in which students were
asked to prepare conceptual questions on the lecture topic to deepen their
engagement with the topic and with their learning. Students asked one another their questions at the end of the lecture to deepen their engagement
with the content and the research reports positive outcomes in this respect. This study does not appear to have made use of technologies for
the interactive approach to engaging students in their learning. However, it
is not difficult to imagine a more hybrid or integrated approach to lecturing
in medical education that could engage students across the duration of the
lecture.

Online teaching is here to stay

Although video conferencing and 'webinars' have been in existence for
many years, the COVID-19 pandemic caused a significant and rapid shift
to teaching online through platforms such as Microsoft Teams® or Zoom®
(see Box 9.3). ► Having emerged out of the 'crisis phase', it is clear that
there has been a permanent shift in technical infrastructure, capability, and
societal attitude in how education and training is delivered. Medical education is realizing the lasting benefit of convenience and service delivery
impact—why require busy clinicians to leave the department, and students
their distributed clinical placements, to meet for a small group tutorial when
it can be done online?

❶ However, educators and learners alike are realizing that with benefits
come costs:

- Educators have an additional skillset to master—online facilitation and
  technical mastery of the software to run the session.
- Educator experience can be compromised—speaking to the 'void' of
  learners without webcams on is not a particularly enjoyable experience!
- Learner experience can be compromised—it is often less engaging and
  more didactic; 'death by *virtual* PowerPoint' is worse than 'death by
  PowerPoint!'
- Reduced sense of belonging—surveys of student experience are
  indicating that the online learning modality has had a serious impact on
  the sense of belonging for university students.

Box 9.3 Hybrid/hyflex modality

Hybrid/hyflex modality

While education institutions are generally exploring the optimal balance of live learning sessions taking place either in-person or online, there are inevitable explorations of a hybrid of the two: Where the educator and some students are in the room physically and some students are online. The benefits of this modality are clear: Students can still participate in the live sessions even if they are isolating due to contagious infection (e.g. COVID-19) or have childcare commitments or live far away or for other reasons. However, the challenges are less obvious but significant:

- Giving high-quality facilitation to both the in-class group and the online group is extremely difficult and stressful, and often requires a second facilitator to manage one or the other;
- The net student experience can be poorer for both groups, particularly the online students; for example, how do the online students engage in group work in those in class?
- The technological demands are greater than those usually available in standard classrooms if the goal is to enable all students to be able to hear and see and participate equally (audio is particularly challenging); this has significant upfront cost implications for education institutions;
- It often constrains the learning activities and tools used resulting in less engaging or creative sessions. This isn't to say it isn't possible, but it is a question of balancing benefits versus costs and, as an educator, judging what is best for the learners overall.

It is not surprising that education institutions, educators, and students are engaged in a lively debate around this topic.

Interactive tools for more engaging teaching sessions

For example, there is a variety of audience response systems (ARS) that enable students to actively engage through interactions—quizzes, polls, free-text responses—during the live lecture. This provides the students with a variety of applications such as preparation for developing and asking their conceptual questions at the end of the lecture. Students could also post their questions and the answers to those questions via the ARS and their responses could be saved for students to review later—a rich learning resource.

According to Moran[3] ARS may facilitate student in-classroom participation and encourage group problem-solving (depending on how the ARS is integrated into the experience). Anonymity in responses allows the learner to engage without fear of embarrassment or being singled out by peers or the instructor. Moran also notes that learners report '*strong positive acceptance, increased attentiveness, and enhanced engagement and enjoyment of the lecture experience*'. Moran also reports on a controlled study that suggests that immediate feedback from the lecturer after students asked their questions through an ARS might improve knowledge condensation (Box 9.4).

Box 9.4 Audience response systems: Benefits

There are many ways that audience response systems (ARS) can be used to benefit learning and teaching:

- Break up a didactic lecture with a short quiz to provide a more interactive learning activity.
- Ascertain the existing knowledge level or experience of the learners at the start of a session so you can tailor the content more specifically.
- Elicit students' opinions and encourage critical thinking by asking open-ended free-text questions.
- Use a standardized multiple-choice questions (MCQ) quiz to test knowledge prior to, and after, a lecture (or a series of lectures) to assess/demonstrate progression of understanding.
- Utilize the motivational aspect of friendly competition by setting a points-based quiz to test understanding.
- Promote collaborative learning by getting students to work in small groups to provide a collective answer—even more effective if there are points involved!
- Use a 'jeopardy' type format to stimulate attempts at defining and understanding terminology (of which there is much in health education).
- Use the 'mark on the image' functionality to assess interpretation of image-based information, e.g. circle the inverted T-wave on an ECG; highlight the parathyroid gland.
- Use a short quiz to obtain immediate student feedback at the end of your session/series.
- Ask students to provide questions *after* the lecture to be addressed between sessions or to be raised during the next lecture.

Export collected responses and provide them as a learning resource for students outside the lecture

❶ Unfortunately, and according to Moran, ARS have shown 'weak or equivocal results in long-term knowledge retention and learning outcomes' and this fact may account for ARS not being taken up on a large scale. Here it should be noted that ARS are not necessarily a part of an institution's technology infrastructure, and the system may well be provided by an external vendor. This may mean a direct financial subscription cost to the institution along with considerations of support demand on training and support, and integration with institutional IT systems and security.

It should also be noted that students' familiarity with the transmissive lectures might provide a barrier to their embracing more interactive forms of teaching and learning.[4] This fact entails that students need to be supported in understanding the benefits of more active approaches to teaching and learning. Indeed, given the large array of engagement tools at the educator's disposal and the myriad ways of using them, it is a key task of the educator to clarify to the learners what the expectations are in the use of these tools and how students are to engage with the tools to maximize the benefit to their learning.

Table 9.1 What is the 'flipped classroom'?

	Traditional approach	Flipped classroom
Primary information delivery	Lecture—*didactic, one way, more passive learner*	Self-directed learning activity (e.g. video lecture)—*student-paced, efficient, repeatable*
Application and discussion	Self-directed learning—*done without the 'expert' facilitator to provide immediate feedback/correction*	Applied learning activities in class—more active, facilitator present to provide immediate feedback/correction, more social learning with peers
Assessment	Unchanged—okay performance [we've been doing it for centuries!]	Unchanged—improved education performance? Improved learning experience? [definitive evidence is yet to be proved!]

The 'flipped classroom' model

'Flipping' the classroom has long been a teaching and learning strategy within education in general and within medical education. This educational approach entails providing students with teaching and learning resources to undertake ahead of the 'classroom' time (asynchronous) which then enables the live (synchronous) session to engage in active learning that utilizes what students have learned ahead of coming to class (see Table 9.1 for a comparison of a traditional and 'flipped' approach). ▶ Instead of using the valuable live session for passive information transfer, the aim is to create an engaging and meaningful learning experience for students in which they are more active in their learning both outside the classroom and inside. This also maximizes the value of the facilitator's live presence to coach learners through applied learning activities and immediate feedback (e.g. getting students to work through clinical case scenarios with benefit from the clinical expert facilitator to correct and explain). Multiple technologies can be used to create learning resources in the flipped classroom approach.

- Screen recording software such as Loom®, Panopto®, or Camtasia Studio® enable the creation of teaching presentations that can include, video, audio, and PowerPoint slides while tools integrated into operating systems such as Windows Voice Recorder® (Windows) or QuickTime® (Apple Inc.) enable audio recordings.
- Communication channels can include the institutional LMS discussion forums where students can pose questions ahead of the interactive teaching session or another platform such as Microsoft Teams® or Zoom® where students can discuss topics in related channels.

According to Moran et al.,[3] web-based learning—which we can understand as students learning online—enables learners to engage with educators as a substitute for, or in addition to, traditional classroom lectures and they recognize that creating these experiences means engaging with a variety of stakeholders including course directors, teaching faculty, and technology experts with these experts often being vital in supporting teaching staff who may not have all of the required technical skills to work with digital technologies.

Web-based learning was perceived as most valuable when associated with 'real-time feedback, self-assessments, a simple user interface, extended time for completion, and topic relevance'. Moran also notes that video-based lectures 'enable trainees to harness repetition, self-paced practice, and active learning'. Video lectures also have the advantage that students can access the recordings at a time and place of their choosing, thereby supporting students with diverse lifestyles and needs. ▶ Moran concludes that multimedia can be transformative in terms of moving away from the traditional lecture to engaging students in discussion and active learning.

Further reading

We can think in terms of three modalities of learning for live (synchronous) sessions: In face-to-face learning students and teachers are co-located in a physical space. In blended learning, there is a combination of face-to-face learning and online learning[4]. In online learning, all learning takes place online with no face-to-face component. Each modality requires the educator to use appropriate pedagogical approaches. Interested readers might like to refer to the following texts:

◆ Ellaway RH. Technology enhanced learning. In: Swanick T (Ed.), *Understanding medical education: evidence, theory, and practice*, 3rd edn. USA: ASME, 2018.

◆ Madden AG, Margulieux L, Kadel RS, Goel AS. *Blended learning in practice: a guide for practitioners and researchers*. Cambridge, MA: The MIT Press, 2019.

Other digital tools for learning in the knowledge domain

There is a growing range of tools available to learners that can support medical students' learning in the cognitive domain, each with varying functions, complexity, and financial demand. Flashcard services present engaging ways of learning terms, definitions, and concepts, typically through multimedia or with a competitive game element (e.g. points, achievements, levels, leader boards) to capitalize on reward and intrinsic motivation. For example, learning functional anatomy definitions through a flashcard points-based game. Collaborative whiteboard services enable the collective contribution of learners to a single digital collection of information that can be utilized across synchronous and asynchronous modalities (see Box 9.5 below).

For example, students can work in groups during a class session to start a case-based disease profile and then continue creating the same digital artefact outside the classroom through online collaboration. There are human anatomy reference resources that provide extremely high-resolution diagrams in a manipulable 3D format, allowing the learner to explore functional anatomy and systems through a variety of multimedia views, typically in a mobile app interface for touchscreen devices. Further, there are digital microscopy software packages that provide large banks of high-resolution histology and histopathology slides augmented with a range of digital functions to maximize learning. However, a barrier to these high-quality resources is the financial cost, either to an institution or to the individual learner (which then raises questions of parity and equality of access).

4 Blended learning is a broad, loosely defined term but it broadly seeks to maximize the affordance of both non-digital modalities (e.g. face-to-face) and digital tools by deliberate pedagogical design. This has been blurred by the increase of live online learning via video conference platforms.

> **Box 9.5 Synchronous and asynchronous interactions**
> *Synchronous vs. asynchronous learning interaction*
> 'Synchronous' teaching and learning activities usually denote those in which the people involved are meeting together at the same time. It might be in a classroom, or it might be on a video call. Activities can be employed that benefit from this resource-intensive opportunity of meeting at the same time and place (physically or digitally). For example, an interactive quiz using an audience response mobile app. Conversely, 'asynchronous' learning activities refer to those in which the people involved engage at different times (often in reference to the synchronous activities). For example, contribution to a chat forum or collaborative group task. This offers the flexibility of individual preference for engagement but lacks benefits such as immediate response/dialogue/feedback with tutor and peers. Some tools span this boundary—being able to be started in class session (synchronous) and continued outside the class time (asynchronous). This matters when you are designing activities since affordances and limitations vary between the two and it is important to be clear with the learners of your expectations of when and how they are to use them.

Quiz banks

Another significant digital tool operating largely in the knowledge domain is question banks—multiple-choice questions (MCQs) or Single Best Answer (SBA) questions delivered through a web or mobile app interface with an indication of performance and progress. There is a significant function of quiz banks in the knowledge domain, and these are often found in mobile apps, e.g. Geeky Medics®, PasTest®, PassMedicine®, BMJ OnExamination®. While these are mostly commercial, revision-focused services, it is important for any medical educator to be aware of them within the learning ecosystem plus to be able to critically evaluate their pedagogical principles and value to utilize their educational benefit.

Quiz banks offer the well-established learning method of self-testing knowledge by quiz questions within the context of a range of additional functions:

- offline capability (important for use while on clinical placement);
- comparison of performance to equivalent peer cohorts;
- spaced repetition (exposing the learner to repeated questions at different intervals based on performance);
- different learning modes;
- adding bookmark or notes;
- peer-to-peer sharing or leader boards.

While these are extremely popular for high-stakes, assessment-focused learning (i.e. exam revision)—and are successfully marketed commercially on such basis—clinical case-based quiz banks can be a valid support for applied learning *during clinical placements*, helping to consolidate learning that is being encountered practically (see the decision-making section below).

The fact that these knowledge-based digital resources are available to learners—either for no direct cost or through range of fees—highlights the demand for a key skill of the medical educator: To be aware of the wider context of our own teaching resources and engage in a degree of critical appraisal:

- Have we identified the pedagogical value of our digital resources in alignment with learning outcomes and assessments?
- What existing resources can we draw on—whether from within our own institution or beyond our institution—instead of reinventing them?
- How will our learners engage with our resources in the ecosystem of all the other resources they have access to?

Similarly, learners need to be equipped more than ever with skills in the critical appraisal of information.

- Do they critically evaluate the source of information presented on professional-looking websites?
- Do they have the capability of assessing whether quiz banks are written authoritatively or at the appropriate level?
- Is the volume of digital learning tools placing a cognitive demand on learners additional to the learning aims of the course?
- Are students judging the use of digital learning resources not just against the costs but also in terms of cognitive demand and time.

Gamification

Gamification is a broad term given to teaching methodologies that employ the affordances of game-like tasks in achieving learning outcomes, such as sequential goal achievement (task completion), competition (against self or others), and rewards (points or progress). They capitalize on theories of intrinsic motivation through goal achievement, active learning, social constructivism, or team-based learning. They typically involve technologies, but not necessarily *digital* technologies and they cover a very wide spectrum of formats.

For example, it could be a physical multiplayer board game with dice and cards for learning about principles in managing an infectious disease outbreak or a single-player quiz game with a competitive leaderboard against peers or a complex 'escape room' format to escape a zombie apocalypse for learning about team behaviours and communication skills. Digital tools and the societal prevalence of computer games have enabled a growing number of creative initiatives for the potential benefit of learning, with the immersive technologies (e.g. virtual reality headsets) growing particularly rapidly.

❶ However, as with any new educational emergence, it is important that medical educators are robust in evaluating the net learning benefit amid the possibility of other drivers such as novelty, and distraction. ▶ This requires further research in the field of medical education to ensure a robust basis around the use of gaming in medical education. It is also important to consider the direct and indirect costs of using gaming in medical education: A physical board game is cheaper to produce/acquire; an interactive online game has significant development costs associated with it; virtual reality requires relatively expensive software and hardware. All of these need a degree of specialist expertise and ongoing support.

Decision-making

Technologies also have a part to play in developing students' clinical reasoning skills both in the educational setting and in the clinical setting. Broadly speaking technologies in medical education for teaching decision-making can include digital learning 'objects' that include content, decision-making pathways, and assessment tasks through to training simulations which can be of various types ranging from actors 'playing patients' through to high-fidelity simulations making use of, for example, specialist mannequins or immersive digital technologies such as virtual reality (VR) or augmented reality (AR).

LMS platforms and other digital tools can also provide clinical case-based scenarios that require deeper thinking and clinical reasoning skills. For example, questions focused on managing a patient scenario are a well-established means of testing clinical investigation, diagnosis, and decision-making, if extensive feedback is provided immediately to maximize understanding of the outcome of decisions (which requires greater input in the authoring and editing stage).

Although a range of commercial revision-focused quiz banks are available to students (see 'Factual knowledge', above), there is a tendency to provide isolated questions rather than more complex case management scenarios that are more effort to author but offer a more applied learning affordance. Sadler et al.[5] recently indicated evidence of a positive association between the use of these case-based apps and learning performance.

Further, there are technologies that can provide more sophisticated ways for students to rehearse their clinical decision-making skills (outside of clinical settings). For example, students can be presented with 'branching' case-based scenarios using a commercial 'adaptive learning' platform, such as Smart Sparrow, or branching scenario software services such as Branchtrack®, H5P, and Open Labyrinth (open source). ❶ There will, however, be direct licensing costs or indirect costs in term of development time.

Students can utilize these technologies to follow a clinical reasoning path and experience the outcome of their reasoning at each stage of the process. In this respect, students' progress along certain learning pathways contingent on their responses to the problem in question: If students reason correctly, then they will progress to a successful patient outcome; if their reasoning is flawed, then they will see the consequences of that flawed reasoning (e.g. decline in patient outcome).

▶ As with any applied learning process, the primary component for education effectiveness on these decision-making tools is the debriefing step—reviewing the choices and learning from the outcomes. Digital tools that lead the student through their decisions and encourage them to reflect on actions for improvement will be more effective for learning.

Authoring branching scenarios can become a technologically and cognitively complex task—increasing the fidelity of possible options available to the learner exponentially increases the complexity of the pathway logic. It is for this reason that high-fidelity commercial services are available but at a high direct cost. As with all educational interventions, all costs (financial cognitive, and time) must be balanced against net benefits.

McGregor et al.[6] report positive outcomes for students' clinical decision-making from making use of simulated clinical scenarios later in medica education. Everson et al.[7] report similarly positive results for the use of simulations in medical education to teach students clinical decision-making and initiating emergency care. However, Everson et al. also report that there was no statistical difference between students who used simulations and those who did not, and, in this respect, they talk about simulations 'showing promise' with more studies required to determine the benefits of simulations in medical education.

Altabbaa et al.[8] report on a study in which simulated scenarios, using high-fidelity mannequins, were used to identify four different forms of bias in medical students' clinical decision-making (momentum bias, confirmation bias, playing-the-odds bias, and order-effect bias). The performance of students in the simulated sessions was recorded using video to enable students to review their 'performance' after their training. ▶ Broadly speaking, various forms of bias were identified in the students' decision-making processes and the post 'performance' review of the videos was successful in helping students 'reframe' their perspectives to remove their biases. ❶ However, there was no follow-up at a later point to determine whether the 're-framing' had remained in place.

Immersive technologies

Technologies that provide a person with a degree of 'immersion' into a digital environment have been around for many years, but we are seeing a resurgence globally as the range of products grows and the relative costs gradually reduce (from a high starting point). The degree of immersion varies and, importantly for education, so does the degree of interaction and engagement (Box 9.6).

A 360-degree video can be viewed with a headset, but the degree of interaction or control of the playback is limited or non-existent. For example, a student can experience the pre-operating theatre patient preparation process from the anaesthetist's perspective as an induction exercise before their first surgical rotation.

This can be taken a step beyond when digital annotations are added to a 360-degree video scenario as the user can interact and even make choices of which action to take and so which path to follow. For example, a simulated scenario for managing an acute patient filmed in a mock or real ward bay using fellow educators or paid actors.

At the other end of the technological extreme, an AR headset can project a view of complex digital artefacts onto the view of the viewer's real physical environment in such a way that allows them to interact with those digital objects and those objects are affected by the physical environment. For example, a group of people with AR headsets in a standard classroom could be tasked with managing a realistic-looking patient digitally projected onto a physical table with additional biometric data in view. No need for occupancy of expensive simulation suites!

As these examples show, immersive technologies have great potential for increasing the fidelity of simulated situations with all the advantages of patient safety, reproducibility, emotional engagement, and ever-greater detail. ❶ However, their educational effectiveness is yet to be fully explored and understood and, as demonstrated with other high-fidelity (and costly) simulation technologies, core pedagogical principles must continue to be applied irrespective of the complexity and fidelity, for example, the value of the debrief.

Box 9.6 Immersive technology terminology

Terminology around immersive technologies in learning

In the rapidly evolving digital world, terminology is often undefined, sub-jective, and transient. However, these are some of the key terms (at the time of writing) around immersive technology and an attempt at defining them:

- **360-degree video**—a video recording that requires a specific video recorder to capture some or all of a 360-degree point of view. Playback requires a capable web page or device. Interactions can be placed within the environment but as an adjunct which operate like clickable objects on a web page.
- **Virtual reality (VR)**—a headset enclosing the wearer's eyes that contains a screen to display a fully digital scene; this could be 360-degree video being played back with no interaction or a fully computer-generated, interactive environment (sometimes designated as 'Interactive VR').
- **Augmented reality (AR)**—the user has a view of the immediate physical environment, but digital artefacts are projected onto it. This might be indirectly (e.g. via a mobile phone camera display) with 3D digital objects projected onto that view or it might be directly (e.g. a headset with glasses) that place 3D digital objects into the field of view.
- **Mixed reality (MR)**—sometimes seen as synonymous with AR and the difference can be subtle and variable. The difference seems to lie in whether the view is indirect (e.g. via a mobile phone screen) or direct (e.g. AR headset) so that a digital object can be manipulated by, or interact with, real-world environment using complex technologies.
- **Extended reality (XR)**—an umbrella term that can encompass VR, AR, and MR.

These technologies also have great potential for negative impacts in a learning context which have also yet to be explored and understood:

- Increasing barriers to accessible and inclusive learning resources as only institutions with the required budget can employ these tools.
- Unequal distribution of access to resources particularly as between wealth distribution across different geographical locations.
- High upfront investment cost with the danger that any technology might quickly become outdated due to rapid technological advancement.
- Highly specialized skills for producing digital content which means having the right expertise and the money to pay for ongoing production.
- The requirement on educators to engage with these new technologies, which entails a steep learning curve on top of their other responsibilities.

Clinical skills development

A traditional and well-known model of clinical skills development in medical education conceives of skill acquisition in terms of:

- understanding the task at hand.

- performing the mechanics of the task, and
- performing the task accurately, efficiently, and safely.

Students can be supported in this process of skill acquisition through explanation and demonstration on the part of their educators, through deliberate practice over time at defined levels of supervision, and through engaging in the task at a highly skilled level once they have achieved competency in the task.

Video and audio

The medium of video is a well-established tool for *demonstrating* a skill or behaviour—► Far more effective than a written description or static diagram (in most situations). While they do take greater effort and collective input (devising the content, persuading your colleagues to act out a scenario, the art and science of editing, and uploading it to a suitable (secure) streaming platform), the reality is that most of us have a high-quality video recording device in our pockets (mobile phone) that can be used to produce an educationally effective video demonstration. It is no longer the preserve of costly video production companies or departments.

► While there is a relatively high upfront development overhead of video learning resources, there are several benefits of the video format that deliver a 'long tail' of benefit:

- **Repeatability**—being able to re-watch and playback at a user-defined speed.
- **Consistency**—students can be exposed reliably to the same instructional content (as opposed to have variation across different sessions/location/instructors).
- **Distribution**—videos con be distributed widely—they are not constrained by room or instructor availability!
- **Accessibility**—closed captions are helpful for learners generally and downloadable transcript can be extremely useful (although automatic speech recognition (ASR) tools are usually about 60% accurate so accuracy must be checked before release).
- **Activity analytics**—most hosting services (including institutional VLEs) will have some degree of activity logging and possibly some analytics. These can be invaluable to the educator, giving potential insight into how many students engage with the material, whether students revisit some points more than others, what this means for future learning sessions or resources.

There are some areas of caution to note:

Video editing is a time-consuming activity that requires access to capable and appropriate hardware and software that isn't usually free or quick to learn. This has time and budget implications that need to be considered.

When video content goes out of date, much more effort is required to change or re-make the video compared to simply changing slides or a document. These 'organizational' costs need to be factored in before creating them, lest students end up with outdated material or staff spend inordinate amount of time working on video collections.

> ### Box 9.7 Sound is powerful
>
> *Sound is powerful*
>
> It is easy to focus on the visual aspect of a multimedia learning resource such as a clinical skill video or a 360-degree video. However, it is the sound that can make the greater impact and thus requires just as much attention, particularly where dialogue is involved. Poor lighting, inauthentic background, and low image quality are all forgiven by the viewer but inaudible dialogue, loud ambient noise, and distracting off-camera sounds can render a decent-looking video unusable. Indeed, the soundscape of a simulated scene (e.g. bedside machine beeps, distant background chatter, low ambient noise) can greatly enhance the fidelity. The power of radio theatre and podcasts is a testimony that sound is powerful! The challenge for educators is that good sound recordings usually require an external microphone (ideally directional; ideally one per person/actor) and cables which increases the variables to manage and the cost.

- Video and audio recordings constitute a 'digital record' in the eyes of most copyright and information governance legislation (see Box 9.7). In the UK, for example, if recordings include any people that are identifiable (and many do), they must be informed how it is going to be used, give formal consent, and that person has the right to request removal at any point. The storer of the information must keep a record of consent, have a retention policy, and store the recordings in compliance with the data protection policy. This is even more important when involving patients and/or children.

Simulation

Patient safety is paramount to clinical education, and the long-standing teaching method of 'see one, do one, teach one' is no longer deemed acceptable by educators. Simulations, therefore, have a key role to play in the training of doctors in an ethically responsible way. Simulations can broadly be thought of in terms of educational experiences that replicate real-world situations that students will encounter in their practice. This is a wide-ranging definition that includes the use of mannequins through to the various sorts of VR environments that we discussed earlier in this chapter.

Simulated learning experiences can therefore range from the use of high fidelity mannequins through to VR experiences in which students are immersed in a learning environment. ▶ An advantage of simulations is that they can be used to present scenarios that medical students might not necessarily encounter on their placements. We can think here of crisis situations that may not be represented during a trainee's time in practice. For example, a holographic patient with an abnormal heart condition can be used to teach students about what a defective heart looks like from a range of different visual perspectives.

Another benefit of digital simulation tools (e.g. holographic patient, 360 degree live-stream video of surgery) is that it crosses physical boundaries extending learning opportunities to students in different rooms, regions or countries, including for those who may not have access to the required medical education expertise for teaching purposes while recognizing the technological infrastructure requirements) and the significant costs associated with these sorts of technology. Interacting with the holographic patient could be supplemented by either a live or recorded presentation from a medical expert in the field of study.

While a recorded presentation would have pedagogical value, a live interaction with an expert using a video streaming platform such as OBS Studio ©, Zoom ©, or YouTube © would provide students with the opportunity to receive immediate expert feedback on their 'performance' with the task at hand. The streaming session could also be recorded so that students could review their performance and feedback after the event.

Simulations have traditionally included a real person acting as a patient but there are more technological versions of simulation including a wide range of facilities from low-fidelity part-task trainers to sophisticated fully digital VR environments where students can interact with digital patients for practising medical procedures.[9] Simulated learning environments now include the use of holographic patients for medical education.

As an example, from medical education,[10] holograms that draw on extensive patient data to provide a rich and detailed visualization of a patient's condition can be utilized to represent a realistic patient to learners. They can interact with the hologram as they practice their clinical reasoning skills for diagnosing a patient's condition, such as detecting a heart defect at an early stage or analysing the function and blood flow of the cardiovascular system.

Recently projects such as Microsoft HoloLens and Google Glass Enterprise provide a glimpse of a future for holographic learning and a web search will provide up-to-date information on contemporary projects. Holographic patients are being used to train future doctors and nurses,[11] in this case in a project between Cambridge University Hospitals (CUH) and the University of Cambridge Faculty of Education. Students take part by donning mixed-reality headsets, which enable them to see each other while also interacting with a multi-layered, medically accurate holographic patient. University of Cambridge students are set to complete several modules using the technology, the first of which focuses on respiratory conditions and emergencies. This involves a holographic patient with asthma, followed by anaphylaxis, pulmonary embolism, and pneumonia.

While simulations of various sorts seem to offer educational benefits to medical students, there are questions about the use of simulations in medical education. ❗ First, there is a question about the 'authenticity' of these simulated environments in terms of, for example, the complexity of the real-world situation, which includes in-the-moment case variants as opposed to a controlled simulation environment.

Another way to put this is that treating a real patient is very different from working with a simulated patient where the parameters of the interaction are necessarily limited due to the nature of the simulated environment. ❗ There is only so much that can be programmed into a simulation and the programming is highly specialized and resource intensive, which means that this sort of technology will be out of reach to many medical schools for the foreseeable future unless costs reduce dramatically.

The research evidence[3] for the benefits of simulations in medical education has yielded mixed findings with respect to developing trainee confidence, performance, and knowledge. That said, trainees have identified positive aspects of simulated learning including the opportunity to receive feedback on their performance, being able to repeatedly practice a skill, the realism of the simulated environment and communicating with a team in a simulated environment. Simulations also actively engage the students in the learning process which is important for knowledge development and for skill development.

Further reading

Readers with an interest in this area might like to look at two critical reviews from McGaghie et al. that report positive educational results for the use of simulations in medical education.

➲ McGaghie WC, Issenberg SB, Petrusa ER, Scalese RJ. A critical review of simulation-based medical education research: 2003–2009. *Med Educ* 2010;44(1):50–63.

➲ McGaghie WC, Issenberg SB, Petrusa ER, Scalese RJ. Revisiting 'A critical review of simulation-based medical education research: 2003–2009'. *Med Educ* 2016;50(10):986–991.

Electronic portfolios and evidence gathering in practice

A key element of the medical profession is the maintenance of a professional portfolio, and a primary component of training programmes is a portfolio demonstrating reflective practice and evidence of achieving the required competencies of the curriculum (see Technology in Assessment below). ∴ undergraduate training programmes increasingly utilize electronic portfolio platforms as a flexible space for students to collect exercises in reflective practice, demonstration of competency in clinical procedures (e.g. the Mini-CEX and DOPS exercises), gathering 360-degree feedback on professional conduct (e.g. Team Assessment of Behaviour (TAB)), and logging attendance at clinical teaching events.

While the specifics of platform functionality vary, these platforms are key in providing students not only with the fundamental principle of portfolio building and evidence of competency in curricular requirements but also some of the digital capabilities required for postgraduate training. ∴ the use of electronic portfolios contributes to the more generic graduate learning outcome of our students being digitally literate and ready to take their place in the workforce.

Electronic 'logbook' solutions enable students to gather evidence of competency in practical skills or attendance at teaching events and include some sort of authentication function by the observing healthcare professional (the all-important 'sign-off'!). Fundamentally, the use of mobile devices and mobile apps has enabled the functional process of obtaining verification 'at the bedside', even in clinical settings where there is no internet connection.

These platforms also offer students and course teams the advantages of secure storage as there is no longer any need for paper logbooks that can be lost. Course teams have instant access for the monitoring of student progress and for providing feedback to students. Electronic portfolios also have advantages in terms of data reporting and learning analytics to 'track students' progress'.

From a student perspective, electronic portfolio systems increasingly utilize functions to place visibility of activity in the hands of the learner rather than the institution. Electronic portfolios typically have a broader purpose or function than logbooks[12] as students can record their personal and professional goals, their achievements, their development over time, and their reflections on their experiences.[2] Electronic portfolios have several advantages over physical portfolios including the fact that they can be easily shared and include multiple forms of media such as audio reflections and video.

❶ The choice of electronic portfolio services available to medical schools also demonstrates common challenges of introducing digital platforms into training interventions involving the healthcare workforce.

- They come at a cost including direct service licensing fees and indirect costs of staff resource in set-up, training, support, and maintenance.
- Students need to be trained in the use of the electronic portfolio platform and this can represent a significant learning curve for students.
- There is a generalizability question meaning how transferable are the principles of each platform to postgraduate training?
- There is service impact with respect to how much time and cognitive load will be placed on the healthcare workforce to have to learn another digital interface.
- Will the data students gather during their training remain in a usable format available after graduation if they wish to refer to their undergraduate learning?
- What interoperability standards are mandated to ensure that different platforms have the capability of useable portable data?

These questions are outside the scope of the individual educator but need to be factored into programme or institution-level decisions that impact students at the start of their professional journey and healthcare professionals supervising them during clinical practice.

Training in electronic prescribing

Another area that has seen the transition from paper to digital (at least in the UK NHS) is in prescribing of medicines. ▶ As NHS Trusts transition to Electronic Prescribing and Medicine Administration (EPMA) systems, it is appropriate to transition training activities from paper prescribing to prescribing electronically. ❶ The challenge is that these EPMA systems are highly complex, active healthcare systems, so allowing access to medical students for learning is limited.

∴ it is helpful for educators to devise simplified versions of EPMA to allow students to learn the principles of prescribing electronically as part of their clinical skills training. However, this can require considerable technical and pharmaceutical expertise to design such a digital learning platform so is not necessarily an easy option. An alternative would be to source an already existing platform but, as with so many technologies, this will likely entail budget implications for the institution.

Patient-centred care

Patient-centred care has been defined in several ways in the literature and has been associated with a range of positive patient outcomes. Key features of patient-centred care from across these different studies include having a holistic perspective on patients, developing a reciprocal and mutually respective relationship with patients, and having a focus on prevention and health promotion.

Further reading

We have synthesized definitions of patient-centred care from the literature. Readers interested in primary sources might like to look at the following references.

⊃ Bejarano G, Csiernik B, Young JJ, Stuber K, Zadro JR. Healthcare students' attitudes towards patient centred care: a systematic review with meta-analysis. *BMC Med Educ* 2022;22(1):324.

⊃ Wilcox M v, Orlando MS, Rand CS, et al. Medical students' perceptions of the patient-centredness of the learning environment. *Perspect Med Educ* 2017;6(1):44–50.

⊃ Rosewilliam S, Indramohan V, Breakwell R, Liew BXW, Skelton J. Patient-centred orientation of students from different healthcare disciplines, their understanding of the concept and factors influencing their development as patient-centred professionals: a mixed methods study. *BMC Med Educ* 2019;19(1):347.

⊃ Henschen BL, Ryan ER, Evans DB, et al. Perceptions of patient-centered care among first-year medical students. *Teach Learn Med* 2019;31(1):26–33.

Positive outcomes can include greater patient satisfaction, improved patient outcomes, and lower healthcare costs. Patient-centred care is, therefore, important in practice and medical schools can teach medical students' patient-centred care behaviours as they develop towards being practising doctors. This focus is particularly important given that evidence suggests medical students become less patient-centred as they progress through their studies.[13–15]

Positive role modelling by supervisors can help students to develop patient-centred care approaches but healthcare professionals have been identified as being negative in terms of adopting patient-centred care approaches.[14] This negativity on the part of clinicians can adversely impact students' adoption of patient-centred care approaches.[15] This means that while teaching patient-centred care in the medical curriculum is important in developing patient-centred care in medical students, there is also a need to ensure that students on clinical placements are supported in practising patient-centred approaches to care.[14]

The challenge ∴ is to deliver a curriculum in which students are supported in developing patient-centred care approaches in their early years and to support students in practising patient-centred care when they are interns. In terms of their pre-clinical years, teaching and learning approaches can include students participating in interprofessional programmes, integrating bio-psychosocial content into the curriculum along with teaching students about moral and behavioural attributes required as practising doctors. ►
Service learning also presents opportunities for developing patient-centred care approaches as does extended community-based learning, and the use of virtual patients.[14]

Technologies have a role to play in supporting students to develop patient-centred care approaches. At a broad level, technologies can support students in learning anywhere and at any time using, for example, video simulations that students can access on their mobile devices. Students can also be recorded during their training in developing patient-centred approaches to care. For example, students can be recorded during simulated consultations with patients, and they then can review and reflect upon their performance.

Simulations can supplement traditional teaching methods to develop patient-centred care approaches in students. In the case of teaching students to deliver patient-centred dementia care[16] the use of simulations which students 'experienced' the effects of dementia led to transformative learning experiences in which students were better able to understand or empathize with the experiences of people living with dementia.

The success of simulations such as this one can be attributed to students having their worldview disrupted by the simulated experience which necessitates re-framing their perspectives based on the simulated experience. Critical reflection is crucial to the process of reconfiguring the student's worldview.

In a study by Kaltman et al.[17] looking at developing patient-centred communication skills in students who were assessing a patient's history of present illness, interactive video simulations were used successfully to develop patient-centred interviewing techniques in medical students including using open-ended questions, providing empathetic responses, and reflecting on their experiences.

This approach to teaching patient-centred communication also has the advantage that it does not place a burden on faculty in terms of time and effort to monitor and provide feedback on student performance with live simulations with standardized patients. Furthermore, video simulations are relatively easy to implement and manage as compared with life-size simulated patient projections or patients in virtual worlds.

Technology in assessment

There are multiple ways to assess medical students contingent on the learning domain that is being assessed and the level of knowledge or performance that is being assessed within the different domains including testing factual knowledge, assessing clinical decision-making, safe competency in procedural skills, communication skills and behaviours, and delivering patient-centred care in a clinical setting.

In a recent publication that recognizes the impact of COVID-19 on the world along with advances in digital technologies in medical education, Park et al.[18] review the multiple technologies that can be used to teach and assess medical students in the context of medical curricula that are designed to graduate doctors suited to a contemporary medical context which requires communication and collaboration skills, the ability to think critically and creatively, and be a lifelong learner.

Expanding the range of assessment modalities

Before we look in detail the use of technologies in assessment, it is worth noting that we may well be on the cusp of an explosion in the debate around assessment in the digital sphere of education first because of the COVID-19 pandemic and secondly because of the emergence of generative artificial intelligence (AI) platforms such as ChatGPT and Google Gemini that are automated 'bot' systems that respond to student input in order to generate answers to their questions and queries by drawing on large language models. In this context, we need to consider:

- How medical faculties can deliver valid, proctored assessments at a distance.
- Managing the changing demand for physical exam halls for large-scale exams.
- How to provide robust hardware and software for large-scale online exams.
- How to address the rise of AI in generating content.

Further reading

♪ JISC Report., Re-thinking assessment. https://beta.jisc.ac.uk/reports/rethinking-assessment

♪ ChatGPT. Optimizing language models for dialogue. https://openai.com/blog/chatgpt/

♪ Google. Bard, experimental conversational AI service. https://blog.google/technology/ai/bard-google-ai-search-updates/

Digital technologies have broadened the assessment methodologies available to educators and they have also sought to bring operational efficiencies for learners, educators, and institutions. ▶ The traditional written assignment can be submitted electronically with a digital receipt proving submission (no more lost essays!), marked electronically (no more illegible hand-written comments!), consistent rubric domain-based marking, and even verbal feedback recorded by the marker for the student.

These 'electronic management of assessment' (EMA) systems typically include features to support academic rigour—checking the content similarity against other students' submissions and some internet sources. This presents academics and institutions with robust data not available without such systems. It also presents a possible line of defence against the growing spectre of AI systems developing the capability of producing academically passable pieces of work. This is a clear reminder that growing technological capabilities require ever more sophisticated counter-capabilities.

As mentioned above, computer-based multiple-choice tests that are integral to all LMSs and other platforms can test factual recall of basic knowledge and provide students with immediate feedback on their learning. There is a clear advantage of not requiring a human to mark the submission. However, learning benefit is dependent on the quality of the question writing and feedback detail which is the time-consuming part.

Testing application of knowledge can be achieved through the LMS using short answer questions[19] and, while not being marked by a human, students can receive immediate feedback in terms of the 'ideal answer' against which they can evaluate their own answer to the question.[15] Earlier in this chapter, we mentioned tools that can be used to engage students in the clinical reasoning process. These can also be applied for assessment purposes.

The prevalence of screen recording solutions and video cameras (webcams, phones) has opened the opportunity for assessment through recorded presentations. This broadens the domains of capabilities beyond a written assignment or quiz. For example, an assessed recorded presentation to test communication skills in both the visual format (presentation content such as slides) and the aural (voice recording +/– other multimedia).

Similarly, assessed tasks can include the creation of a digital artefact—a patient information website, a functional anatomy animation, a video demonstration of a procedure—that offer a broader assessment toolset and can be more engaging for the learner. These digital assessments can also incorporate the assessment of digital capabilities that are required for the medical practitioner.

Examinations

High-stakes, summative assessments such as end-of-year written exams and Objective Structured Clinical Examinations (OSCEs) present both opportunities and challenges in terms of their scale, their impact, and their resource demand. Paper-based mark sheets have been replaced by computer-based examinations which dramatically speed up real-time data gathering and interpretation for the organization, and less waiting time for the student to receive results with detailed feedback.

They also increase the rigour of analysis of question performance (and examiner performance!) and electronic question banks can increase the efficiency and rigour of exam management. ❶ However, the challenges are significant.

- Physical space has always been difficult for proctored exams but the practicalities of having hundreds of students in one large room each with laptops or tablet devices are often unavailable physically or technologically to achieve a fail-safe solution.
- Similarly, tablet-computer OSCE marking solutions demand far greater technological infrastructure and capital outlay for organizations. The greater the complexity of the system, the greater the potential for points of failure.

Portfolio assessment

Digital portfolios and logbooks have been mentioned above and these are typically included in summative assessment purposes in medical education, either through constituent parts or wholly as an assessed entity.[19] Postgraduate training places heavy emphasis on portfolio assessment and thus medical schools typically introduce students to this concept. However, a summatively assessed portfolio raises a common barrier for learners and a challenge for educators. Seeking to engage learners to use a portfolio for honest reflection of knowledge, skills, and behaviours as a summative demand is inherently disruptive to honest reflection and a barrier to engagement.

Robust assessment design—what are you really testing?

While the increase in assessment modalities and methodologies afforded by digital tools offers a broader toolset to educators, there is a risk of decreasing the specificity and validity of the assessment through the introduction of digital tasks. For example, you design the assessment to be a recorded video presentation on a topic – —is this assessing the knowledge of the topic? Is it assessing competence in producing a presentation? Is it assessing competence in recording a video and uploading successfully to a streaming service? If these digital capabilities are indeed part of the explicit learning outcomes and stated assessment criteria, then they are valid. 0 However, it can be easy to inadvertently introduce assumed digital requirements that are not part of the assessment design but will unfairly increase the demand on the learner.

Health information technologies

Han et al.[20] recognize the changing nature of healthcare provision and the need for curricula to change to graduate doctors ready to take their place in contemporary medical practice. Changes to healthcare provision include an increasingly digitized healthcare environment in which doctors and patients have access to substantive amounts of biomedical information, an exponential increase in medical knowledge requiring that doctors be able to continuously source up-to-date information and AI to support the diagnostic process.

The utilization of data generated from patients' wearable devices also represents a new dimension to patient care.[21] This means ∴ that medical students need to be prepared to work in a highly technologized environment but also that patient-centred care will be vitally important as technology cannot replicate a patient-centred approach to the provision of healthcare. As with the argument for considering pedagogy before technology, so doctors must consider the care of their patients ahead of the use of a technology.

Healthcare students, therefore, need to be prepared to work with, and make the best use of, health information technologies.[21–23] This fact has been recognized in the UK in the Topol Review,[24] a government-commissioned report published in 2019 that focused on the potential advantages for healthcare offered by genomics, digital medicine, AI, and robotics. Amid the comprehensive set of recommendations were those with an explicit focus on actions to support a digitally enabled workforce including that '*education providers must ensure that students gain an appropriate level of digital literacy at the outset of their study for their prospective career pathway*'.

This means ∴ that the case can be made for incorporating teaching about health information technologies into the curriculum so that students are prepared to work in a contemporary medical environment. However, there are practical considerations here including, for example, how to incorporate technologies into teaching medical students along with which technologies to teach given the rapidly changing nature of the technology environment. For example, teaching students about health information technologies in the traditional lecture along with providing hands-on experiences in simulated environments. Students might also be presented with elective opportunities that focus on health information technologies.[21]

▶ It has long been known by educators and by educational design experts that we cannot simply assume that our students will be competent in the use of a technology whether this be the LMS or a sophisticated simulated learning environment. This entails that there is a need to incorporate training in the use of information and communication technologies into the curriculum. Students can be taught how to use their mobile devices to search for information[25] to provide evidence-based answers to clinical problems presented by the lecturer. Students can also learn to evaluate data sources with respect to the reliability/integrity of the data that they are sourcing.

For example, making use of UpToDate® for sourcing clinical evidence, MedScape® for news and resources, and Epocrates® for point-of-care information. Students might also be expected to make use of bibliographic tools such as Endnote® or Mendeley® to reference their answers to clinical problems presented by the lecturer. These are skills that will be essential not just in their studies but also in their medical practice.

❶ Finally, one should not make assumptions about one's learner population. Rather, one should undertake an assessment with respect to students' levels of competence with the use of technologies to be utilized in the learning process. For example, the fact that the cohort consists of eighteen-year-old students does not necessarily entail that they are going to be digitally enabled or digitally inclined. This is something that needs to be examined to identify students' levels of confidence and competency with technologies that are going to be utilized in learning. If students do not have the requisite skills, then they need to be provided with supports to develop their competency.

Data, learning analytics, and information governance

With the growth in formal learning platforms and the use of digital learning resources, there has been an exponential growth in the amount of data produced and stored in these systems. This has given rise to the focus on learning analytics—interrogating these multiple data streams to draw meaning that can benefit the learner's educational outcomes and thus benefit the faculty and organizations. For example:

- Log-in activity in the LMS.
- Participation in online activities.
- Engagement with digital library resources.
- Attendance in lectures and on clinical placements.
- Clinical placement activity logbooks (sign-off).
- Assessment performance.

All these, and more, can be aligned and analysed to gain a general picture of individual student engagement which can contribute to earlier indications of students falling behind and thus earlier remedial action. This can be provided to the student for them to take primary responsibility and or by faculty to action. Clearly, the storage and use of data in such a way also give rise to necessary moral and ethical considerations: Are students aware of this data collection activity and how it will be used? Who has access to it? What happens when they leave the institution?

Personal and sensitive data must be managed in an ethical and legally compliant manner. Although institutions carry some responsibility, any access to, and storage of, these data by educators also carries responsibility so we need to be aware of these and handle identifiable learner data accordingly. Information Governance is typically part of the core medical training curriculum and ongoing healthcare continuous professional development (CPD) requirements. You should be able to find guidance and the person responsible for information governance at your employing institution. See, for example, this helpful collection from NHS England: ✎ https://digital.nhs.uk/data-and-information/looking-after-information/data-security-and-information-governance

Conclusions

We opened this chapter by arguing, broadly, that teaching and learning considerations need to 'drive' the use of technologies in medical education. In this respect, we reviewed the TPACK model along with the three domains of learning. We have taken a comprehensive look at the use of technologies in medical education across students learning factual knowledge, developing their clinical reasoning skills, and cultivating a patient-centred care disposition. We have also considered how technologies can be used to enhance the assessment process. Finally, we discussed health information technologies in the patient care landscape.

This chapter should provide interested readers with a comprehensive grounding in the use of technologies in medical education, a foundation from which they can research further in terms of our suggestions for further reading. In this respect, the foundations for teaching and learning approaches tend to be something of a constant. However, the rate of technological change is rapid remaining current with the technological landscape requires time and effort. Assistance in this respect is very often available from learning designers within faculties who, by the very definition of their role, do dedicate their time to keeping across new and emerging technologies.

Finally, the question of research evidence for the effectiveness of technologies in medical education is important in two respects. There is a substantive research base in medical education that teachers can draw upon to inform the choices that they make about the use of a technology in their teaching. This can include learning about how to implement the technology in a way that is most likely to lead to positive learning results. Secondly, there is the question of teachers researching their own practices. This 'research' can range from reflective practice on the efficacy of a technological intervention through to a full-scale research project with the aim of publication.

Further reading

Our aim in this chapter has been to provide a pedagogically grounded and comprehensive overview of the use of technologies in medical education. The literature in this respect is vast and, for those interested in reading further we would recommend the following texts. The first is highly regarded book that has recently been updated. The others may appear to be a little dated in this digital era, but they are still considered to be foundational texts in medical education.

➲ Dent JA, Harden RM, Hunt D (Eds.). *A practical guide for medical teachers*, 6th edn. Amsterdam: Elsevier, 2021.

➲ Ellaway R, Masters K. AMEE Guide 32: e-learning in medical education part 1: learning, teaching, and assessment. *Med Teach* 2008;30(5):455–473.

➲ Masters K, Ellaway R. AMEE Guide 32: e-learning in medical education part 2: technology, management, and design. *Med Teach* 2008;30(5):474–489.

➲ Mehta B, Bhandari B. Engaging medical undergraduates in question making: a novel way to reinforcing learning in physiology. *Adv Physiol Educ* 2016.;40(3):398–401.

References

1. Davies DJ, McLean PF, Kemp PR, et al. Assessment of factual recall and higher-order cognitive domains in an open-book medical school examination. *Adv Health Sci Educ* 2022;27(1):147–165.

2. Ahmed I, Ishtiaq S. Assessment methods in medical education: a review. *ISRA Med J* 2014;6:95–102.

3. Moran J, Briscoe G, Peglow S. Current technology in advancing medical education: perspectives for learning and providing care. *Acad Psychiatry* 2018;42(6):796–799. doi:10.1007/s40596-018-0946-y

4. Luscombe C, Montgomery J. Exploring medical student learning in the large group teaching environment: examining current practice to inform curricular development. *BMC Med Educ* 2016;16(1):184.

5. Sadler J, Wright J, Vincent T, Kurka T, Howlett D. What is the impact of apps in medical education? A study of CAPSULE, a case-based learning app. *BMJ Simul Technol Enhanc Learn* 2020;7(5):293–296.

6. Mcgregor C, Paton C, Thomson C, Chandratilake M, Scott H. Preparing medical students for clinical decision making: a pilot study exploring how students make decisions and the perceived impact of a clinical decision making teaching intervention. *Med Teach* 2012;34:e508–517.

7. Everson J, Gao A, Roder C, Kinnear J. Impact of simulation training on undergraduate clinical decision-making in emergencies: a non-blinded, single-centre, randomised pilot study. *Cureus* 2020;12(4):e7650.

8. Altabbaa G, Raven AD, Laberge J. A simulation-based approach to training in heuristic clinical decision-making. *Diagnosis* 2019;6(2):91–99.

9. McGaghie WC, Issenberg SB, Petrusa ER, Scalese RJ. Revisiting 'A critical review of simulation-based medical education research: 2003–2009. *Med Educ VO-50* 2016;(10):986.

10. Haleem H, Javaid M, Khan IH. Holography applications toward medical field: an overview. *Indian J Radiol Imaging* 2020;30(3):354–361.

11. Cambridge University Hospitals. Hologram patients to help train future doctors and nurses. Cambridge University Hospitals, NHS Foundation Trust. 2022. https://www.cuh.nhs.uk/news/hologram-patients-to-help-train-future-doctors-and-nurses/

12. Tan R, Qi Ting JJ, Zhihao Hong D, et al. Medical student portfolios: a systematic scoping review. *J Med Educ Curric Dev* 2022;9:238212052210760.

13. Henschen BL, Ryan ER, Evans DB, et al. Perceptions of patient-centered care among first-year medical students. *Teach Learn Med* 2019;31(1):26–33.

14. Rosewilliam S, Indramohan V, Breakwell R, Liew BXW, Skelton J. Patient-centred orientation of students from different healthcare disciplines, their understanding of the concept and factors influencing their development as patient-centred professionals: a mixed methods study. *BMC Med Educ* 2019;19(1):347.

15. Wilcox M v, Orlando MS, Rand CS, et al. Medical students' perceptions of the patient-centredness of the learning environment. *Perspect Med Educ* 2017;6(1):44–50.

16. Meyer K, James D, Amezaga B, White C. Simulation learning to train healthcare students in person-centered dementia care. *Gerontol Geriatr Educ* 2022;43(2):209–224.

17. Kaltman S, Talisman N, Pennestri S, Syverson E, Arthur P, Vovides Y. Using technology to enhance teaching of patient-centered interviewing for early medical students. *Simul Healthcare* 2018;13(3):188–194.

18. Park JC, Kwon HJE, Chung CW. Innovative digital tools for new trends in teaching and assessment methods in medical and dental education. *J Educ Eval Health Prof* 2021;18:13.

19. Tabish SA. Assessment methods in medical education. *Int J Health Sci (Qassim)* 2008;2(2):3–7.

20. Han ER, Yeo S, Kim MJ, Lee YH, Park KH, Roh H. Medical education trends for future physicians in the era of advanced technology and artificial intelligence: an integrative review. *BMC Med Educ* 2019;19(1):460.

21. Aungst TD, Patel R. Integrating digital health into the curriculum—considerations on the current landscape and future developments. *J Med Educ Curric Dev* 2020;7:238212051990127.

22. Al Sayed I, Al-Saiyd N. The impact of information technology in medical education. In: International Conference in Technological Trends in Engineering and Medical Sciences (ICTTEMS). 2019. doi:10.1016/S2589-7500(21)00005-4

23. Tuma F. The use of educational technology for interactive teaching in lectures. *Ann Med Surg* 2021;62:231–235.

24. Health Education England. Preparing the healthcare workforce to deliver the digital future. 2019. https://topol.hee.nhs.uk/the-topol-review/

25. Boruff J, Storie D. Mobile devices in medicine: a survey of how medical students, residents, and faculty use smartphones and other mobile devices to find information. *J Med Library Assoc* 2014;102(1):22–30.

Research, evaluation, and scholarship in medical education

John Sandars, Rakesh Patel, Kevin McLaughlin, and Megan E.L. Brown

Medical education research

Medical education research is a process of inquiry into the education and training of health professionals. The purpose of this inquiry is to answer a question about what is happening, how it is happening and why it is happening. The broad term 'medical education research' encompasses the concepts of research, evaluation, and scholarship in medical education. These concepts are often used interchangeably but they do differ.

What is research?

Research 'seeks to deepen the knowledge and understanding of learning, teaching, and education'.

📖 Ringsted C, Hodges B, Scherpbier A. 'The research compass': An introduction to research in medical education: AMEE Guide No. 56. Med Teach 2011;33(9):695–709.   https://www.tandfonline.com/doi/abs/10.3109/0142159X.2011.595436?journalCode=imte20

Examples of research questions are:
- What is the effectiveness of using standard textbooks compared with online resources for learning about cardiac arrhythmias?
- How does professionalism develop through the use of body painting within anatomy education?

What is evaluation?

Evaluation is the 'systematic determination of the merit or worth of an object'.

➡ Scriven M. The methodology of evaluation. In: Tyler RW, Gagne RM, Scriven M (Eds.), Perspectives of curriculum evaluation (pp. 39–83). Chicago, IL: Rand McNally, 1967.

Examples of evaluation questions are:
- What is the impact on learning of a flipped classroom approach to teaching biochemistry?
- What is the satisfaction of learners with the use of blogging to teach rheumatology?

What is scholarship?

Scholarship of teaching and learning is 'systematic inquiry into student learning which advances the practice of teaching by making inquiry findings public'.

📖 Cleland JA, Jamieson S, Kusurkar RA, Ramani S, Wilkinson TJ, van Schalkwyk S. Redefining scholarship for health professions education: AMEE Guide No. 142. Med Teach 2021;43(7):824–838.

Examples of scholarship questions are:
- How can I improve the feedback that I give clinical students on my gastroenterology placement?
- How can I develop self-directed learning in students during my histology class?

Similarities and differences

The three activities of research, evaluation, and scholarship use similar research methods, such as questionnaires and interviews, but ▶ their intended purposes are different.

Table 10.1 The differences between research and service evaluation, adapted from the HRA decision tool: http://www.hra-decisiontools.org.uk/research/docs/DefiningResearchTable_Oct2017-1.pdf

Research	Service evaluation
The attempt to derive generalizable or transferable new knowledge to answer questions with scientifically sound methods including studies that aim to generate hypotheses as well as studies that aim to test them, in addition to simply descriptive studies.	Designed and conducted solely to define or judge current practice.
Quantitative research—can be designed to test a hypothesis as in a randomized-controlled trial or can simply be descriptive as in a postal survey. Qualitative research—can be used to generate a hypothesis, usually identifies/explores themes.	Designed to answer: 'What standard does this service achieve?'
Quantitative research—addresses clearly defined questions, aims, and objectives. Qualitative research—usually has clear aims and objectives but may not establish the exact questions to be asked until research is underway.	Measures current service without reference to a standard.
Quantitative research—may involve evaluating or comparing interventions, particularly new ones. However, some quantitative research such as descriptive surveys, do not involve interventions. Qualitative research—seeks to understand better the perceptions and reasoning of people.	Involves an intervention in use only. For example, in clinical settings the choice of treatment, care or services is that of the care professional and patient/service user according to guidance, professional standards and/or patient/service user preference.
Usually involves collecting data that are additional to those for routine practice but may include data collected routinely. May involve interventions additional to routine practice. May involve data collected from interviews, focus groups, and/or observation.	Usually involves analysis of existing data but may also include administration of interview(s) or questionnaire(s).
Quantitative research—study design may involve allocating participants to an intervention. Qualitative research—does not usually involve allocating participants to an intervention.	No allocation to intervention: for example, in a clinical setting, the care professional and patient/service user have chosen intervention before service evaluation.

Research focuses on creating new knowledge that can inform national or international policy and practice, whereas evaluation is concerned with improving quality within a local context. The UK Health Research Authority highlights the main differences between research and evaluation (See Table 10.1).

These differences are critical, as they influence whether ethical approval is necessary. Research normally requires ethical approval, whereas service evaluation usually does not. Remember to check with your local ethics board to be sure.

Scholarship of teaching and learning has a focus on improving practice and is usually concerned with creating new, local, practitioner knowledge.

Perspectives and research methods in medical education

Medical education is an interdisciplinary field, informed by the social sciences. As discussed in ➲ Chapter 2, paradigms (shared assumptions, beliefs, values, and practices) inform how medical education research is designed, conducted, and interpreted. Research may be conducted from the following perspectives:

- A **positivist paradigm**, where researchers assume that we can come to know about the world around us objectively through careful, bias-free observation, and experimentation
- A **post-positivist paradigm**, where researchers assume that we should strive to obtain objective knowledge about the world around us, though acknowledging that this knowledge will always be imperfect, as humans introduce their own perspectives and error into observation and experimentation
- An **interpretivist paradigm**, where researchers assume that our ways of knowing about the world around us are tied to our experiences and social contexts. There is not one world that can be objectively known, rather our experiences of the world are multiple, and there are multiple knowledges that are related to sociocultural, and sociopolitical contexts
- A **realist paradigm**, where researchers assume that we can come to know about the world around us through considering the mechanisms at work within that world that connect our context (setting, our characteristics) with the outcomes we observe. Though there are multiple ways of knowing, there is a real world that is independent of our interpretations
- A **pragmatic paradigm**, where researchers focus on solving practical problems, and ways of viewing the world and knowledge can shift within research, as researchers seek the most practical and efficient way to answer their questions of interest

There are two main 'approaches' to research that the above perspectives (ways in which we view the world) draw upon to design and direct the research methods used in research, evaluation, and scholarship inquiry projects:

- A **qualitative approach** is most typically used by interpretivists and realists. Qualitative research methods are used to understand how individuals think, feel, or behave in particular situations. The value of qualitative research is the in-depth understanding of individuals, or groups of individuals, by using methods that include interviews, focus groups, and observation.
- A **quantitative approach** is most typically used by positivists and post-positivists. Quantitative research methods are used to count or measure the object that is the focus of inquiry. The value of quantitative research is that a numerical measurement of the characteristics of individuals, or groups of individuals, can be obtained by using methods that include surveys and assessments.

Both qualitative and quantitative perspectives and research methods can be combined in an inquiry project, by using a mixed-methods approach. For example, an initial questionnaire survey can be used to identify a group of individuals with a particular characteristic and then more in-depth study of this group can be performed through interviews.

Mixed-methods research can be conducted from multiple paradigms (where different ways of viewing the world inform quantitative and qualitative components), though careful consideration must be given to how approaches and paradigms interact and inform one another. Mixed-methods research can also be conducted from a pragmatic paradigm.

Designing an inquiry project

All research, evaluation, and scholarship inquiry projects have several phases:

- Choice of topic and development of a clear focus with a specific question
- Consideration of appropriate paradigm, and how this relates to, or should shape, your question of interest
- Consideration of the feasibility and the need for funding
- Consideration of the ethical aspects and obtaining ethical approval (if required)
- Choice of the most appropriate approach and research method/ methods to answer the specific question
- Data collection using the chosen research method/methods
- Data analysis of the collected data
- Making sense of the results, including an assessment of the quality of the use of research method /methods
- Presentation of the results to others, e.g. academic audiences, organizational leaders/policymakers, patients, and the public (sometimes referred to as 'dissemination')

Research topic and feasibility

Finding a topic for inquiry is an essential first step! There may be an opportunity to choose the topic—did something surprise you and do you want to find out more? Are you dissatisfied with what you are doing, and do you want to change the way that it is done? However, often the topic has already been chosen, such as when you are enrolled on a higher degree, or there is funding for a specific project.

Most researchers hope that the findings from their inquiry will have an impact, such as changes in practice or policy. ▶ Achieving this impact is more likely if the concerns and answers of the potential users of the findings can be identified and answered at an early stage within a research project.

Once the topic has been broadly identified, it is time to consider your focus, feasibility, and funding.

Focus

The broad topic of interest, such as the use of reflection by undergraduate medical students, needs to be further refined into a question or aim, such as 'why do undergraduate medical students not engage with reflective learning?'

A narrower focus is recommended, with the development of objectives, since these are more specific aspects of the inquiry and will require an appropriate paradigm, approach, and research methods to be chosen.
For example:

- What are the views of learners on reflective writing within an undergraduate medical course? This suits an interpretative paradigm, and a qualitative approach and research methods are most appropriate, such as a focus group.
- What is the correlation between year group and engagement with reflective writing on an undergraduate medical course? This suits a positivist or post-positivist paradigm, and quantitative research methods are most appropriate, such as questionnaires with statistical data collection and analysis.

Consideration of feasibility and funding

❶ Many projects fail because of a lack of early consideration of feasibility and the need for potential funding.

Feasibility

A major consideration is the time constraints for involvement of both the potential participants and the researcher. Many projects are too ambitious, with plans to involve large numbers of participants, numerous time-consuming interviews, and the use of control groups. For clinical medical education researchers, the time commitment required for research usually has to be balanced against the high time demands of clinical service. For all researchers, time commitment has to be balanced alongside teaching, or other academic roles. All researchers should generally consider whether they have the appropriate skills and experience in your research team for the given project.

Funding

Involvement in any project usually has some financial cost. For participants, answering questions requires time away from other activities, and it is important to ensure that their employers have given their approval. For researchers, there are similar considerations, but it is also essential to consider additional costs, such as specific software required for data collection and analysis, transcription of audio recordings, travel, and preparation of training materials. Consider local sources of funding, and national sources, e.g. grants from organizations which support medical education.

Ethical aspects

All inquiry projects, including research, evaluation, and scholarship, must ensure that the ethics of the project have been clearly and carefully considered. The British Educational Research Association (BERA) highlights the importance of ensuring that the rights of the individual are always considered, but there are wider responsibilities to the sponsors of the research and the wider community of educational researchers.

℘   *https://www.bera.ac.uk/wp-content/uploads/2014/02/BERA-Ethical-Guidelines-2011.pdf?noredirect=1*

For example, an interview may trigger memories associated with a painful or stressful experience in participants, and it is essential to ensure that participants are fully informed about the type of questions they will be asked. Any unforeseen consequences must be mitigated as much as possible (for example, having a protocol in place for if a participant does become distressed and communicating this with participants prior to their sign up to the interview).

The specific requirements for deciding whether a project is considered to be research can be confusing for early career researchers in medical education. Advice from an experienced supervisor or mentor, and consulting with an institutional ethics review board is recommended at the earliest stage of any project. Even for work considered to be evaluation or scholarship, medical education academic journals usually require formal ethical exemption or approval by a review board. For projects that are considered to be research, formal ethical approval is essential and must be obtained before the research project commences. Failure to comply with this process can have major professional and legal implications. Obtaining research ethics approval can be a long and protracted process, and it is important for the application to be reviewed by an experienced researcher to avoid multiple resubmissions.

The importance of the literature review

A review of existing literature is essential for all research and is also important for evaluation and scholarship. ▶ A literature review should be performed at the earliest stage in planning any project.

A literature review has several functions:

- Summarizing current knowledge to establish what is already known about a topic and the need for further research.
- Identification of the strengths and limitations of the research methods that have been previously used in studies.
- Identification of conceptual and theoretical models that have been used to inform research in previous studies.

Once completed, the literature review is the basis for the justification of any research project and is essential for the background section in a research proposal, such as for funding applications, and when writing up the research to share with others, or for publication.

A well-performed literature review may also be suitable for publication. An important organization that can offer guidance on performing high-quality systematic literature reviews for medical education is the BEME (Best Evidence Medical Education) Collaboration ℅ *http://bemecollaborat ion.org/Home/*

Types of literature reviews

There are a variety of ways in which the existing literature can be summarized.[1] Broadly speaking, literature reviews can be descriptive or integrative.

- A **descriptive** review describes the methods, outcomes, and conclusions of each study separately
- An **integrative** review categorizes the existing literature based upon similarities in methods, outcomes, and findings in an attempt to draw conclusions that are reproducible and generalizable or transferable

For example, if there are limited studies about a topic then embarking upon an integrative review, such as a meta-analysis, may be inappropriate. Similarly, if there are already one or more systematic reviews then another review is likely to be unnecessary, so an updated review or a 'review of reviews' would be more appropriate. An initial scoping review is often performed to gauge the extent and types of previous studies or reviews on a topic.[2]

When dealing with qualitative outcomes, or literature where there is significant heterogeneity in methodology and/or results, a descriptive review is typically more appropriate. This review can take the form of a narrative overview or a systematic review. In both of these the goal is to critique and summarize each article included in the review, but narrative and systematic reviews differ in the degree of scope and purpose.

Within clinical medicine, systematic reviews are understood to represent 'stronger' evidence than narrative reviews, as they involve detailed searches of the literature, and appraisal of included study quality. Within medical education, what separates systematic and narrative reviews is not the strength of the evidence those reviews offer, but the intended purpose of the review. Indeed, many narrative reviews within medical education now include systematic search strategies. Narrative reviews and systematic reviews adopt different epistemological positions—by this, we mean that how knowledge is created, and what this knowledge can do, is different between narrative and systematic reviews. A more detailed discussion of epistemology can be found in Chapter 2.

- **Systematic reviews** adopt a positivist ontology and epistemology—as one, objective reality exists that we can know through bias-free science, evidence quality is critical in knowledge creation. The purpose of systematic reviews is, ∴, to synthesize high-quality (i.e. neutral, bias-free) knowledge which tells us about our singular, objective reality
- **Narrative reviews** embrace ontological and epistemological plurality—they recognize that there are multiple versions of reality, and ways of knowing, which depend on individuals' experiences and sociocultural settings. Quality of evidence is not as important as context, and how the authors interpret the findings of the studies they use. Narrative reviews place focus on the author's experience, and the authors are often experts in their area, or practitioners of the approach being reviewed. The purpose of narrative reviews is to explore the impact of context and integrate evidence and experience.

The choice of methodology for the review should be based upon:

- The amount of literature that already exists
- The types of outcomes reported in the literature
- The purpose of the planned research project
- Whether or not there is an intention to publish the review

Table 10.2 lists common review types and the questions they are best placed to answer within medical education.

Table 10.2 Common review types within medical education, and the questions they might focus on

Type of literature review	Questions the review can answer
Narrative review	What are the main concepts and new ideas regarding a topic of interest? How can context and expert experience influence interpretation of disparate evidence?
Systematic review	What is known about a specific research question through an approach that aims to minimize bias?
Meta-analysis	How can the results of similar studies identified within a systematic review be quantified?
Meta-ethnography	What are the shared themes, interpretations, and experiences across qualitative studies on a topic? How can these studies be synthesized to generate new insights or theories?
Scoping review	Quantity, quality, and direction of the research? What review or research is now needed?
State-of-the-art review	What is the current state of knowledge, and what are the current priorities?
Rapid review	How much literature is published, and what is the quality and direction?
Realist review	What works, for whom, under what circumstances, and why?

When studies included in a review are similar with regards to participants, interventions, outcomes measures, and methodologies, there may be an opportunity to integrate the findings of individual studies. This process can increase statistical power and improve the precision and generalisability of results for quantitative data and improve the depth, dependability, or confirmability of qualitative data.

For example:

- Quantitative data can be pooled so that a systematic review can be enhanced by the addition of a meta-analysis
- Where outcomes are qualitative, data can be synthesized narratively, or explored in depth within a meta-ethnography
- Where outcomes are both qualitative and quantitative, findings can be pooled in a realist synthesis, narrative synthesis, or thematic analysis

An important type of review, especially to make sense of the complexity of interventions in social sciences and education, is the realist review which seeks to identify what works, for who and in what circumstances.[3]

Performing a literature review

There is an increasing number of studies in medical education, both published and unpublished, which are widely dispersed across several databases. Since medical education is a social science, published studies are often found in education, psychology, philosophy, and sociology journals.

Seek early advice of a librarian on the search strategies for different databases such as:

- PubMed (biomedical literature)
- Ovid MEDLINE (biomedical and life sciences literature)
- Excerpta Medica Database (EMBASE) (biomedical and pharmacological literature)
- Scopus (life, social, and physical sciences literature)
- Education Resources Information Centre (ERIC) (education literature)
- Journal Storage (JSTOR) (humanities, social sciences, and sciences literature)
- Education Source (education literature)
- PsycInfo (behavioural and social sciences literature)
- Cochrane Library (systematic reviews)
- Web of Science (science, social science, arts and humanities literature)
- Cumulative Index to Nursing and Allied Health Literature (CINAHL) (nursing and allied health professions literature)
- African Journals Online (AJOL) (medicine and medical education)
- Latin American and Caribbean Health Sciences Literature (LILACS) (health sciences and medical education)
- SciELO (multidisciplinary, Latin America, the Caribbean, Portugal, Spain, South Africa)
- Index Medicus for the Eastern Mediterranean Region (medicine)
- Indexing of Indian Medical Journals (INDMED) (medical journals)
- KoreaMed (medical, dental, nursing, nutrition, and veterinary journals)
- CORE (multidisciplinary, aggregates open access papers)
- 'Grey literature' databases (containing conference abstracts or PhD theses, which may not be found in the previously listed databases) e.g. EThOS (e-theses online service), The Grey Literature Report, OpenGrey, and ProQuest Dissertation & Theses Global.

Grey literature may be appropriately searched in other ways, including through the use of web searches, and Google Scholar. A librarian can offer guidance on the strengths, limitations, and use of each approach to searching grey literature.

The use of data management software is recommended, for example: Covidence, RevMan, or Rayyan. Some of this software is free, some requires a subscription. Check if your institution offers any access to paid services.

Conceptual and theoretical frameworks

Both quantitative and qualitative research are guided and shaped by a study's conceptual and theoretical framework. Though the terms conceptual and theoretical framework are often used interchangeably within medical education, they do differ.

What are conceptual frameworks?

Conceptual frameworks convey why a research project or study is required; they establish the investigation's methodological underpinnings, describe what is known about a topic, and highlight any areas in which existing knowledge may be built upon. A research paper's introduction often includes a description of the conceptual underpinning for the inquiry. Most usually, conceptual frameworks are written or visual (they may be synthesized as a graphic), and communicate the relationships between the key factors, concepts, or approaches in a study to justify its position in wider academic literature.

A conceptual framework can be developed from issues identified from an initial scoping interview with open-ended questions, from issues identified from a literature review of the topic, or from the previous experience of the researcher.

Why are conceptual frameworks important?

Conceptual frameworks inform the design and delivery of research—without a clear idea of what concepts are of interest (and why) and how these concepts connect, a project's research questions, methodology, and methods may not achieve the intended aims of the study.

Given the diversity in definitions of many key concepts within medical education, it is important to make clear how concepts within a study have been conceptualized (defined and understood) to allow those who read about the research to understand how it might (or might not) apply to their own experiences, contexts, and understandings.

Further, conceptual frameworks help map how a project will contribute to existing knowledge on a topic. Given scarcity of resources (such as research consumables, faculty time, participant time, and grant funding), ▶ clearly establishing the intended contribution (and the value of that contribution) within a project's conceptual framework is an ethical issue (Box 10.1).

What are theoretical frameworks?

Theoretical frameworks are a synthesis of ideas from one or more theories. Researchers use theoretical frameworks to organize medical education research (including to inform study design, data analysis, and the discussion of a research paper).

Why are theoretical frameworks important?

Theoretical frameworks are critical within medical education research, as they connect what's already known and well-established within educational, social sciences, psychological (etc.) theory to the findings of a project. Using theory helps us to build on existing knowledge and increases the transferability of qualitative research.

> **Box 10.1 Example of a conceptual framework**
>
> A research team wishes to explore variation in degree awards across the United Kingdom. Though UK medical degrees are technically unclassified, some universities provide academic awards such as 'pass with honours'. This topic has been informed by members of the research teams' experience regarding the awarding of application points to degree classifications within postgraduate training, when medical schools seem to adopt different approaches to classifying degrees. International literature suggests that, in the US, for example, there are differences in admissions to honours societies between medical schools, and these differences are biased (in that those from minoritized backgrounds are least likely to receive honours). There is no UK data on the approaches to degree classification different medical schools take. As an assessment outcome which informs career progression, understanding the current system of degree classifications, and possible variations within this system, within the UK is an issue of equity and of the consequential validity of the awards.
>
> Read more in the published paper: ✎ Byrne, M.H., Yale, S.E., Glasbey, M., Revell, E. and Brown, M.E., 2023. All medical degrees are equal, but some are more equal than others: An analysis of medical degree classifications. Medical Education, 57(8), pp.732–740. https://onlinelibrary.wiley.com/doi/10.1111/medu.15019

How are theoretical frameworks used within medical education research?

Theory can be used at many different points within a study—there is no one right way to employ or draw on a theoretical framework—but clarity when describing one's approach is key.

Theory can be used:

- **Deductively**, where a study tests a theory or some aspect of a theory; and
- **Inductively**, where theory is approached at a later stage within analysis to inform data interpretation and the study discussion

Theoretical frameworks might be described in the methods of a research paper, if theory has been used to shape study design or analysis or in the introduction of a paper, if the study concerns deductive use of theory. Across all approaches, theory is a common character within the discussion section of research papers, where it can be used to contextualize findings and highlight novel insights.

Increasingly popular is the use of theory as a **'sensitizing concept'** within qualitative data analysis. Sensitizing concepts are most commonly associated with constructivist grounded theory. This is a research approach that focuses on developing a theory to explain how something works using qualitative data. Within this approach, it is acknowledged that each researcher applies their prior knowledge and experiences (or sensitizing concepts) to theory creation.

Increasingly, sensitizing concepts are also used within thematic analysis. Thematic analysis is an approach to qualitative research that involves identifying recurring patterns within qualitative data. These patterns, once connected, tell the story (through 'themes') of the study data. Sensitizing concepts in thematic analysis are identified as relevant within analysis—as researchers analyse data, they identify core concepts that appear repeatedly in the data which resonate with existing concepts or theories in the literature. Researchers then undertake a period of theoretical immersion in associated theory and background literature to better conceptualize and understand relevant facets of their data. These insights are applied to the data and may shape the report produced. Varpio et al. refer to this approach as 'theory-informing inductive data analysis' (Box 10.2).

Box 10.2 **Example of a theoretical framework**

A research team is exploring medical student experiences of clinical practice during the COVID-19 pandemic. They discussed experiences in focus groups with the students, adopting an inductive approach to data collection and analysis given a lack of knowledge at the time regarding experiences as a volunteer. As they collected data, they began to realize that students were telling stories of how difficult or challenging events and situations had led to significant shifts in their perspective of who they were as future doctors, and who they were aiming to become. As educational researchers with postgraduate qualifications in medical education, the team were aware of Kegan's developmental model of identity. This theory describes how social experiences affect individuals' cognitive perceptions of their identity.

Shifts in identity are often in response to 'disorienting dilemmas' that cause them to re-evaluate their own stance. When students spoke of their role, values, and shifts in understanding of what it was to be a doctor, this alerted the team to a connection with the concept of professional identity—the idea of who one is, and who one is seen to be, in relation to occupational role. Kegan's model and identity development have been previously connected. The team used Kegan's model as a theory to conceptualize how shifts in professional identity occur and consider the impact of attending clinical clerkships during COVID-19 on identity. Kegan's model was used as a 'sensitizing concept' within thematic analysis of the focus group data, and informed theme construction, and definition.

Read more in the published paper: ✍ Brown, M.E., Lim, J.H., Horsburgh, J., Pistoll, C., Thakerar, V., Maini, A., Johnson, C., Beaton, L., Mahoney, C. and Kumar, S., 2022. Identity development in disorienting times: the experiences of medical students during COVID-19. Medical Science Educator, 32(5), pp.995–1004. https://link.springer.com/article/10.1007/s40670-022-01592-z#Sec2

Qualitative research methods

All qualitative research methods seek to obtain a 'rich' understanding of how individuals, or groups of individuals, think, feel, or behave in particular situations, such as the perceptions of learners about reflective writing. The 'richness' requires in-depth data collection (of interview audio and transcripts, field notes, diaries, videos, and/or images), usually from a small number of participants. The large amount of data must be analysed, interpreted, and then presented. There is no singular approach to qualitative analysis and data presentation, though we present some common approaches in 'qualitative data analysis', below. What is key between approaches is that ▶ analysis and presentation should accurately represent the 'richness' of the data that has been collected.

Selection of participants

A random sample can be obtained but, usually, participants are selected to broadly represent individuals within a specific context, such as third-year undergraduate medical students with a mandatory reflective writing task. ▶ An important approach to sampling for qualitative research is purposive sampling, in which individuals are selected based on their particular characteristics so that they can provide greater insight of the topic of research. An illustrative example is the selection of students that enjoy reflective writing tasks and those that dislike this task.

There is no specific size for the sample, unlike quantitative research methods where a sample size (power) calculation can be performed. Instead, necessary qualitative sample size depends on a project's methodology, methods, intended aims, and the data that is collected itself.

❶ Given this, it can be difficult to decide on the size of a qualitative sample prior to data collection, and decisions regarding when a sample is sufficient are often made during data collection, or during analysis.

There are several concepts that researchers can consider to guide discussions of when qualitative sampling and data collection should cease:

- 'Saturation' of qualitative data—medical education researchers used to discuss data 'saturation' as the point at which data collection should end. Data were 'saturated' when no additional data were being collected that added new depth or insight to a research question. ❶ However, 'saturation' has fallen out of favour, in recognition that it was variously used and difficult to determine and justify. Further, the concept is critiqued on the basis that the richness and multi-faceted interpretations of qualitative data mean that data also has more to give, it is never fully 'saturated'. Those wishing to use 'saturation' must discuss their methodological orientation, as the concept is contemporarily seen as most suited to use within grounded theory studies and justify how they reached the decision that their data were saturated.

- 'Sufficiency' of qualitative data—▶ many researchers have now shifted to describing their data as 'sufficient' in answering their research question of interest. Sufficiency also depends on the rigour of qualitative analysis. Sufficiency acknowledges that there isn't an objective point at which there is no more to learn from data, but there is a point at which research needs to stop, and that point should be when analysis is sufficiently robust, and data are sufficiently rich, to respond to or answer the study research question. 'Theoretical sufficiency' is used within grounded theory studies to describe the point at which the theory created by the research project is sufficient in explaining the phenomenon under study.

This being said, often ethics applications and grant applications require provision of an intended sample size. Malterud et al.'s concept of **'information power'** can be used to help estimate the necessary size of a qualitative sample. 'Information power' is distinct from 'statistical power', and depends on five variables:

1. **Study aim**—if the aim of a study is specific and narrow, a smaller sample size can achieve this aim.
2. **Sample specificity**—if the participants required for the study are specific (in that they meet several specific criteria or share several specific characteristics), a smaller sample size is justifiable.
3. **Whether theory is used**—using established theory situates a study amongst what is already known, and so fewer participants are required.
4. The **quality of dialogue** within collected data—at the ethics/grant/planning stage, this may be speculative, or retrospective if reviewing the information power of a study following or during analysis. Studies with rich interview dialogue require fewer participants.
5. **Plans for analysis**—longitudinal data analysis and in-depth approaches (for example, phenomenological analysis of participants' lived experiences) require smaller samples than studies that describe and compare processes, phenomena, and experiences across participants (e.g. interpretative description). Guidance exists (❶though it is just that, guidance, rather than hard and fast rules) regarding sample size for various approaches to analysis that can act as prompts for discussion (e.g. phenomenological research usually requires fewer than 10 interviews; whereas interpretative description usually requires 15–20 interviews).

Reviewing others' studies through the lens of information power can also help structure discussions in research planning and contribute to an estimated qualitative sample size.

Data collection

The intention of data collection in qualitative research methods is to obtain a rich understanding of a topic. The two main approaches can be described as fieldwork and deskwork.

Fieldwork

Data collection occurs 'in the field' from new sources of data. The main methods are interviews and focus groups:

- **Interviews**—a one to one in-depth discussion about an individual's thoughts and views about a topic. The data is attributable at the level of the individual.
- **Group interviews**—Group interviews are any interviews that bring together a group of individuals for questioning during a research project. This may be done for convenience, and if the focus is on collecting data from individuals within a group setting, rather than

discussion, the umbrella term 'group interview' is used. Focus groups are a type of group interview, where discussion is facilitated between members of a group of individuals about their thoughts and views about a topic. If there is adequate focus on discussion within the study research question, and within analysis, data is attributable at the level of the group since the comments are the consequence of the socially constructed collective thoughts and views of the focus group.

Interviews can be structured, semi-structured, or unstructured. The nature of the interview determines how an interview is conducted, and the types of questions asked.

- **Structured interviews**—predetermined questions are asked in a specific order. Researchers cannot deviate from the list of questions, or the order in which they are asked.
- **Semi-structured interviews**—the research interview is guided by a list of predetermined question stems (usually generated from background literature, theory, and sometimes pilot research). Unlike structured interviews, researchers can diverge from the question stems to explore the experiences participants volunteer in greater depth. Stems usually include both open and closed questions.
- **Unstructured interviews**—questions are not predetermined in advance of an interview, though there may be general topics provided to a researcher to cover during the interview. There are no specific questions, no agreed question order, and the interview unfolds like a conversation would.

The type of interview selected depends on the study's aim, and the type of data required to meet this aim.

- Structured interviewing is most common in survey-based approaches and is often conducted from a positivist or post-positivist orientation with the intent of comparing participants and their answers directly.
- Semi-structured interviewing is the most common approach to qualitative interviewing within medical education, as it provides some guidance on relevant questioning/prompts but offers flexibility to explore participants' experiences in greater depth. ▶ Semi-structured interviewing is particularly useful in research where some degree of comparison is desired, but the subjective nature of participants' experiences (and so the value of stories and incidental comments) is embraced.
- Unstructured interviewing is most typical in in-depth approaches to qualitative research that focus on lived experience (e.g. phenomenological research) and, because they are more participant-guided, ▶ can be particularly effective in establishing rapport and comfort when discussing sensitive, difficult, or emotional topics.

Across all approaches to interviewing (individual or group; and structured, semi-structured, or unstructured), the researcher will need to develop an interview topic or question guide. This is a list of the main questions to be asked, prompts to encourage discussion, or topics to consider within an unstructured interview. In structured and semi-structured approaches, each question or prompt has a probe to obtain more information and elicit deeper discussion (Box 10.3).

Box 10.3 Example of an interview probe
Main question: 'What is your opinion about work-based assessments on clinical placements?'
  Probe: 'Why do you say that?'

In semi-structured approaches, the sequence of questions may be guided by the responses to the initial question but usually questions are asked in a structured sequence that is informed by the researcher's conceptual framework of the topic of interest.

The responses to the questions are usually audio-recorded and then transcribed to produce a text-based transcript for analysis. It is important to remember that the recording should be of high quality to allow accurate transcription—the use of a separate microphone or dictaphone is recommended. Good ethical practice in data handling is to anonymize and securely store the file containing the audio-recording as soon as possible and to delete any files that are on the mobile audio recorder.

Another fieldwork data collection method is observation (often called ethnography), such as observing teamwork in an operating theatre.

Deskwork

Data collection occurs 'at the desk' using pre-existing sources of data. An example is the review of existing documents, such as policy statements, or images, such as photographs used in press releases about the latest advances in healthcare.

Qualitative data analysis

The focus for the analysis of qualitative data is to make sense of the large amount of data that has been collected. The main approaches are inductive, deductive, and hybrid.

● Inductive approach

The inductive approach uses a 'bottom-up' process to progressively reduce the data into a series of codes and categories, from which a small number of themes can be identified.

The process: The researcher reads through the transcript several times to identify words and phrases that give meaning to the messages that the participant is presenting to the researcher. These words and phrases are the codes, such as 'Everyone was so busy on the ward' or 'All of the patients were so ill that they were not suitable'. There may be several hundred codes but these can be reduced into a smaller number of categories, such as 'busy wards' or 'ill patients', that contain several codes with a similar meaning. Finally, the categories can be reduced into a smaller number of themes that represent the main messages of the participant and connect codes in a way that helps explain meaning in your data, such as 'time pressures negatively influence student perceptions of competency' or 'severity of patient illness influences student involvement in care'.

One common methodology within inductive qualitative approaches is grounded theory methodology. The name 'grounded theory' was created because, in this methodology, understanding of the phenomenon under research ('theory') is emergent ('grounded') from the data that has been collected. However, an essential aspect of the 'grounded theory' process is the repeated cycles of refinement that require going forwards and backwards through the data to ensure that the codes, categories, and themes comprehensively represent the data. This process is called 'constant comparative' data analysis.

● Deductive approach

Deductive approaches to qualitative research use a 'top-down' process to place data into a small number of predetermined themes.

The process: The researcher initially develops a template which contains a small number of specific themes. These themes require an existing 'theory', or conceptual model, of understanding the phenomenon under research. An illustrative example is the conceptual model of force-field analysis to understand change, with helping and hindering factors that influence change. The researcher reads through the text several times to identify data that represents the themes of helping and hindering factors, and the data is placed into these template themes.

One approach to analysis that can be deductive (but isn't always) is 'framework analysis', which is especially useful where data gathered are highly structured, such as in a policy document. In deductive approaches, a framework is created either from existing theory, or from established concepts and prior research findings relevant to the topic of analysis.

● Hybrid approach

A hybrid approach to data analysis is frequently used, combining aspects of both an inductive and deductive approach. A purely inductive analysis can be time-consuming, but a purely deductive approach can be too restrictive and not fully represent all of the data. As above, framework analysis is not always deductive—it can also be hybrid. Frameworks can also be created from inductive analysis of one or more cases of data from within the study.

The process: There are several stages and at each stage there is a systematic and transparent process that is shown within an analytic 'framework'.

1. Data management—the researcher becomes familiar with the data through reading and re-reading the transcript to identify several codes and categories that are used to develop a coding matrix of several initial themes, with each theme being supported by illustrative examples. The initial themes are usually informed by the researcher's conceptual model that has guided their interview questions and are related to the research question. Researchers may not wait until all their data is collected before beginning analysis—analysis can occur alongside data collection, and inform subsequent data collection, as researchers might identify areas of their framework requiring further development.
2. Descriptive accounts—the initial themes are refined by seeking associations between the themes, with each theme being supported by illustrative examples identified from the diversity of data.
3. Explanatory accounts—conceptual patterns across the themes are developed and attempts are made to explain these patterns, with illustrative examples of the explicit process.

▶ Framework analysis has the advantage of developing a series of themes at an early stage that can be iteratively refined (refined throughout the process of a research project, as data collection and analysis occur alongside one another, and inform one another) and each of the several stages of the process can be explicitly described. Overall, there is a systematic, transparent, and justified approach to data analysis.

❶ Qualitative data analysis is often confusing to novice researchers and the use of the various qualitative analysis software (e.g. Dedoose, Quirkos, NVivo, Atlas.ti), which are designed to ease the handling of data, does not overcome the need for the researcher to perform the actual analysis. Similarly, the rise of large language models, which some researchers are exploring (with explicit participant consent) for their ability to summarize and describe data, does not mean researcher interpretation isn't needed. Making connections between data in a research project and making meaning from these connections to tell the story of the data, requires researcher interpretation. Training is advised for novice researchers, with supervision by an experienced qualitative researcher.

Making sense of data and data presentation

The presentation of data is mainly as a series of themes, with each theme accompanied by an illustrative comment (quote) from a participant. Some studies choose to present quotes in tables, separate from the description of the themes, though ❶ this risks removing the quotes from context and negatively influencing readability. Themes should be integral components of a wider conceptual model that provides an overall way of presenting the associations between themes. This conceptual model provides the message to the readership—for example organizational barriers to work-based assessments in clinical contexts.

An essential aspect of the presentation of the overall findings of the inquiry is to discuss the rigour, or trustworthiness, of the research. This notion is considered differently to the concepts of validity, reliability, and generalizability within a quantitative perspective.

Quantitative research methods

Quantitative research methods study outcomes that can be observed and measured. The measured outcomes are then subjected to statistical modelling so that the relationship between [independent] explanatory variables of interest and [dependent] outcome variables can be quantified.

Types of quantitative studies

Each quantitative study has a clear question that the researchers are attempting to answer or a hypothesis that they are testing. ▶ The appropriate study design is selected depending upon whether the goal is to answer a question or test a hypothesis.

• Descriptive studies

Descriptive or observational studies are designed to observe associations between explanatory and outcome variables and answer the questions 'Is [explanatory variable] x associated with [outcome] y?'

Demonstrating an association in an observational study does not imply causation since the direction of the association cannot be inferred reliably. For example, if we design a descriptive study to answer the question 'Is exposure to simulation training associated with improved clinical skills?' and then demonstrate a statistically significant association, our results could be explained by the fact that simulation training is an effective tool for improving clinical skills or that learners with better clinical skills are more likely to seek out opportunities for simulation training.

• Experimental studies

In contrast to descriptive studies, experiments manipulate exposure to explanatory variables in an attempt to support the claim of a causal relationship. For this reason, experiments are designed to test hypotheses and since the researchers control exposure to the explanatory variable, finding a significant association under these circumstances supports the hypothesis that the exposure causes the outcome.

In order to support a causal relationship with greater confidence, researchers design their experiment to reduce the risk of bias on the relationship between explanatory and outcome variables. There are many potential sources of bias and techniques to mitigate these, but among those most commonly encountered in quantitative studies are:

• **Selection bias**—error in assigning individuals to groups (such as volunteer bias where volunteers aren't representative of a population, and sampling bias where participants selected by researchers aren't representative of a population) leading to differences which might influence the study outcome. Can be reduced by random allocation of participants to different interventions

• **Performance bias**—where individuals change their behaviour because they are conscious of being observed or receiving a particular type of intervention. Can be reduced by blinding of participants +/− researchers to the study hypothesis and nature of the interventions

In observational studies and in experimental studies where it is not possible to eliminate extraneous variables, multivariate statistical analyses (e.g. multiple regression) can quantify the impact of other variables on the outcome variables. ▶ Expert statistical advice is recommended to ensure appropriate analyses are performed.

Quantitative data analysis

It is important to recognize that all statistical tests have assumptions that must not be violated. For this reason, the selection of the appropriate statistical analyses should not be an afterthought. Instead, statistical analyses should be planned at the same time as decisions are being made about the appropriate study design. The assumptions of statistical tests primarily relate to the type of outcomes being measured, the number and type of explanatory variables, and the study design.

Selecting appropriate statistical analyses

Questions to consider when selecting statistical tests include:
- Is my outcome variable continuous, dichotomous, or time-to-event?
- If continuous, is my outcome variable normally distributed or skewed?
- Is my outcome variable measured only once or repeatedly?
- How many groups/interventions are being studied?
- Is there one explanatory variable of interest or more than one?
- Is there possible interaction between explanatory variables?

For example, an independent t-test assumes a comparison of two groups with no other explanatory variables and a normally distributed continuous outcome variable that is measured only once.

Interpreting the results of quantitative studies

The results of quantitative studies are usually presented as a collection of numbers in a graph or table. An understanding of what these numbers denote is essential for appropriate interpretation (Box 10.4). Each of these numbers conveys valuable information:
- The **mean** is the average outcome for each group and is used to describe outcome data that are normally distributed
- **Standard deviation** is a standardized measure of the variance of the outcome data around the mean
- The **p-value** is the probability of incorrectly rejecting the null hypothesis. It is the probability of measuring a difference when in reality, there is no difference between groups (which is the null hypothesis). A cut-off p-value is established prior to quantitative studies (the most frequently used cut-off is $p < 0.05$, which means that there is a 95% chance there is a true difference between the groups and a 5% chance the measured difference was due to chance). Whenever the calculated

---

Box 10.4 Example quantitative study results

An experimental study found that when students were randomly allocated to a simulation scenario that included exposure to the murmur of mitral regurgitation they were more likely to recognize the features of mitral regurgitation when examining a real patient than students allocated to a scenario without a cardiac murmur. The mean diagnostic performance of students in the first group was 74.0% (standard deviation = 36.4%) compared to 36.8% (standard deviation = 33.1%) in the second group. The calculated p value for this comparison was <0.001 and the effect size (Cohen's d) was 1.07.[4]

p-value is less than the stated threshold, the null hypothesis is rejected in favour of the alternative hypothesis that states that there is a difference between groups
- The **effect size** quantifies the strength of the observed difference. There are many ways to calculate effect size, and one of the most frequently used is Cohen's d statistic. For ease of interpretation, effect size can then be categorized as small (d = 0.2), medium (d = 0.5), or large (d = 0.8).

Other commonly reported numbers include:
- **Proportion**, which quantifies the number of participants experiencing the outcomes compared to the total number of participants.
- **Confidence intervals** express the degree of confidence that the true population parameter that we are trying to estimate lies within the range of values stated. Since our study participants represent only a sample of a larger population, we cannot actually measure the true population mean, but when we provide 95% confidence intervals we are implying that if we repeated our study on multiple different samples then the true population parameter would be captured within the stated intervals 95% of the time.
- **Odds ratio**, which quantifies the strength of association between explanatory variables and dichotomous outcomes. As the name suggests, the odds ratio is used to compare the odds of an outcome with exposure to the explanatory variable to the odds of an outcome without exposure to the explanatory variable. An odds ratio that is significantly higher than 1 supports an association between explanatory and outcome variables, and the higher this number then the stronger the association.

Tips for using quantitative research methods
- Based upon the review of the existing literature, decide whether the aim of the proposed study is to answer a research question or test a research hypothesis
- Seek advice and/or further training on study methodology to ensure that this is appropriate to answer the research question or test the research hypothesis
- Seek advice and/or further training on quantitative statistics, including the use of statistical software
- Pilot and improve the tools that will be used to gather data during the study and establish validity of these tools prior to the main study
- Perform a sample size/power calculation prior to starting the main study

Evaluating the quality of qualitative and quantitative research methods

An essential aspect of making sense of the findings obtained from a project is a judgement about the overall quality of the process of inquiry, especially the methods that have been used to collect and analyse data.

Many of the concepts will be familiar to early career researchers in medical education and are based on a quantitative perspective, such as internal and external validity, reliability, and bias. These concepts are still useful at times, but ▶ a wider view of quality is important, recognizing the increasing use of qualitative research and mixed-methods research. In Table 10.3 below, readers will see the increasing number of qualitative-specific markers of quality now used within medical education.

Table 10.3 Quality in qualitative and quantitative research

Qualitative marker of quality	Quantitative marker of quality
Credibility	*Validity*
The extent to which the findings are believable and this depends on the richness of the information gathered, rather than the amount of data gathered. Credibility can be achieved by several approaches, including prolonged engagement with participants, and seeking a wide range of participants who may have diverse opinions.	The research and any associated measurement tools utilized within the course of the research measure the characteristic (e.g. knowledge, skills) that they intended to measure.
Dependability	*Reliability*
The findings and approach to the research project should be consistent and logical. The data collection and data analysis need to be made explicit and transparent through clear documentation, e.g. through auditing the research process.	The reproducibility of the research—the probability that the research would gain the same results if it was conducted again with the same participants under the same conditions.
Transferability	*Generalisability*
Involves three components: applicability, theoretical engagement, and resonance. Concerns the impact of qualitative research findings beyond the context in which data were collected. Applicability is the degree to which findings can be applied in another context and requires detailed description of study context and layers of meaning within data. Theoretical engagement offers a shared language for researchers that promotes transferability. Resonance is the degree to which the research and its presentation evokes a sense of familiarity, shared experience, or embodied understanding.	The findings of the research can be extrapolated to a larger, wider population. To do so, the research sample must be representative of the population from which it was drawn.

Table 10.3   (Contd.)

Qualitative marker of quality	Quantitative marker of quality
Confirmability Involves clearly establishing the connection between the interpretation of data, and study findings (including the justification of themes by providing illustrative codes, such as quotations made by the participants). Also involves clear explanations regarding the rationale behind methodological decisions and analytical choices.	*Objectivity* Research which is free from bias and conducted by researchers adopting a neutral perspective.
Internal coherence Alignment between the philosophical orientation of the study, research design, methods of data collection, data analysis, and the tenor of the data interpretation. Critical part of logical decision making within project design and execution.	
Reflexivity Essential within qualitative research. Awareness of the extent to which beliefs, opinions, and past experiences of the researcher(s) influence study design, data collection, and analysis. Researchers need to reflect on their perspectives, make these clear, and then embrace these to deepen data analysis and interpretation. This can be achieved through keeping a reflective diary throughout the inquiry process, regular discussions with a peer group of researchers, and critically discussing the potential influences on the inquiry process in the final write-up and presentation of the project so that readers can make their own decisions about the interpretation of presented findings.	*Reflexivity* We would suggest that reflexivity is also important within quantitative research (though not all scholars would agree with us). Particularly if research is conducted from a post-positivist paradigm, the possible influence of the research team is noted to be important. As with qualitative research, reflexivity involves an awareness of the extent to which beliefs, opinions, and past experiences of the researcher(s) influence study design, data collection, and analysis; alongside a written description of this in project outputs.

Disseminating findings and impact

The way in which the outputs from data analysis are presented are just as important as the collection and analysis of the data! The presentation of data rarely involves just reproducing the outputs following the process of analysis—the findings should be tailored to the audience.

Dissemination

Dissemination is the sharing of a study's findings and recommendations with key interested parties (e.g. other educators, clinicians, organizational leaders, patients) that the study is likely to have an impact on. ▶ Ask yourself: who do you want to know about your work, and who do you want to act on these findings? The answers to this question should inform the way in which you share, or disseminate, your findings.

Though dissemination of a research project is an essential final stage, especially since there are many instances where research is undertaken and the findings are not communicated, dissemination should be considered at the start of the investigation (as part of the design of a research project). ▶ Early engagement with the people you wish your research to be read, and considered, by can maximize later impact. Important parties can be involved in project development, design, and act as a sounding board for ongoing data analysis throughout the lifespan of a project. Further, the requirements of peer-reviewed publications may directly influence the study design, especially for randomized-controlled trials, systematic reviews, or meta-analyses—where publishing guidelines are strict. ▶ Early consideration of routes to dissemination may help you work towards the deadlines for specific events and conferences at which your target stakeholder audience will be in attendance.

There are a variety of routes through which you can disseminate your research. Which route(s) you choose depends on the audience you're trying to reach. Routes of dissemination include:

- Academic journal publications.
- Academic conferences—most specialties hold specialty specific conferences, but there are also medical education conferences within the UK (including the Association for the Study of Medical Education or ASME annual conference), and internationally (including the Association of Medical Education or AMEE conference).
- Press releases—if you are affiliated with a university, universities have teams responsible for communicating cutting-edge findings with news teams for reach to the general public.
- Newsletters and blogs—academic institutions and organizations often run blogs and newsletters and invite submissions to these. Find out what's available in your area and publicise the findings of your research through these established channels.
- Social media—sharing findings on social media, particularly social media which you use for professional purposes, and the links to any publication of your research, can broaden your reach and increase paper citation counts. Make use of relevant hashtags, and tag leaders influential in your field or area of interest. Producing graphics or videos to share on social media can increase the impact of your posts.

- Snowballing—word of mouth can be a powerful way of sharing research findings (this approach can generate project momentum, like a snowball rolling down a hill). Reach out to colleagues interested in the area you are working in and share your findings. There may be heads of department or influential educators you can connect with and ask to amplify your findings.

How you will communicate your findings, as well as where, is an important consideration when planning project dissemination. Different target audiences may respond to different approaches, and different language. For press releases and social media posts, for example, clear jargon-free language is best. Leading with one headline finding or take-home message can increase impact. For journal publications, and conference presentations, jargon may be more appropriate.

Conference presentations are often an expected part of project dissemination. Careful abstract preparation is key to improving your chances of acceptance (Box 10.5). Below are several important principles for effective abstract preparation, which also apply to peer-reviewed publications and conferences presentations.

Impact

One aim of an effective dissemination strategy is enhancing the impact of a research project. Impact within medical education research is variously defined but what unites many definitions of impact is the sense that research should create positive changes in practice. Positive changes may manifest for a variety of stakeholders including patients, students, trainees, qualified practitioners, and managers (some impact literature refers to 'beneficiaries' to acknowledge the idea that impact should be positive).

Impactful medical education research should have practical applications to the environments research is conducted in, processes within education and training, policy, or educational and training outcomes. As it is easier to measure and demonstrate, documented impact usually concerns the process of education and training (for example, influencing guideline creation; informing changes in policy; promoting professional debate; informing a new model of training).

Box 10.5 Abstract preparation top tips

1. Align any abstract to the wider themes running through the conference programme
2. Make the findings relevant and interesting to the intended audience
3. Clearly highlight the main message that you want the audience to take away from your publication or presentation. It is often useful to write a short structured draft abstract to focus thoughts
4. Seek feedback from an experienced mentor with a track-record of publications in peer-reviewed journals and presentations at conferences before any submissions
5. Take every opportunity to write or present the findings to peer groups—and act on their feedback!

Within the UK, research impact is measured formally through the UK Research Excellence Framework (REF), a process through which UK universities submit the outputs of their researchers for evaluation of those outputs' impact. Not all universities submit medical education research to the REF. Where medical education research is submitted to REF, impact case studies can be developed using approaches which combine quantitative insights (e.g. paper downloads, policy downloads, Altmetric scores which capture media attention), and qualitative insights (e.g. interviewing stakeholders to examine any changes in practice as a result of the research, collecting emails from stakeholders regarding the impact of the work).

Researching interventions within medical education

In addition to deciding the content of a learning intervention it is essential to consider both how and where the intervention will be delivered. Important considerations are:

- At what stage are the learners in the novice-expert development continuum?
- To what extent is learning instructor-directed or learner-directed?
- Do all the instructors provide identical interventions to all learners?
- Is feedback provided and, if so, how, and when is this done?
- Who decides when the training ends (learner or instructor)?

Comparing interventions across groups

When designing a study to evaluate the effectiveness of a novel educational intervention, a competing intervention may be considered so that a comparison can be made between the learning outcomes associated with both interventions. ❶ However, adequate randomization across the groups can be impossible due to individual differences in instructors and learners, as well as differences in contexts. Randomization and the presence of a control group are not essential when researching the value and impact of an intervention within medical education. New programmes of teaching, for example, can be considered from the perspective of student, teacher, and wider stakeholder experience, and outcomes.

Choice of outcome measures

There are a variety of outcome measures that can be used to evaluate the effectiveness of educational interventions. One model that can be used is Kirkpatrick's model (Figure 5.1)[5]:

- Level 1—Reaction, which is the degree to which learners consider the training to be engaging, beneficial, and relevant

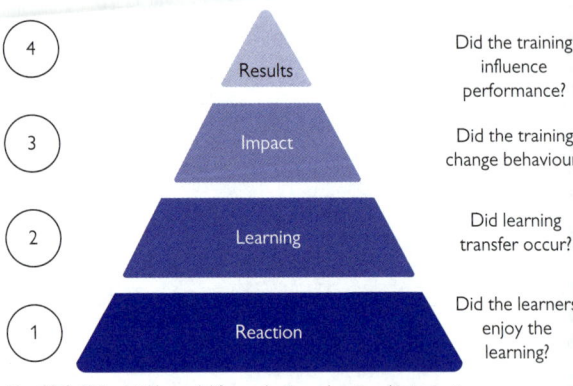

Fig. 10.1 Kirkpatrick's model for evaluating educational interventions.

- Level 2—Learning, which is the gain in knowledge, skills, and/or attitude experienced by learners
- Level 3—Behaviour, which is the degree to which learners subsequently apply learning in their real-life practice
- Level 4—Results, which is the degree to which clinical outcomes are improved (e.g. healthcare outcomes for patients)

Although the outcome measures increase in importance, they also become more difficult to attain since these outcomes require transfer of learning to actual professional performance and practice. Medical education has typically focused on reaction (did learners enjoy an intervention, or do they feel more confident) and the effectiveness of interventions (how well learners perform or how valuable an outcome is) but it is likely that in the future there will be greater emphasis on efficiency (which considers the resource utilization, including the time required to achieve competency and financial costs). Within medical education research, it is increasingly understood that learner satisfaction and confidence are poor outcome measures—though they may be useful within the local evaluation of an intervention, they are not understood to be high-quality outcomes within formal research.

Understanding the processes that influence educational interventions

Interventions that we think will improve learning outcomes frequently have little or no impact on learning outcomes! This finding has led to an increasing interest in understanding the process of learning interventions. These interventions are dynamic and typically involve a series of interactions (processes) that can have an impact on learning outcomes. These processes include:

- Interaction between learner and learning content (including learner's motivation, preferred learning style, preparation for learning, and prior knowledge)
- Interaction between learner and teacher
- Interaction between learners

The use of action research

Action research may not be familiar to many medical educators, but it has been widely used in other education contexts, from primary to higher education, to effectively achieve change in complex educational systems—for example, the introduction of new teaching interventions and curriculum development. The action research perspective considers that effective change is not possible unless there are dynamic cycles of action/research/action. An initial cycle of the intervention (the action) is applied to a situation and there is critical reflection on the resultant effect (the research). The insights from critical reflection lead to a refined intervention, which is then applied to the situation. Through the repeated cycles, effective change in the organizational system and the intervention occurs by having greater understanding of the complex factors that influence the implementation of the intervention. An important aspect of action research is the involvement of all stakeholders, including administrators, teachers, and learners, in all phases and cycles.

Finding support

Finding support whilst in the process of conducting any inquiry project, whether research, evaluation, or scholarship is important, but within medical education there are particular challenges.

Firstly, the dominant perspective in medicine is that of biomedical science with a positivist view of the world. Many potential sources of support, including people and availability of financial resources, tend to be geared to this perspective. Secondly, a substantial amount of training is required for the effective use of both qualitative and quantitative research methods. However, there are a number of short courses available as well as taught Master's programmes for individuals committed to a career in medical education research.

Finally, finding a mentor as well as a peer group or network is important for those who are novices to research, evaluation, or scholarship. The following organizations can be helpful.

ASME (Association for the Study of Medical Education)
℞ https://www.asme.org.uk
JASME (Junior Association for the Study of Medical Education)
℞ https://www.asme.org.uk/jasme
TASME (Trainee Association for the Study of Medical Education)
℞ https://www.asme.org.uk/tasme
NIHR Incubator for Clinical Education Research
℞ https://clinicaleducationresearch.org/
AMEE (Association for the Study of Medical Education)
℞ https://amee.org/home
IAMSE (International Association of Medical Science Educators)
℞ http://www.iamse.org/
AoME (Academy of Medical Educators)
℞ https://www.medicaleducators.org/
AMA (American Medical Association)
℞ https://www.ama-assn.org/
ANZAHPE (Australia and New Zealand Association for Health Professional Educators)
℞ https://www.anzahpe.org/
CAME (Canadian Association for Medical Education)
℞ https://www.came-acem.ca/

Further reading

⊃ Akman M, Wass V, Goodyear-Smith F. *How to do primary care educational research: a practical guide.* Boca Raton, FL: CRC Press, 2021.
⊃ Cohen L, Manion L, Morrison K. *Research methods in education*, 8th edn. Abingdon: Routledge, 2017.
⊃ Eva KW. Medical education research approaches. *Med Educ* 2018;52(11):1100–1102.
⊃ Gray DE. *Doing research in the real world*, 4th edn. London: Sage, 2017.
⊃ Hess GR, Tosney KW, Liegel LH. Creating effective poster presentations: AMEE Guide no. 40. *Med Teach* 2009;31(4):319–321.
⊃ Newcomer KE, Hatry HP, Wholey JS. *Handbook of practical program evaluation*, 4th edn. Chichester: John Wiley & Sons, 2015.
⊃ Ritchie J, Lewis J, Nicholls CM, Ormston R (Eds.). *Qualitative research practice: a guide for social science students and researchers*, 2nd edn. London: Sage Publications, 2013.
⊃ Stringer ET. *Action research*, 4th edn. Thousand Oaks, CA: Sage Publications, 2013.
⊃ Tavakol M, Sandars J. Quantitative and qualitative methods in medical education research: AMEE Guide No 90: Part I. *Med Teach* 2014;36(10):746–756.
⊃ Tavakol M, Sandars J. Quantitative and qualitative methods in medical education research: AMEE Guide No 90: Part II. *Med Teach* 2014;36(10):838–848.

References

1. Cook DA. Tips for a great review article: crossing methodological boundaries. *Med Educ* 2016;50(4):384–387.
2. Arksey H, O'Malley L. Scoping studies: towards a methodological framework. *Int J Soc Res Methodol* 2005;8:19–32.
3. Wong G, Greenhalgh T, Westhorp G, Pawson R. Realist methods in medical education research: what are they and what can they contribute? *Med Educ* 2012;46(1):89–96.
4. Fraser K, Wright B, Girard L, Tworek J, Paget M, Welikovich L, McLaughlin K. Simulation training improves diagnostic performance on a real patient with similar clinical findings. *Chest* 2011;139:376–381.
5. Kirkpatrick DL, Kirkpatrick JD. *Evaluating training programs*. Oakland, CA: Berrett-Koehler Publishers, 1994.

The medical educator portfolio: Documenting achievements and communicating scholarship

Zareen Zaidi, Helen R. Church, Marian C. Limacher, Ellen M. Zimmermann, and Elisa A. Zenni

Introduction

Portfolios have been used to showcase artists' work in the visual and performing arts for decades and were later used in educational settings to assess student performance. Their use to demonstrate and evaluate educators' accomplishments emerged in the 1980's and has steadily increased.[1] An Educator Portfolio (EP) is a document that catalogues and describes teaching accomplishments and educational innovations. It details the range, quantity, quality, and scholarly nature of educational work beyond a standard curriculum vitae.[2]

Similarly to artist and student portfolios, an EP can be started at any stage of a medical educator's career but, in our opinion, the earlier, the better. For many medical school faculties, the core elements of a person's EP may be included in one's professional curriculum vitae. However, as this chapter explains, as educational interest and experience out-grows the sub-division it is often afforded within a professional curriculum vitae, an ▶ EP provides a dedicated, purposeful space to collate, reflect upon, and develop an educational career.

What are the different types of educator portfolio?

EPs can be categorized as *developmental* or *promotional*.[2]

A developmental EP tracks educational activities, helps with goal setting, can provide evidence on which to discuss career planning with mentors, and serves as a basis for eventual promotion. The document is formative, flexible, and dynamic—an ever-growing evidence base of educational activity and reflection.

In contrast, a promotional EP is more focused, aligned to the specific criteria laid out in an institution's promotional guidelines, and forms a more summative, 'fixed' document for submission to a promotion panel. Promotional EPs are likely to be created through drawing on evidence stored within the developmental EP; by purposefully selecting presentations, reflections, and evidence of scholarship, a promotional EP ∴ creates a narrowly focused snapshot.[3]

Table 11.1 summarizes the comparison between the two portfolios.

Early EPs were paper collections, but current formats are typically electronic. Some are a simple text document, while others use more sophisticated electronic platforms, using images, audio, video, animation, and

Table 11.1 Comparison of developmental and promotional educator portfolios (adapted from Baldwin et al.[2])

	Developmental educator portfolio	Promotional educator portfolio
What is it?	A comprehensive repository containing a broad perspective on all educational activities.	A focused document highlighting and summarizing key educational achievements.
Why is it useful?	Aids the educator to reflect on completed educational activities, to identify future goals and strategies to meet said goals. Provides an evidence base for discussions with mentors/supervisors Evidence can be purposefully selected to populate a promotional EP.	Provides a structured, organized approach to presenting evidence for career advancement opportunity, with specific examples, timelines, and outcomes.
Who needs it?	All those with educational roles. Encouraging early-career academics to establish their developmental portfolio will serve them well throughout their subsequent career.	Educators applying for promotion or advancement (e.g. promotion application/job interview).

Table 11.1 (Contd.)

	Developmental educator portfolio	Promotional educator portfolio
When is it updated?	Either at specific times of the year, or sporadically after major educational activity. Having dates in one's diary to review and update the portfolio at regular intervals is encouraged to maintain an up-to-date record.	During preparation for career advancement opportunities, where selected data is drawn from the developmental EP to evidence the criteria being assessed for the career advancement opportunity.

internet technologies to build a digital collection of educational work that demonstrates both competence and reflection. ▶ The key is to establish a place to compile evidence—digital or analogue—which is easy to organize, accessible as required, and aids the user in updating/creating the desired portfolio output.

Creating an educator portfolio

A successful EP requires time, planning, and organization. An understanding of the underlying principles for documenting educator activities and a knowledge of available or required templates will help lead to the creation of a portfolio that effectively displays the educator's strengths and accomplishments.

EPs are often speciality-specific with headings and sub-headings that reflect the diversity of educational experiences. Some general principles apply that form the foundation for an EP that can then be customized to reflect medical specialty activities.[4,5]

Educator portfolio templates

While compiling evidence is important ▶ a portfolio must demonstrate both the breadth and the impact of activities undertaken by the educator. With this in mind, the Association of American Medical Colleges (AAMC) identified two guiding principles for educators documenting their activities across the EP categories, known as the 'Q2Engage' model (Quality, Quantity, Engage):[6]

- **Excellence**, including both the quality and quantity (how much, how often, with whom) of educational activities. Given the wide range of activities that an educator performs in their role, categorizing similar activities and 'filing' them together is helpful for both compiling the evidence in a systematic way, and when finding and accessing evidence to serve a specific purpose.
- **Engagement** with the education community, showing that the activity was grounded within and/or contributed to the wider educational community. An example of this might be utilizing journal articles or other academic publications to demonstrate that the activity was informed by the current literature in that field, or by directly contributing to the literature on the chosen topic through presentation and/or publications.

Imagine the portfolio as a filing cabinet. The different-coloured folders within represent different activity categories, and inside each of these, relevant evidence is collated and contextualized.

Template 1: Promotional educator portfolio

Here is an example of the 'folders' which might be featured in a promotional EP filing cabinet:[6–9]

- Teaching and facilitating learning

Teaching is defined as any activity with the intent of fostering learning. Concise details of years, hours devoted to the activity, and numbers and types of learners demonstrate the quantity of teaching. Quality may be shown through learner evaluations (● though we appreciate that learner evaluations alone are not a robust way of evaluating teaching quality because of the presence of bias in evaluations, teachers may wish to selectively synthesize helpful evaluations to offer constructive insights as part of a broader picture of teaching competence), peer reviews, other statements from students, and description of teaching awards. Educator reflections would also be welcomed here, with the potential for peer discussions to be documented through written or audio modalities.

- Learner assessment

Learner assessment includes any activity which aims to evaluate learners' knowledge, skills, and attitudes. It may include assessment of learners in areas in which the faculty teaches, as well as areas separate from the teaching activities (e.g. writing national exam questions). The faculty should state their role in the assessment (e.g. being an examiner/moderator, development, or implementation of a specific assessment tool), the numbers and types (e.g. under/postgraduate) of learners involved, and when possible relate the assessment results to evidence of teaching effectiveness and/or record feedback on assessments from learners.

- Curriculum development

Curriculum development is a longitudinal programme that includes more than one teaching session or presentation of educational activities and has been evaluated.[6] The topic and type of curriculum, number, and types of learners, educator's role (designing, delivering, evaluating the curriculum), and location of delivery (e.g. department, institution, regional, national, etc.) can be included. Curricula may be described using the GNOME (Goals, Needs, Objectives, Methods, Evaluation) framework[10] to demonstrate quality:

- Goals—appropriate for learners and context, with specific and measurable objectives
- Needs assessment of learners—used to determine and refine the goals and objectives
- Objectives—how learners will achieve the goals of the programme—stepwise approach to achieving the desired outcomes
- Methods of teaching/learning—should be aligned with the learning objectives, and appropriate for the type(s) of learner(s)
- Evaluation—both learner assessment and feedback and curriculum/programme evaluation. Assessment methods should be reliable, valid, and feasible, and be used to refine the needs assessment of the learners and adjust the goals, objectives, and teaching methods.

- Mentoring and advising

Mentoring is defined as a *'sustained, committed relationship from which both parties obtain reciprocal benefits'*,[6] whereas 'advising' involves a more limited relationship in both length of time and scope. Documentation would include details regarding the number of individuals (including names if appropriate), time and duration engaged, and accomplishments or outcomes of the mentees or advisees.

- Educational management, leadership, and administration

Educational leadership involves achieving results through directing others and transforming organizations by demonstrating the value of work through evaluation, dissemination, and maximization of resources. Specific details about the time involved, numbers and types of learners impacted, and duration of role, help to document the depth of involvement and impact. ► This is a particularly important category for those working clinically, particularly if they also supervise clinical students or trainees (in a formal capacity or otherwise).

- Educational research and scholarship

Evidence-based education is relevant to all educators, be that within an active researcher/supervisor role, or as a consumer of scholarship which might influence educational practice. Either way, documenting this engagement and demonstrating its impact might be done through listing publications, presentations, or academic posters presented at conferences, or through reflection on articles of interest which have led to a change in educational delivery. We would encourage educators to also think more broadly about impact and consider changes others have made as a result of your research/scholarship, e.g. colleagues, changes of practice within your department, public outreach, and community engagement events.
• Recognition of excellence

This evidence might be woven throughout the other categories according to its context, or alternatively compiled within its own category. Either way, collating and reflecting on awards and prizes should be showcased.

Template 2: Developmental educator portfolio
Developmental EPs would closely resemble the promotional categories of evidence as above, but in addition may also include a statement of educational philosophy, five-year educator goals, and emails or letters of gratitude from learners, where the latter might be filed within the 'Recognition of Excellence' category.
• Statement of educational philosophy

The statement of educational philosophy describes the educator's approach to teaching. It should be rooted in educational theory or principles (see ➲ Chapter 2 of this handbook, particularly the content on grand theories), demonstrate application to the teacher's experience (through examples of teaching and professional development courses), include self-reflection on educational strengths and practice, and provide specific examples of how the philosophy translates into educational practice. The statement can be brief but aims to serve as a reminder of one or more foundational beliefs which underpin the overall aims of the educator's teaching approaches: *what* the educator wishes to provide and/or impart to their students in the broadest sense of learning and *why* this is important to their educational development. Given that this philosophy is likely to evolve with increased educational experience, educational philosophy statements are dynamic and require intermittent review and updating.
▶ Dalton et al. (2018)[8] provide practical advice for those getting started with their teaching philosophy statement to ask one's own educational mentor or supervisor to share their statement as an example, and to request them to review a first draft of the philosophical statement itself.
• Medium/long-term career plan

A medium/long-term career plan, such as a 'five-year plan', must strike the balance between ambitious educational goals that allow the educator to grow and realistic, and clear steps to how such objectives might be achieved.

Personalizing the portfolio
While categories have been suggested above, educators should note that specific templates may vary from institution to institution, often combining or splitting some of the sections and furthermore, that personalization is

often the key to ensuring engagement with a portfolio. Similarly, some evidence may be better housed in different categories than the suggestions above and categories might widen their remit to include evidence not listed above.

Systematicity and standardization are key to ensuring an organized, accessible portfolio, but the 'folders' within the filing cabinet are as individual to the educator as the evidence that they contain.

Peer review

A recently created EP by an early career educator usually benefits from expert review by a senior colleague. Such review is particularly valuable for EPs destined to be submitted for promotion or other academic milestones or posted online.

Expert review prior to submission was one of the twelve tips for creating an EP, as recommended by Little-Weinert and Mazziotti.[9]

Challenges in using educator portfolios

Given that there are many different templates for EPs, ❶ their subjectivity has been criticized and the need for clear guidelines and standards has been highlighted.[1]

∴ Tools exist which measure both the quality and educational impact of the activities listed in an EP, such as one developed by Chandran et al. (Figure 11.1).[10,11]

The EP analysis tool in Figure 11.1 has seven sections paralleling those in the EP template, including the 'Measures of Educational Scholarship' section that is designed to holistically evaluate the whole EP. The tool encompasses 18 quantitative items and 25 qualitative items. The developers of the tool encourage faculty to keep the quantitative measures simple and not just focus on the quantity, e.g. number of teaching activities, but also quality, e.g. diversity of teaching methods. In order to simplify the qualitative items on the tool and to provide 'competitive equivalence', a three-level scoring system (one: novice, two: intermediate, three: expert) is utilized.

Acceptability of educator portfolios

EP models often describe the need for balanced EPs, which incorporate an emphasis on structure as well as social interactions. Personalized coaching and meetings with peers to review portfolio content and personal development plans were noted to be key to the success of an EP. ❶ Faculty users have criticized that EP assignments as being too directive or rigid. Others caution that the EP 'should not serve as an exhaustive repository of teaching activities, but should be tailored to the needs of the teacher by being a selective and purposeful collection of materials that allows for critical reflection'.[12] Teachers appreciate the opportunity to select their own coaches, as rapport and trust are fostered when teachers choose their own personal coaches.[13]

Development of electronic educator portfolios

Portfolios vary in their format and can be paper-based or electronic. Research from undergraduate education shows that medical students do not find electronic portfolios labour intensive; this is because most of today's students are arguably more familiar with, and adaptable to, utilizing newer digital technologies.[14] Current standards that exist within institutions (where institutions require educators to keep portfolios) may adhere to paper-based portfolios, and therefore some faculty resistance to electronic EPs might be simply down to the systematic difficulties of introducing a new 'system'. ▶ Acceptability and use in continuing professional development of electronic platforms has been shown to be influenced by technical support and ∴ provision of such support is an important factor to consider in the implementation of EPs. Some higher degree courses include an EP as part of its curriculum.

Additionally, institutions should establish a process for the faculty to update portfolio contents, paying attention to the fact that contents should be updated throughout the academic year rather than at the end of each calendar year. It would be helpful to provide the option for the faculty to be

Educator Portfolio Section	Evaluation Items	Quantitative Score	Qualitative Rating*
EDUCATIONAL PHILOSOPHY	1. Self-reflection, self-appraisal		X
	2. Philosophy *both* rooted in theory or principle *and* applied to experience		X
	3. Evidence of philosophy applied throughout EP		X
FIVE-YEAR GOALS	4. Goals set appropriately high		X
	5. Focused and realistic plan		X
1.1 Teaching	6. Learner number score	X	
	7. Teaching hours	X	
	8. Teaching Impact Score	X	
	9. Variety of teaching strategies		X
1.2 Assessment of Learners	10. Roles in learner evaluation	X	
	11. Learner assessment strategies		X
	12. Balance of methods at upper level of "Miller's Triangle"		X
	13. Results of evaluations of learners		X
1.3 Evaluation of Teaching	14. Teaching evaluation score	X	
	15. Multiple sources and types of evaluations		X
	16. Response to evaluations of the candidate's teaching		X
II. Curriculum Development	17. Curriculum Impact Index	X	
	18. Curriculum Role Score	X	
	19. Quality of goals/objectives		X
	20. Quality of needs assessment		X
	21. Quality of methods		X
	22. Quality of evaluation		X
III. Mentoring/Advising	23. Number of mentees/advisees	X	
	24. Mentee productivity: Publications, awards, grants	X	
	25. Mentee professional advancement: Promotions, leadership roles	X	
	26. Quality of mentoring		X
IV. Educational Leadership/Administration	27. Program Leadership Index: Number, geographic impact, and duration of leadership	X	
	28. Committee Leadership index: Number, geographic impact, and duration of leadership	X	
	29. Membership on educational committees: Number and duration of involvement	X	
	30. Quality of leadership role		X

Fig. 11.1 (*Contd.*)

V. Other Information	31. Reviewing or Moderating Index	X	
	32. Awards: Geographic impact level	X	
	33. Personal professional development in education	X	
MEASURES OF EDUCATIONAL SCHOLARSHIP (Whole EP evaluation)			
A. SCHOLARLY APPROACH TO EDUCATION	34. Application of an accepted model or a structured approach		X
	35. Glassick's Criterion 1: Clear goals		X
	36. Glassick's Criterion 2: Adequate preparation		X
	37. Glassick's Criterion 3: Appropriate methods		X
	38. Glassick's Criterion 4: Significant results		X
	39. Glassick's Criterion 5: Effective communications		X
	40. Glassick's Criterion 6: Reflective critique		X
	41. Overall Scholarly Approach (Total 34-40)		X
B. PRODUCTS OF EDUCATIONAL SCHOLARSHIP	42. Scholarly Productivity Index (Peer-reviewed publications [print or electronic]. Peer-reviewed/Invited presentations and workshops; Non-peer-reviewed publication/presentation; Books; educational Product Dissemination score)	X	
	43. Grants Index (PI or Co-PI; No.; geographical impact, $$)	X	
ITEM COUNT		18	25

Fig. 11.1 Academic Paediatric Association educator portfolio (EP): Analysis Tool Item Summary; *Qualitative ratings: 1 = Novice; 2 = Intermediate; 3 = Expert (elaborated with comments, as needed). Reproduced with permission from Latha Chandran, Maryellen Gusic, Constance Baldwin et al., Evaluating the performance of medical educators: a novel analysis tool to demonstrate the quality and impact of educational activities, 2023, Wolters Kluwer Health Inc.

able to grant access to selected peers or mentors to their EP, for feedback purposes. Finally, institutions must ensure that they are using the best-suited technology platform.[15]

Outcomes of educator portfolios

Research from higher education shows that while educators feel that that EPs are useful resources to document and reflect upon educational activity, ❗ they have concerns about the time demands required to develop and maintain their EP.[16] In medical education, researchers have shown an increasing use of EPs at institutions. This has been followed by efforts to develop EP evaluation standards that describe what constitutes excellence in teaching, productivity, or evidence of critical self-reflection on teaching to drive continued professional development. As described in the section on standards for documentation earlier in the chapter, EP evaluators are encouraged to use a described evaluation framework, which emphasizes not just quantity but also quality, scholarly approach, and reflection by faculty.

❶ To date, there is little evidence to support or refute the value of EPs in professional development.[17] Beecher et al. interviewed 10 faculty who prepared EPs for promotion. Faculty indicated that reflection about education had occurred, resulting in:

(a) surfacing of dilemmas in practice
(b) seeking support
(c) reformulating educational practice
(d) transformation of educational practice.

The authors concluded that EP preparation resulted in reflection on educational practice, which promoted faculty development.[18] Pinsky et al. interviewed 48 medical school faculty who were awarded distinguished teaching awards. The faculty commented on reflective practice being integral in planning and anticipation of teaching. They described the reflection process as beginning in the planning stages of teaching activities, i.e. anticipatory reflection. During this phase, they considered how they would involve learners, innovate while designing the session, create a positive atmosphere for learning and engage learners, while preparing adequately and limiting content. They also noted reflection in action, described as a response to dynamic changes in the teaching encounter by maintaining flexibility during the session. Further reflection-on-action was described as a thoughtful analysis of what went well, how it could go better, and how could they improve their teaching ability in the future.[19]

Emerging conceptual frameworks for educator portfolios

While the quality of teaching and learning has been a focus of attention for many decades, Boyers's work draws attention to ▶ 'teaching as scholarship' in contrast to 'teaching versus research' and subsequently Glassick's definitions of 'excellence in scholarship' have set standards for assessing scholarship.[20] Glassick's six standards (listed in Figure 11.1) focus on excellence in scholarship and provide a useful tool to assess the quality of scholarship. Philosophers like Dewey and Schön have described the importance of reflection, emphasizing that teaching is a form of action research where practice, reflection, and reaction on teaching practice give way to new knowledge, building on the concept of 'reflection-on-action' and 'reflection-in-action'.[21] More recently, Trigwell et al. use Glassick's standards and Dewey and Schön's concepts of reflection to provide a framework incorporating such deliberate practice to assess the extent to which teachers are engaging with scholarship:[22]

(1) *The Informed Dimension* is the extent to which the teacher engages with scholarly contributions of others, including the teaching and learning literature both in a general sense and also in specific reference to their field;

(2) *The Reflection Dimension* focuses on the educator's reaction to their own teaching practice and their students' learning;

(3) *The Communication Dimension* focuses on how the educator effectively communicates aspects of practice and theoretical ideas about teaching and learning, both pertaining to grand educational theories, and more nuanced ideas relating to their specific field;

(4) *The Conception Dimension* focuses on their conceptions of teaching and learning, whether the focus of their activities is on student learning and teaching or mainly on teaching.

This model can be useful for teachers, EP coaches or facilitators, and promotion committees who are assessing and providing feedback on EPs. While Glassick's criteria focus on the quality of scholarship, this model focuses more globally on multi-dimensional aspects of the 'scholarship of teaching'. The three-level scoring system (one: novice, two: intermediate, three: expert) proposed by Baldwin et al.[23] can be used for this model as well to allow EP coaches and promotion committees to assess EPs. While the theory and the dimensions serving as the foundational model for an EP seem clear, ❶ the practical aspects of collecting relevant data remain challenging for modern faculty. Still, recent data suggest that the process of completing the EP promoted self-reflection on educational practices, serving as a compelling rational for its important role in medical education.[24]

Areas for future research

There remain gaps in the literature regarding the benefits of implementation of EPs, i.e. does the use of an EP help educators become more thoughtful, reflective, and deliberate about their pedagogical practices and research? Do EPs become a checklist or a repository for educators? Do EPs end up as 'busy work' for already busy clinicians, i.e. do they view EPs only as an essential task for promotion? The near-perfect storm of pressures on physicians to increase patient care-billing, along with the challenges of tele-medicine, and increasing electronic health record documentation burdens contribute to job dissatisfaction and physician burnout. In this environment, it is increasingly important to firmly establish the positive benefits of EPs for clinician educators in terms of clarity of their personal career goals, sat-isfaction with their professional development, and readiness for successful promotion.

The impact of EPs on professional development needs to be established using methodologically sound research. Studies evaluating the degree of transformative change secondary to use of EPs are needed. It is well-established from research in undergraduate education that students need to be coached while using portfolios. Similar evidence is emerging from the lit-erature on faculty EPs. The assessment rubrics available for EPs need valid-ation studies, with further thought on how to assess transformative change.

Conclusion

The EP is a valuable tool for recording educators' activities and accomplishments. It can be used to assist in evaluation, development of individual learning plans, and promotion of reflection and professional growth. Many institutions adopt the use of EPs to assist the decision-making process during promotion opportunities, and therefore more general guidance pertaining to what constitutes excellence in educators is required to allow individual institutions to set fair standards for evaluating educator performance. The need to provide EP coaches may become a useful strategy for successful implementation within a given institution.

References

1. Simpson D, Hafler J, Brown D, Wilkerson L. Documentation systems for educators seeking academic promotion in U.S. medical schools. *Acad Med* 2004;79(8):783–790.
2. Baldwin CD, Gusic M, Chandran L. Leadership lesson. The educator portfolio: a tool for career development. Association of American Medical Colleges. 2013. https://www.aamc.org/professional-development/affinity-groups/gfa/faculty-vitae/educator-portfolio-tool
3. Simpson D, Fincher RM, Hafler J, Irby DM, Richards BF, Rosenfeld GC, Viggiano TR. Advancing Educators and Education: Defining the Components and Evidence of Educational Scholarship. Proceedings from the Association of American Medical Colleges Group on Educational Affairs Consensus Conference on Educational Scholarship, 9–10 February 2006, Charlotte, NC/ Washington DC: AAMC 2007.
4. Thomas JV, Sanyal R, O'Malley JP, Singh SP, Morgan DE, Canon CL. A guide to writing academic portfolios for radiologists. *Acad Radiol* 2016;23(12):1595–1603. doi:10.1016/j.acra.2016.08.015.
5. Sidhu NS. The teaching portfolio as a professional development tool for anaesthetists. *Anaesth Intensive Care* 2015;43(3):328–334.
6. Simpson D, Anderson MB. Feature: Educational scholarship: how do we define and acknowledge it?. AAMC, 2006. https://www.aamc.org/members/gfa/faculty_vitae/148580/educational_scholarship.html
7. Kuhn GJ. Faculty development: The educator's portfolio: its preparation, uses, and value in academic medicine. *Acad Emerg Med* 2004;11(3):307–311.
8. Dalton CL, Wilson A, Agius S. Twelve tips on how to compile a medical educator's portfolio. *Med Teach* 2018;40(2):140–145.
9. Little-Wienert K, Mazziotti M. Twelve tips for creating an academic teaching portfolio. *Med Teach* 2018;40(1):26–30.
10. Chandran L, Gusic M, Baldwin C, et al. Evaluating the performance of medical educators: a novel analysis tool to demonstrate the quality and impact of educational activities. *Acad Med* 2009;84(1):58–66.
11. Chandran L, Gusic M, Baldwin C, et al. APA educator portfolio analysis tool. *MedEdPORTAL* 2009;5:1659.
12. Sidhu NS. The teaching portfolio as a professional development tool for anaesthetists. *Anaesth Intensive Care* 2015;43(3):328–334.
13. Tigelaar DE, Dolmans DH, de Grave WS, Wolfhagen IH, van der Vleuten CP. Participants' opinions on the usefulness of a teaching portfolio. *Med Educ* 2006;40(4):371–378.
14. Tan R, Qi Ting JJ, Zhihao Hong D, et al. Medical student portfolios: a systematic scoping review. *J Med Educ Curric Dev* 2022;9:23821205221076022.
15. Lewis KO, Baker RC. The development of an electronic educational portfolio: an outline for medical education professionals. *Teach Learn Med* 2007;19(2):139–147.
16. Tucker PD, Stronge JH, Gareis CR, Beers CS. The efficacy of portfolios for teacher evaluation and professional development: do they make a difference? *EAQ* 2003;39(5):572–602.
17. Mann K, Gordon J, MacLeod A. Reflection and reflective practice in health professions education a systematic review. *Adv Health Sci Educ Theory Pract* 2009;14(4):595.
18. Beecher A, Lindemann JC, Morzinski JA, Simpson DE. Use of the educator's portfolio to stimulate reflective practice among medical educators. *Teach Learn Med* 1997;9(1):56–59.
19. Pinsky LE, Monson D, Irby DM. How excellent teachers are made: reflecting on success to improve teaching. *Adv Health Sci Educ* 1998;3(3):207–215.
20. Glassick CE. Boyer's expanded definitions of scholarship, the standards for assessing scholarship and the elusiveness of the scholarship of teaching. *Acad Med* 2000;75(9):877–880.

21. Schon DA. The new scholarship requires a new epistemology. *Change* 1995;27(6):26–34.
22. Trigwell K, Martin E, Benjamin J, Prosser M. Scholarship of teaching: a model. *High Educ Res Dev* 2000;19(2):155–168.
23. Baldwin C, Chandran L, Gusic M. Guidelines for evaluating the educational performance of medical school faculty: priming a national conversation. *Teach Learn Med* 2011;23(3):285–297.
24. Deshpande S, Chari S, Radke U, Karemore T. Evaluation of the educator's portfolio as a tool for self-reflection: faculty perceptions. *Educ Health (Abingdon)* 2019;32(2):75–78.

Challenges
in medical education

*Marcus A. Henning, Iain Doherty, Megan E.L.
Brown, and Mataroria Lyndon*

Introduction

There are innumerable challenges in medical education, as with any educational process in any discipline. The profession of medicine requires training beyond graduation which inevitably involves further challenges and complexities in addition to undergraduate teaching and learning. The learning and teaching of medicine revolves around ensuring that high-stakes competencies are achieved, and this involves several interconnected constructs, such as best practice in clinical care, attaining a comprehensive knowledge base, and developing a professional attitude and identity.

To ensure medicine is taught efficiently and effectively, several components need to be considered, including:

- using suitable medical educational theories, strategies, and principles
- ensuring the curriculum is fit for purpose
- utilizing a range of instructional methods that optimize learning
- providing a wide range of appropriate learning environments and opportunities
- ensuring assessments are aligned with the learning outcomes and that they are reliable, valid, authentic, and practicable
- ensuring educators are adequately trained in the facets of medicine as determined by their practice specialty, and
- making best use of technologies including, but not limited to, the learning management system to support students in achieving learning outcomes and to support the delivery of authentic assessments.

In this chapter we start by describing the context of medical education, and highlighting the broad areas that challenge its efficacy. Next, we focus initially on the challenges associated with recruitment and admission, followed by those associated with the curriculum and its constituent parts. Finally, we draw attention to the major areas within medical education that require continued and timely attention.

Admittedly, we cannot cover all of the possible challenges in medical education, but we aim to highlight those that appear to be significant and pertinent to the global medical education community today. Uncertainty will always pervade speculation on future challenges and, indeed, the recommendations we offer should be read as a product of the state of medical education in 2022 and viewed sceptically through the lens of each reader's own context and moment in time. For, as Kelli Russel Agodon, an American poet considering the uncertainty of forward thinking in her poem 'I Don't Own Anxiety, But I Borrow It Regularly', put it:

> 'We cannot plan a party for the apocalypse
> because friends of the apocalypse know
> the apocalypse always shows up
> uninvited with a half-eaten bag of chips.'

The context of medical education and broader challenges

There are a variety of wide-ranging challenges that impact medical education both internationally, and within the UK.

▶ The major issues affecting UK doctors are those linked to increasing mobility and movement of doctors both within the UK and across global boundaries. This has implications for continuing medical education and involves decisions related to societal, political, technological, and professional issues. One clear example, indicating the need for global unity amongst doctor educators and rapid, accurate communication between professionals, are the early adaptations and lasting changes that have been instigated in response to the COVID-19 pandemic which disrupted the education sector as a whole, including face-to-face teaching in medical schools worldwide. Lessons learnt overseas can inform all doctors, no matter their geographical location. Moreover, doctors often work or travel overseas to gain educational knowledge and skills, and this has implications in terms of approving or accrediting the gains achieved. The global movement of doctors must be accounted for within online learning, and questions should be asked regarding how doctors can relate learning achieved abroad to continuing medical education and professional development portfolios.

In this subsection, we unpack the societal, political, technological, and professional issues facing doctors globally.

Overarching, contextual issues

Societal factors

These factors include addressing the social determinants of health and health disparities, and the increasing demands for healthcare due to chronic disease and an ageing population. Some of the emerging issues in medical education include the changing face of ethical conduct, patient safety, learning interactions, and the changing nature of the healthcare environment.[1]

Political factors

These factors centre around the health systems that are in place, healthcare reform in terms of service sustainability and integration of services, and the need to provide accessible healthcare. Health systems throughout the world are constantly changing as they grapple with the wider changes impacting health performance and the capacity of the healthcare system to meet the needs of a changing society. Challenges include the financial implications associated with ageing populations, increasing healthcare costs, meeting the needs of the workforce (including within training, and in relation to pay), coping with advances in medical science and technology, and meeting the expectations of patients as a consumer group.

In the UK, politics often goes hand in hand with medical education, especially given that the National Health Service explicitly and implicitly affects the delivery of medical education across the country. For example, there are major medical education implications in terms of selection, training, and retaining doctors who can deliver effective patient care within this overarching system. Brice and Corrigan[2] provide a useful and extensive discussion on the full extent of these implications.

Technological factors

Increasingly, issues within modern education concern working with big datasets of information, coping with new information generation and cognitive overload, synthesizing expertise with the learning demands of technology, and keeping abreast of emerging technologies such as the use of artificial intelligence, as well as augmented, alternative, and virtual realities.

'Big data' is an increasingly common term within healthcare and medical education. It refers to data that possesses the '3V's'; high-volume, high-velocity, and high-variety, and is usually beyond the data management and analytical capabilities of standard database software.[3] Much health data is now 'big data'. The utilization of this data has substantial potential, but judicious management of personal data is critical as 'big data' is vulnerable to online security breaches. The key to managing online security is the early detection and remediation of Botnets and malware through utilizing machine learning techniques like 'clustering'.

A further issue relates to increased availability of information for clinicians through electronic health records and the accessibility of information around diagnosis and treatment. There are inadequate numbers of clinician educators who are versed in informatics and data science to teach trainees analytic techniques and data-driven decision-making. In addition, there is an increasing need for teaching technology skills and data science to learners because of the increasing digitization of healthcare.

Professionalism factors

These elements are usually related to both desired graduate competencies, and the need to provide an exemplary service to the communities that doctors serve. There have been recent changes in educational priorities, and medical education has shifted from a focus on knowledge retention and recall to demonstrating clinical competence.[4]

In the UK, the General Medical Council (GMC) regulates doctors and sets standards for the professional conduct of both undergraduate learners, and postgraduate clinicians (including those in training, and those undergoing revalidation).

The GMC's professional capabilities framework stresses the importance of the continual development of professional values and behaviours, professional skills, and professional knowledge.[5] There are transferable needs and priority areas within this document, likely to also be of interest to a global audience:

- the development and value of utilizing standardized patients before students are exposed to patients in the 'actual' clinical environment
- learning in seemingly 'chaotic' and intense clinical environments
- coping with major environmental challenges (i.e. COVID-19) including how this affects professional conduct, e.g. managing the rise of racism
- the need for lifelong learning
- provision of exemplary information systems to ensure the progression of learning
- awareness around self-care and workload issues (such as compassion fatigue and burnout)
- developing efficient and accurate health management information systems

- the need to ensure equitable representation of minority and disadvantaged groups
- working with diverse communities in a culturally safe manner
- the need to ensure training programmes are accessible and relevant for the needs of key stakeholders.

Though each country's context (and so their social, political, technological, and professional climates) is unique, there are issues within medical education that span global boundaries. These include flexible means of working, rapid changes in technology and its provision, impacts on global and local economic markets, and ever-changing political landscapes.[2] All of these challenges have been exacerbated during the COVID-19 pandemic.

Recruitment and admissions

Before we examine the challenges of undergraduate and postgraduate medical education, we must first consider the recruitment and admission processes, which shape selection into, transition to, and progression within the medical workforce.

Recruitment can be considered in reference to students' admission into medicine, but what is often neglected is that it also pertains to the recruitment of sufficient numbers of competent *educators*. These educators are needed to implement curriculum change, as well as manage the training and development of healthcare workers. In the current era of medical education, the pace and face of medical knowledge is changing quickly, necessitating that curricula adapt to this change. For example, it is increasingly critical that medical school curricula focus on frailty, given the ageing population.

There are two fundamental questions we should ask of recruitment and admissions within medical education:

- Firstly, how do institutions and governing bodies attract students and clinical teachers into the learning of medicine and how does this influence the delivery of medical education?
- Secondly, what are the fundamental underlying issues of admission and the associated challenges within this process? How can we ensure that the best students are admitted, and the best qualified teachers are employed?

Recruitment and admissions: Central issues

● *Are medical schools admitting the best students, who will graduate to be the best doctors?*

In the UK, one of the key issues is the 'selection ratio' when there is a relative abundance of medical schools for a given number of applicants. This provides more choice for students in terms of where they would like to apply to study, but less certainty for medical schools with respect to recruiting the best students. This inevitably affects selection criteria and creates more competition between medical schools with the view to attracting the best students (and likely the best clinical teachers to teach those students). But in the long-term, the concern here is whether these students will actually become the 'best doctors' in terms of having an optimal set of personal and professional skills that meet the needs of patient care.

Cohen[4] states there are six potential ways in which students could be selected to study medicine:

1. We prescribe measures of prior educational gain through appraising, for example, the Medical College Admission Test (MCAT) scores within the US, or the Graduate Medical Schools Admissions Test (GAMSAT) scores within the UK. The scores can be viewed as a threshold measure. Admission then becomes a two-step process— first, applicants must achieve the academic threshold before being progressed to a further admission process which evaluates humanistic qualities such as desire to serve others. One way to measure these humanistic and leadership qualities is the Multiple Mini-Interview (MMI). The MMI approach tends to reduce interviewer bias as prospective

students are assessed using several stations that can capture their responses to a set of humanistic dimensions or challenging scenarios.

2. We select purely on personal characteristics first, and then on the academic thresholds mooted above. In this way, students who have compelling personal characteristics might warrant further investigation to assess whether they did not achieve the academic threshold based on doing poorly in isolated exams, or because of sociopolitical inequality affecting the support they have received.

3. We could create preferential entry for mature students who see medicine as their 'true calling' as long as they are academically able to cope with the medical programme.

4. We could remove academic criteria in relation to average academic scores (such as MCAT) and create a more refined system of gauging entry. Increasingly, medical schools are evaluating approaches to ensure that medicine is accessible to those from minoritized backgrounds (often referred to as 'widening participation'). Some widening participation admission strategies include acknowledging contextual offers that may take into account grade reductions below standard academic score requirements, where students meet pre-set eligibility criteria demonstrating that they have been disadvantaged socio-politically. There is a more expansive discussion of equity issues within recruitment, below.

5. We could comprehensively evaluate applicants' academic and non-academic past histories and credentials.

6. We could devise more complete systems with more valid weighting on each of the admission measures.

Changes need to be informed by longitudinal research to determine the most valid approach to selection.

∴ More evidence is required to support more diverse approaches to selection, such as using informed self-selection, academic achievement, general cognitive ability, as well as measuring personality and interpersonal skills.

Equity issues in recruitment.

Equity (fairness) is a difficult balance to achieve. In the UK, one of the aims of current practice is to select students who are likely to complete medical study, but at the same time increase the diversity of the medical school population and consequently the clinical workforce. However, these aspirational aims are not easily implemented in practice, as learners face barriers to progression once admitted to medical school. For example, there are concerns around gender imbalance within various areas of the clinical workforce. Gender bias, gender stereotyping, and the pressure placed on women to be primary caregivers to loved ones, pushes women towards certain specialities (such as primary care, and psychiatry) rather than other specialties (e.g. surgery). Lack of representation of women within certain specialities, and within positions of seniority and leadership in medical education is a complex, multi-layered issue, which includes obstacles such as a lack of mentors and role models, tacit messaging regarding the role of women, and lack of funding for those with less-traditional career paths.[6]

▶ In terms of encouraging diversity within the medical workforce, it is important to remove social and legal barriers to medical school access, challenge educational barriers associated with the poor treatment of medical students from minoritized backgrounds within and beyond medical school, to continue to raise awareness of how diversity benefits everyone, and work to develop a culture of inclusion across the continuum of medical education which embraces diverse perspectives.

Despite the importance of diversity, and the emerging efforts of many medical schools in exploring the challenging issues within their organizational culture that act as a barrier to equity, organizational policy often falls short. In Canada, Razack et al.[7] analysed the language used on medical school websites aimed at promoting inclusion within selection processes. They found that the messaging regarding equity within the school's selection processes were unclear. The drive to acknowledge and rectify past social injustices was not noticeably articulated and, thus, the schools were not adequately addressing their obligations to marginalized societies and communities. Diversity and inclusion issues are complex and globally relevant, although each geographical region will have its own unique challenges that need to be acknowledged and addressed.

There are numerous articles concerned with the under-representation of minoritized groups in the practice of medicine.[6–9] Learners and educators may be minoritized as a result of their ethnicity, their socioeconomic status, their sexuality, disability status, their gender, age, and other demographic factors. Racism is a particular concern and is pervasive within medicine and medical education. In the US, Rodríguez and colleagues[8] soberingly note that 'racism, promotion disparities, funding disparities, lack of mentorship, and diversity pressures exist and affect minority faculty in academic medicine'. Under-representation of minoritized people, including Indigenous and ethnic minority groups within medical education contributes to the continued marginalization of these groups, and adversely impacts the processes and outcomes of healthcare. The Black Lives Matter Movement, catapulted into the public eye during 2020, highlights the abhorrent racism and inequality experienced by Black people. Within medicine, there have been repeated calls since to action practices and policies to challenge the issues the movement drew, and continues to draw, attention to.[9] Without such advocacy which, in many places both nationally and internationally is lacking, a lack of diversity (both regarding racial and ethnic diversity), but also in respect to other demographic characteristics, means that healthcare is likely to fail to address the future health needs of all demographic levels of the community.

The importance of representation within the medical workforce is also linked to the development of cultural consciousness (understanding and communicating with people from diverse cultures), competency, and safety. Many countries throughout the world have heterogeneous populations, with diverse populations within populations. Working as a doctor or studying as a medical student involves a commitment to serve patients, who may belong to diverse community groups. Doctors and medical students must learn to interact respectfully and effectively with people from diverse cultures, who they are likely to encounter during their practice.

Diversification also requires decolonization of old or entrenched ideas that may create explicit or implicit bias. Decolonization is the practice of addressing the devastating impact and ongoing violence that European empires have perpetuated against others.[10] Ways in which we may decolonize medical education curricula are discussed in the section on potential solutions, below.

How do medical schools attract minoritized students into their programmes?

There are different pathways into medicine and each pathway has its own criteria and merits. At the University of Auckland in New Zealand different pathways into medicine exist, and therefore potential students are recruited at one of the following stages depending on their personal educational journey:

- after one year as a biomedical student; or
- graduate entry or when a student has completed their first degree; or
- preferential admission schemes which are available for domestic students only—via a Regional Rural Admission Scheme or Māori and Pacific Admission Scheme (MAPAS).

How do medical schools attract the best teachers, what are the inherent qualities required to be an effective teacher and what are the optimal training and development initiatives required?

It is important to attract teachers who not only have expertise but are also motivated to teach students. The essential characteristics of a clinical teacher are[11]:

- expert medical knowledge
- good patient rapport
- provision of a good context for learning
- inclusion of learners
- adherence to general principles of teaching, and
- utilization of case-based teaching scripts.

In addition, in the current teaching climate, expertise must extend to having technological knowledge, pedagogical knowledge, and content knowledge. That is, teachers must know their subject and discipline knowledge, how to teach their subject most effectively, and how to make use of technologies to enhance teaching and learning. The technological, pedagogical, content knowledge (TPACK or technological pedagogical content knowledge) model suggests that medical educators could view their teaching through these three concurrent lenses to ensure currency with discipline knowledge and appropriate teaching and learning methods for teaching medical education. This requires purposeful use of technologies such as adaptive learning tools to support students in the development of clinical reasoning skills.

One of the challenges to medical educators and for those training medical staff as teachers, is, 'Can these attributes be taught?'

Selection into specialty programmes has implications related to meeting the needs of the population.

With an increase in the ageing population there is a greater need for increases in the workforce both generally and within certain specialties to care for this vulnerable population.

In addition, we are mindful that a divergence has evolved between primary and secondary care in many countries, especially in the area of diagnostic purpose and role. The hospital-based specialist aims to minimize uncertainty and error and to explore possibility. In contrast, the general practitioner is a mediator between the predicament of the patient and what bioscience can offer. Therefore, the general practitioner copes with uncertainty, explores probability, and minimizes peril. This division of purpose not only impacts patient care, but the way students perceive and measure the suitability of different discipline careers options. A potential consequence being that deficiencies have been noted in the workforce due to this divergence of purpose. There are not enough people who are interested in taking on a career in primary care, general internal medicine, geriatrics, and family medicine. Certain factors appear to be important in selecting a subspecialty, namely educational experiences, the nature of patient care, income, and lifestyle, together with aspects of the hidden curriculum which influence career decisions due to culture and attitudes within the faculty.

Recruitment and admissions: Potential solutions

To meet the numbers of medical students required to sustain a well-resourced clinical environment, it is crucial that medical schools attract students who are well-motivated and see the learning of medicine as a 'high priority'. One possible solution is, rather than lower entry standards across the board, which may lead to lower retention, medical schools might target students early, pre-higher (or pre-tertiary) education, and provide students with the right subject knowledge and skills to be able to cope with medical education. Contextual admissions, which aim to better account for challenges students from minoritized backgrounds might have experienced, are another possible solution.

Some of the key factors influencing the choice of medical school, against which organizational leaders may wish to evaluate their institutional strategy, are:

1. curriculum factors (e.g. teaching methods and quality of teaching and patient access)
2. academic and non-academic reputation of the school
3. personal contact (e.g. communication accessibility and influence of partners and family)
4. location (e.g. physical accessibility, appeal of the location, and university social life)
5. facilities (e.g. access to a large hospital and teaching centre)
6. reputation for teaching, mentorship, research, and other support mechanisms, and
7. affordability and availability of scholarships.

Equity issues in recruitment

As previously stated, a diverse workforce is critical in meeting the health needs of the communities that it serves. Representation of all genders, ethnicities, and socioeconomic backgrounds, for example, benefits both those within medical education and patients. Medical students must also be equipped with the skills to interact with patients from diverse cultural backgrounds. Those responsible for shaping admissions processes and policies need to consider equity and representation to ensure the medical workforce is as inclusive as possible, and well-prepared to respond to the needs of the communities it serves.

Rodríguez and colleagues[8] put forward several recommendations for meeting the challenges of minority under-representation in medicine in the US. For example, increasing minority student enrolment can be maximized through employment of pipeline programmes aimed to cultivate competitive Black and Latinx medical school applicants (e.g. Science Students Together Reaching Instructional Diversity and Excellence

🔗 https://med.fsu.edu/sstride/home). They also propose providing useful resources to reduce student debt and inculcating a more culturally accessible curriculum.

In New Zealand, similar initiatives have been implemented, such as the Māori and Pacific Admission Scheme (MAPAS 🔗 https://www.auckland.ac.nz/en/fmhs/study-with-us/maori-and-pacific-at-the-faculty/maori-and-pacific-admission-schemes.html) which aims to enhance diversity within medicine through actively challenging the predominant medical school student characteristics (white, male, upper middle class with university-educated parents). The MAPAS scheme provides a mechanism to address previous biases in selection and supports greater representation of minority groups within the health professions in New Zealand. The MAPAS pathway involves entry into courses and these enrolled students are eligible for additional academic (group tutorials, study space, academic progress tracking) and pastoral (access to a support advisor, peer networking) support.

In Australia, similar Indigenous entry programmes have aimed to address the disparities that exist related to low numbers of Indigenous doctors (@⁺ Sadler K, Johnson M, Brunette C, et al. Indigenous Student Matriculation into Medical School: Policy and Progress. The International Indigenous Policy Journal. 2017;8(1):5 https://ojs.lib.uwo.ca/index.php/iipj/article/view/7507); estimates suggest that only 0.18% of the medical profession is Indigenous compared with 2.4% of the Australian population being Indigenous.

Targeted support to encourage admissions from groups that are underrepresented within medicine is critical. Collaboration with community stakeholders is key to designing recruitment and admissions processes, and supportive structures, which advance equity for minoritized groups. Through meaningful collaboration, in which community voices are respected, prioritized, and heard, pipeline programmes can be designed, which aim to address the cultural and financial barriers to participation that are present within medical education institutions.

There is also ongoing work within medical education to challenge colonial ideology. There are three core approaches to decolonizing curricula:

1. **Focusing on content**: what values and skills the curriculum and educators transmit; what knowledge is taught; where this knowledge is from: centring non-European voices, perspectives, experiences; and diversifying teaching resources, like anatomical models
2. **Focusing on structure**: what forms of support are offered for students from diverse backgrounds within the curriculum; is there compulsory education on decolonization; can students take electives in other disciplines that might help them to appreciate diverse perspectives
3. **Focusing on process**: shifting power relations to actively recognize students as knowledge-creating agents of change; appreciating the intersectional identities that students bring to learning; valuing and lifting up student voices, perspectives, and lived experiences; rather than teaching, accompanying students in their learning, embracing their agency, and what they bring to the table

Figure 12.1 offers examples of ways in which one might begin to decolonize the content, structure, and process of teaching or curricula.

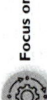

Focus on content

Examples:

- Diverse anatomical model
- Literature from outside of the global West
- Medical humanities, e.g. using film to explore colonialism, poetry to explore diverse lived experiences

Focus on structure

Examples:

- Culturally competent student support policies and services
- Compulsory decolonisation education within medical studies
- Offering electives which focus on ways of knowing within other disciplines, e.g. medical history, anthropology

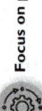

Focus on process

Examples:

- Establishing psychologically safe small group, discussion-based teaching
- Valuing student voice in curriculum design
- Adopting an intersectional approach to education
- Employing initiatives to develop students' professional identities

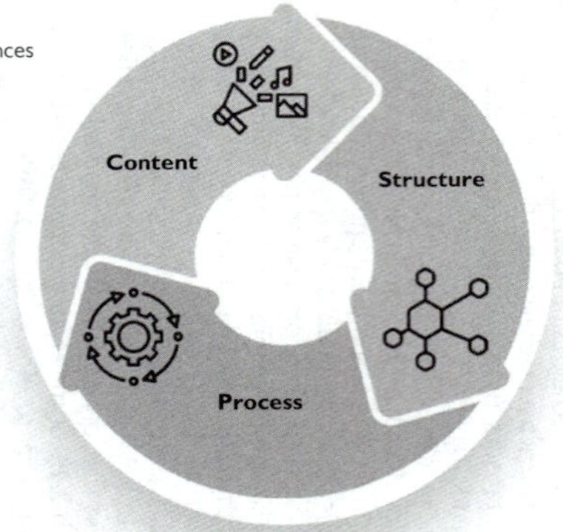

Fig. 12.1 Exemplar ways to begin decolonizing the content, structure, and process of medical education.

There are also various toolkits available for educators and medical students interested in decolonizing their approach to education, or their educational institution. These provide an extremely useful synthesis of relevant literature, and a starting point in regard to evaluating one's own teaching and approach. Mbaki, Todorova, and Hagan's framework for self-assessment and resource toolbox is a useful start for educators,[10] whilst Becoming a Doctor's Decolonising Guide for Medical Students is an excellent resource for learners.

@* https://issuu.com/soyouwanttodecoloniseyourmedicalschool/docs/so_you_want_to_decolonise_your_medical_school_v2_

How do medical schools attract students into their programmes?

In the US, a new initiative that is being trialled in one medical school (the University of Louisville) is to provide a Guaranteed Entrance to Medical School (GEMS) programme, which occurs prior to university. (To read more about this programme, please see: *Coffey JA. Addressing the Distinctive Needs of Guaranteed Entrance to Medical School (GEMS) Students. 2004* or @* https://louisville.edu/medicine/admissions/programs/gems). These programmes are used to attract highly motivated and academically able students and aims to minimize their educational expenses as well as unnecessary worry regarding eventual entry into medical school. The GEMS programme (not to be confused with the use of the GEMS acronym within the UK, where the term GEMS most often refers to graduate entry medicine) provides strong support systems to ensure student success and aims to guide them in their chosen career in medicine. One area of caution with guaranteed admission is related to locking in a defined career at such a young age. Students may also be pressured (e.g. from their families) to remain in their prescribed course of study even though, as they mature, they may realize that other study options suit them better.

When comparing graduate (those who already have a higher education/tertiary qualification) versus undergraduate entry programmes, the assumption is that graduate-entry students will be more mature and capable than their latter counterparts. In their study, Dodds et al.[12] found that there was a marginal advantage in academic performance, with graduate-entry students performing better on assessments of bioscience knowledge and clinical skills over 2 years. However, they asserted that the effect was small, and this difference would unlikely translate into a substantial subsequent difference in terms of medical competency. Feeley and Biggerstaff report that changes in medical school entrant demographics within the UK (i.e. an increasing number of graduate-entry students) has not altered approaches to learning, including student motivation.[13]

It is difficult to answer the questions mostly asked when considering academic faculty requirements. For example, how do medical schools attract the best teachers and what are the inherent qualities required, and what are the optimal training and development initiatives required? However, in part-response, it can be useful to consider the reasons why clinicians want to teach. The top 10 reasons as to why teachers are motivated to teach medical students have been quoted and ranked as[14]:

1. I teach because I want to help my students become good doctors
2. I like the challenge of teaching students as effectively as possible
3. I teach students to show them the correct way of clinical practice in my specialty

4. I enjoy spending time with students in small groups
5. I teach because I have been inspired to teach by my mentors
6. I teach to ensure the students appreciate my specialty in a favourable way
7. I teach to be challenged in my established views
8. The teaching I had as a medical student has inspired me to want to teach
9. I teach because I feel responsible for the student learning outcomes of my efforts, and/or
10. I teach because I can enhance my knowledge and understanding of resident doctors.

When attracting teachers—it will likely be important to select candidates using these criteria and consider other models of best practice.[11] Further questions that need to be answered are: How do we gauge the ability of teachers to teach? What professional development might be required to ensure engagement in lifelong learning for teaching?

The issue of lifelong learning is crucially linked to faculty development. The GMC professional capabilities document could provide useful guidelines as to how to promote development and auditing in this area. They propose a framework based on several domains, such as professional values and behaviours, which includes facets related to professional integrity, ensuring accountability, demonstrating emotional resilience and situational awareness, being cognisant of patient safety concerns, being aware of limitations and implementing practices to rectify these, and so forth.[4]

In 2006, Steinert and colleagues[15] conducted a systematic review to review the quality of evidence regarding the impact of faculty development interventions on knowledge, attitudes, and skills with respect to medical educators and the educational systems they serve. Some of the key features raised by the review were the value of such educational interventions in terms of being involved in experiential learning, being exposed to the provision of feedback, and creating effective peer and collegial relationships. However, they suggested that methodological limitations in the literature impacted the quality of evidence in this area. Further research is likely necessary to determine the efficacy of varied faculty development interventions at both individual and organizational levels.

There are several formal educational initiatives that aim to enhance faculty development in relation to medical education. Many institutions globally now offer courses of postgraduate study on the topic of medical education for clinicians. In the wake of COVID-19, many of these courses now run exclusively online, or in a blended model, and involve the provision of regular and informative feedback, include engaging in formal assessments, and provide their participants with access to innovative learning experiences. In line with the recommendations from Steinert et al.'s[15] systematic review, one of the challenges of medical education is to ensure that such postgraduate courses of study are fit for purpose. Many of the evaluation methods used in universities are aimed at reaction (how learners feel about the course of study) or learning (how well they do in assessments). It is important to consider levels of behaviour (how learners apply what they learn), results (organizational benefits), and the impact these courses have on the wider community, including on patient care. However, organizations' current focus is understandable, as these latter three criteria (levels of Kirkpatrick's model) are very difficult to measure due to issues related to the mobility of the workforce and willingness of a representative sample to engage in rigorous longitudinal research. (↪ See Chapter 8: Evaluation and feedback).

Curriculum

A curriculum is more than simply a syllabus or a document describing the content that people must learn. It describes all the constituent parts that allow for optimal teaching and learning to take place. Learning in a specialized context can be described as a process in which knowledge of a particular discipline is assimilated and implies that new knowledge is added to existing knowledge.[16] Evidence of learning implies that new knowledge has been stored and understood, even if the level of understanding is rudimentary. In the medical sciences, knowledge acquisition and retention are relatively more important in the early medical years but, as learners progress, they need to show evidence of application of these knowledge and skill areas, such as in the area of clinical reasoning, and the ability to solve complex problems. The curriculum scaffolds students through to applying knowledge and skills they have learned and to then applying these to clinical practice once they qualify.

The learning process encompasses learning outcomes, content, educational strategies, learning opportunities, assessment, and the educational environment. ▶ Each component has its challenges, and the ultimate challenge is getting the balance right to graduate health professionals who are ready to meet the challenges of patient care and to create an optimally balanced workforce. This requires careful consideration of the integral parts of the teaching and learning environment, then a curriculum is developed by synthesizing the foundational and applied sciences as they relate to the practice of medicine.

Many medical postgraduate and undergraduate curricula are either transferring to online platforms or are taught with a combination of face-to-face teaching with online resources supporting the lecture-based or small group teaching environments. For example, the University of Auckland medical programme staff have developed a medical portal, which provides extensive access to associated learning resources and management systems. Informal discussions with students suggest that such portals are information-rich but suffer the problem of coping with multiple platforms and the ever-expanding knowledge domain, ease of navigation, and making assessment information more transparent. The advent of e-assessment improves efficiency in marking and allows for extensive feedback. Clearly utilizing more e-assessments and more integrated online learning platforms are the way to the future, given their inherent flexibility with delivering collaborative and creative curricula methodologies, as well making audit systems easier to manage. With greater WiFi access, online approaches are further relevant in terms of enabling doctors and students living and working in remote areas by providing more access to training and development opportunities.

The key elements of curriculum and their challenges are discussed below.

Learning outcomes

There are pros and cons to using learning outcomes. The way in which learning outcomes are used within curriculum design and assessment is discussed in ➋ Chapter 6, Assessment principles. One issue with learning outcomes is their congruence between curriculum designers, teachers, and learners. Hussey and Smith[17] state that learning outcomes are purported to be precise, as they require explicit statements that are linked to objective assessments. However, some aspects of education are not so easily observed and measured. For example, in the clinical learning environment, opportunistic learning occurs, which is likely to be unplanned, and thus may deviate from the intended learning outcomes of a particular clinical teaching session.

However, opportunistic learning in the clinical environment is incredibly valuable. Though clinical learning can be very structured, teaching sessions often make use of patients available on the day and at the time learners are present. One example of this is in the outpatient clinic which provides unique educational opportunities, such as management of chronic diseases, and allowing time for informed discussion between teacher and student.

As Hussey and Smith[17] state, ► good teachers welcome unique opportunities rather than sticking steadfastly to 'predetermined' learning outcomes. Nevertheless, in an ideal educational setting, clear outcomes are necessary to ensure that students can be assessed as having the appropriate knowledge, skills, and attitudes to graduate as doctors. Learning outcomes are also a useful benchmark for learners to check and review their own progress. At the same time, we can accept that students will engage in informal learning opportunities. With respect to the latter, we need to know that they are aware of what they are learning and how they are integrating knowledge gained in this way with knowledge gained through formal learning.

Formal and informal learning

Eraut[16] makes a distinction between **formal** and **informal** learning. Formal learning is more suited to the achievement of learning outcomes. It requires a prescribed learning agenda involving the use, and prior planning, of an organized learning session. It requires the presence of a teacher, or if conducted online it requires a learning structure. Credit is usually provided for completion of the task and there is often an explicit connection with external specialization or professional outcomes. In contrast, informal learning is a residual process that occurs outside formalized teaching and can involve opportunistic teaching and learning. In many cases, informal learning may be as impactful as formal learning, especially when learning to cope, adapt, and thrive in a clinical learning environment.

The hidden curriculum

The hidden curriculum occurs outside the formal curriculum. It involves the acquisition of values, attitudes, beliefs, and related behaviours that are considered important in medicine and concerns the replication of the culture of medicine.[1] The term *hidden curriculum* is often used interchangeably with the term *informal curriculum*, though the terms differ. Although both types of curricula are ad-hoc, the informal curriculum is learnt within unscripted interactions within teaching sessions or clinical education, whereas the hidden curriculum is communicated at the level of the organization, through cultural norms and ways of working.[1]

Through their immersion in the world of medicine, students receive various messages through the hidden curriculum. The hidden curriculum can be positive (for example, students might perceive a culture of kindness that in turn influences their own behaviour towards peers and patients or affirms some element of their professional identity in some way), or negative (there might be haphazard teaching suggesting a lack of educational prioritization, or institutional bias). There may also be messages communicated through the hidden curriculum that are open to students' interpretation and their impact—be that positive or negative (i.e. the importance of hierarchy and getting ahead by being competitive).

Despite the possibility for the hidden curriculum to communicate messages that are positively received, these may be antithetical to the ideas and values being learned in the clinical environment through an intense socialization process. Due to the conflicting values that medical students are exposed to outside of the formal curriculum, they may become confused by conflicting messages, they may internalize some of the values they are exposed to in the clinical settings, and their barometer regarding morality and ethical guidelines may become compromised.[1] One way ahead is to utilize the power of the hidden curriculum within teaching (confusing elements of the hidden curriculum may be discussed in supportive spaces), and to focus on studying how the positive facets of it work, rather than focusing only on the negative ones.

Content

Several issues are highlighted as challenges when considering the type and amount of content to be taught within a medical curriculum, whether this be at the undergraduate or postgraduate level. We begin this section by discussing issues related to the prioritization of content—ensuring that the amount and level of knowledge being taught to clinicians and students prepares or meets the needs of clinical environments and patients.

Prioritizing content is an integral part of the curriculum design process and auditing phases are required when establishing a course. One way to achieve this, is to determine the correct balance between what is needed to be taught and what students are able to optimally learn.[18] Content is one of the key elements of curriculum design and in the design of a curriculum it is crucial to define the content of the course and to align this with a blueprint of the assessment strategies that are in turn, aligned with certification or professional accreditation standards. ▶ It is also crucial to acknowledge the importance of defining teaching and learning approaches (constructive alignment) so that students can achieve the learning outcomes and fully integrate the content being disseminated. This means students' achievements can be assessed in line with the course's learning outcomes.

One way to plan the selection and use of content is to specify what is mandatory, versus what is optional. The decisions behind determining what content should be included in a curriculum relate to what are the essential aspects for each discipline or subject area, what is required for competent practice, and areas of study that can apply to different disciplines. Core elements need to be determined based on the importance of the topic and its relation to how key decisions are made, the prevalence of the problem being studied, and the transferability within medicine across subject areas.

❶ With the exponential increase in information seen in recent years within medicine, medical educators are faced with several problems. First, the defined boundaries of curriculum and time and the increasing amount of knowledge needing to be imparted. This is not an easy equation to solve. This may lead to students being taught information at a faster, more 'efficient', rate which leads to information overload. Second, the growing increase in information requires challenging decisions to be made regarding what should remain in the curriculum and what should be removed. Often those responsible for these decisions have their favourite areas of study that they may prioritize at the expense of other critical areas.[19]

∴ This leads to problems of defining the core curriculum versus deciding on the optional content matter. A further issue that has arisen relates to whether clinicians are adequately trained to meet the evolving needs of the clinical environment. Norman and colleagues[19] suggest that there is a gap between what learners perceive as being essential and the priority identified by educational bodies for continuing medical education. The authors recommend several methods for ensuring the requirements of knowledge and skills are maintained at acceptable levels. They suggest conducting periodic internal audits by using electronic office records, implementing audits through comparing practice with comparative current literature or practice guidelines, benchmarking with exemplary peers, and utilizing auditing tools developed by academic units for continuing medical education.

▶ *Cognitive Load Theory* is a concept that has great relevance for medical education.[20] For example, the design of simulations as an instructional tool can be enhanced if learning material is aligned with learners' cognitive capacity, especially in terms of optimizing their use of critical thinking skills. The proponents of this theory suggest that the brain utilizes complex memory systems, which involve aspects of information processing and decision-making, such as sensory, working memory (which can only process a limited number of information elements at any given time), and long-term memory.[20] Figure 12.2 displays the way in which Cognitive Load Theory hypothesizes that these memory systems are connected.

If the student is cognitively stretched, there is a risk that they may experience cognitive overload. Hence, the skill of the educator is to include the appropriate amount of content and to create tasks that extend the student but do not overload them, i.e. scaffolding students through a course or unit of study. Some methods for creating a balanced educational system and working within the constraints of cognitive load include maximizing the transfer of knowledge that is linked to the learning of essential knowledge and skills, and minimizing the transfer of non-essential information.

This type of deliberative learning requires that learning be designed including the explicit signposting of teaching and learning approaches. The

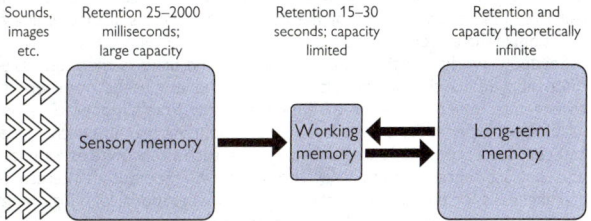

Fig. 12.2 The connections of sensory, working, and long-term memory in cognitive load theory.

explicit nature of the process activates cognitive strategies in learners to ensure the procurement of the essential aspects of medicine. The crucial and pragmatic intention is to guarantee greater patient safety. Some instructional techniques include:

- simple-to-complex sequencing of learning tasks based on authentic and real-life tasks
- eliminating extraneous material and stimuli (e.g. visual overload occurs when slides are busy and students don't have time to read them; students may find it more difficult to concentrate when a ward environment is noisy, or there are many interruptions)
- supporting students to develop 'schemata'—knowledge structures in their long-term memory (e.g. by teaching illness scripts such as the core characteristics of angina, and its management; or by using mnemonics) which help them to store and process information and reduce working memory load
- highlighting essential material
- promoting the learning process through corrective and immediate feedback; and
- providing opportunities for relevant and repetitive practice for selected aspects of a complete task.

For a comprehensive guide to instructional techniques that manage cognitive load, see ℘ Young, Van Merrienboer, Durning, and Ten Cate's Association for Medical Education (AMEE) guide on cognitive load theory.[20]

Educational strategies

Educational strategies are based on medical education theory and became popular on the basis of their perceived use and impact. The theories often used within medical education strategies include adult learning theory, work-based learning theories, and the theory of educational development. To discuss each one of these in depth would mean writing a textbook on each theory, hence we briefly point out the limitations associated with each approach.

Firstly, adult learning theory, as proposed by Knowles and others, describes the attributes of an idealized learner. The guidelines proposed by these theorists, such as Knowles' theory of andragogy, are thus useful as an ideal but need to be cautiously considered in line with contextual variables, e.g. many adult learners are motivated by extrinsic demands and values such as the need to make money or achieve learning credits. Adult learning theory suggests a difference between the way in which adults and children learn, a foundational premise of the theory that scholars are increasingly questioning the evidence of Kolb and Schön.[21]

Secondly, workplace theories, such as Kolb and Schön's theories,[21] are often applied to clinical workplace settings and are useful frameworks to engender reflection. Some of the criticisms of Kolb's model focus on its defined experiential categories and the confusing way in which these categories are positioned along polarizing axes, such as concrete experience and abstract conceptualization. ● Though Schön's theory is an interesting starting point for thinking about the praxis of organizational learning, there is a lack of empirical research to support the claims made.

Thirdly, one of the most often-cited developmental theories in medicine is the model of skill acquisition attributed to Dreyfus and Dreyfus.[22] According to this theory, learners develop through several learning stages. Using this framework, educationalists assume that students advance according to a linear developmental process and, therefore, education strategies are put in place to simulate this stage theory. This developmental model creates an intuitive notion of learning development but may not fully acknowledge the complexity of the learning process.[22] For example, clinical reasoning is a skill that is depicted in the model that develops over time, from a novice position to ideally an expert one. However, within a systems approach, experts not only differ from novices in terms of automaticity but also in terms of their deep understanding mapped onto a rich cognitive schema, which can be consciously or unconsciously accessed.[23] Clinical reasoning also requires a complex interplay between the implicit and explicit aspects of understanding. ▶ Thus, the reliance on intuitive aspects of decision-making implied in the Dreyfus' model needs to be considered with caution.[22]

❶ These limitations evidence the need to take the theories underpinning educational strategies not as positions of fact, but as perspectives and frameworks that need to be adapted to the educational workplace in question.

It can be useful to consider the purposes of medical education, as these can inform the educational strategies, and corresponding theories, selected for use in curriculum development. Some refocused educational principles that can be applied to medical education may include:

1. Medical education should be a continuous learning process, known as lifelong learning
2. Training and development initiatives should be based on identifiable needs with definable outcomes
3. Training and development should include aspects of process (e.g. clinical reasoning) as well as gains in content knowledge
4. Learning methods should be relevant and each method depends on the specified learning outcome (e.g. self-directed learning, computerized educational programmes, and hands-one learning)
5. Educational activities and content transfer should be driven by evidence-based practice
6. Inclusion of interdisciplinary education is crucial
7. Outcome-based approaches should be the driver behind the design of educational initiatives

Technology and learning

Synthesizing technology advances with learning theory is the way ahead, and a challenge, for clinical learning development initiatives. For example, Goodyear[23] makes reference to a more modern approach to the notion of educational design. The two core elements consist of:

1. Consideration of a 'pedagogical framework' and how this relates to the real-world setting
2. Addressing the educational setting which depicts the activities, processes, people, and artefacts involved in a learning activity

Both of these elements work within an organizational context, such as within a medical school. There is an inevitable exertion of influence from the organization that impacts the design and management of the educational setting and the way in which the pedagogical framework integrates with the educational context. Goodyear, thus, emphasizes the underlying philosophy of learning (how educators think people learn), a high-level pedagogy (a broad approach such as problem-based learning), a pedagogical strategy (e.g. online problems or an online debate) and pedagogical tactics (the detailed activities teachers engage in everyday (e.g. facilitation of problem solving or debates). This approach could easily be applied to the medical context, which embraces different philosophies of learning that are applied at different stages of learning (e.g. a first-year undergraduate as compared with a final-year student).

When theory is integrated with technology, it is crucial to develop and design pragmatic educational strategies to enhance learning. For example, use of technologies and an online interface often promote learning and accessibility. Nevertheless, they may present some challenges.

For example, Lazda-Cazers[24] designed a course utilizing a collaborative wiki, which was seen as highly educational, but several challenges emerged in the educational process. The challenges for learners were to learn a reasonable level of technological literacy and research skills so that they could inform and develop pertinent learning content. Some of these skills are not formally learned during a medical degree. Some of the challenges for both teachers and learners were linked to:

* designing and effectively using the wiki
* learning how to use the technology
* removing systems of teacher-centred teaching to more task-oriented teaching
* establishing agreed guidelines around group-based behaviour
* the creation of learning content, and
* developing and designing an equitable system of assessment of the diverse wiki entries

The shift from teacher-centred teaching to facilitating learning has been talked about, and deliberated on, for a long time and is key in removing systems of teacher-centred teaching to more task-oriented teaching.

Learning opportunities

The idea of learning opportunities is that the learning is not prescribed and formally planned. So, when opportunities occur, they are noticed and acted upon without preparation. As we have seen from previous discussion in this chapter, learning opportunities often occur in the clinical environment and may involve the use of patients who present with an interesting or instructive perspective or illness that can then be discussed between a teacher and student. To emphasize the learning gains from learning opportunities, teachers may need to use improvised teaching and learning practices, which can heighten individual attention levels. Learning gains and opportunistic learning within clinical environments are also integral to the development of students' professional identity, which is crafted through social interaction.

Eraut[16] has described the various levels of learning that could easily be applied to the learning that occurs within medicine. These levels propose a continuum from implicit learning to deliberative learning. Implicit learning occurs even when the learner has no conscious awareness that learning has taken place. This involves the acquisition of tacit knowledge—'we don't know why we know it, we just do'. In contrast, deliberative learning occurs when a specific time and place are set aside for learning to take place.

Between these two categories is reactive learning, which describes when learning occurs explicitly but also spontaneously. In reactive learning, the learner is aware that information transfer is operating but the learning situation is unplanned. This type of learning appears to be akin to the idea of learning opportunity. Learning opportunities can occur at any time during any teaching session, either a lecture, a small group learning session, or online such as on an e-learning discussion board. Once the problem is observed and noticed, a discussion can ensue.

Learning opportunities can present a challenge when prescribing learning outcomes.

❶ In addition, there are challenges associated with learning opportunities. If the learning opportunity is not fully explained, it may involve the inculcation of tacit knowledge rather than explicit knowledge, and this may create confusion as the acquired knowledge is not connected with deliberative knowledge. Eraut[16] suggests this may create problems when working with people in certain contexts, such as the development of unwarranted assumptions based on an atypical dataset or knowledge based on a one-off encounter with an atypical patient. Hence one of the major issues associated with learning opportunities is to put the knowledge into perspective and to create informed links with evidence-based reasoning and deliberative learning.

Assessment

Assessment is a vast subject on its own and is a crucial indicator for determining whether teaching and learning has effectively taken place. Assessment in medical education is essential, but ❶ there are numerous threats to the validity and reliability of existing assessments, especially those associated with workplace assessment, such as the perennial problem of assessor bias.

Consequently, one of the critical assessment challenges in the modern era of medicine is the measurement of competency. The increasing emphasis on competency based medical education (CBME) has highlighted the need to assess doctors and students so that they are able to cope with modern medical workplace environments. These environments are 'characterised by increasing interdependence among healthcare professionals, the recognition that patient safety is everyone's responsibility, and an expectation of transparency and accountability'.[25]

Lockyer and colleagues[25] assert that graduates need to be ready to provide safe, effective, patient-centred care. Therefore, assessments need to be multifaceted and comprehensive to assess all the key elements of training to ensure optimal practice is the most likely outcome.[25] Assessment of prescribed training is the first step to ensure competency-based medical education is achieved. To be meaningful and lifelong, Lockyer and colleagues stress the importance of the following ideas:

- Timely ongoing assessments with audit systems in place
- Use of multiple assessors, reliable rubrics, and assessments to ensure assessment processes are comprehensive and fit for purpose
- Data can be collected from various sources to ensure competence is present and active
- Faculty development needs to occur at all levels of the organization
- Formative feedback systems need to be in place for all key stakeholders
- Assessors need to be trained and assessments need to be evaluated and researched in reference to their psychometric properties for various settings and participants

One system that has been promoted to ensure assessments are inclusive of all factors involved in the training process is a programmatic approach to assessment.[26] The aims of a programmatic approach are to maximize learning from assessment, whilst also allowing educators to make robust decisions about learners' progress, which can inform high-stakes decisions regarding learners' competency. The key components of the model of programmatic assessment include consideration of the following:

1. *Learning activities* and tasks need to be aligned with the core principles of instructional and curriculum design. The compendium of tasks needs to be multidimensional in order to meet all the various stages and levels of learning development

2. The *assessment tasks* also need to be multidimensional and meaningful. The main idea is that a single data point will likely only provide a blurred vision of the learners' progress and competency. Data points in programmatic assessment and multiple, and assessment is usually carried out longitudinally. This is often difficult given that many assessments need numerous assessors to ensure the test is valid and reliable, such as when using the miniCEX

3. *Supporting activities* need to be factored into the model, such as guaranteeing opportunities for reflection based on feedback and other acquired assessment data which can inform the revision of existing, flawed tasks and the generation of new, valid learning tasks
4. At the end of each defined assessment stage or period *intermediate evaluation* processes need to be implemented. This is followed by the *final evaluation* of the learner's progress

Certain challenges with this model have been discussed,[26] although the benefits outweigh the limitations. The first challenge is the financial cost of implementing the process, although the cost of making a mistake about a learner's progress needs to be considered. The second challenge is to ensure that all the stakeholders are clear about their role in the programmatic systems to avoid making the process 'trivial' or 'ambiguous'. A third challenge is to convince traditional university systems that may favour unitary measures of achievement, such as course grades or credits, to change their approach. The last challenge is to convince managerial personnel that feedback can be sourced from all-inclusive assessment sources, which at times may require a willingness to consider subjective information and judgement, in addition to more traditional measures of competency.

Epstein and assessment

❶ As a final overview, Epstein[27] has listed several challenges in assessment in relation to medical education. The first relates to the assessment of new and evolving domains of medical education. These can include areas such as measuring effective teamwork in ensuring quality of care and patient safety. Although there are validated measures of effective teamwork, such as using observer-based ratings of teamwork skills, these assessment methods appear to have good reliability and validity with respect to only simulated or classroom settings. A recent systematic review[28] was designed to identify available assessments used to measure competencies of teams working in 'real-world' emergency care settings. The authors reported that the final 16 articles concentrated on areas of leadership, teamwork, communication, and situation awareness. However, only one article from the 16 had developed and reported substantive psychometric validation of information. Therefore, more research is required for the integration of well validated assessment instruments used in simulated environments and their applicability for assessment in 'real-world' clinical environments. i.e. assessing empathy and communication with regard to patient care.

Second, as we have discussed above, with the emergence of multiple methods of assessing competence and the emergence of programmatic assessment,[27] Epstein suggests that new ways are needed to integrate qualitative and quantitative methods of assessing competence. The development of portfolios within medical education has generated useful discussion concerning how to formulate valid measures of attainment, using effective benchmarking, comprehensive assessor discussion, and development of holistic scoring rubrics using global performance descriptors.

Third, Epstein considers the problem of standardization between medical schools within the US. The issue of standardization and maintaining high standards of quality medical education across institutions can be extended to the global stage. Assessment principles can be developed globally, through worldwide collaborations across medical schools, and must support the desired outcomes of medical education. These outcomes should consider the unique existing cultural contexts of each institution, and their local community.

Fourth, Epstein restates the mantra that 'assessment drives learning' but also makes the point that assessment can have intended and unintended consequences—it doesn't only drive learning, a more accurate mantra might be 'assessment influences learning', alongside other things. One of the challenges in medical education is to make sure that both the intended and unintended outcomes of assessment translate into greater competence. The unintended behaviours on the part of students that need to be avoided relate to cramming and superficial learning. A further area that is crucial is the unintended consequence of dishonesty and cheating, which can arise due to highly competitive and stressful learning environments, in which burnout may be an issue. Addressing and acknowledging quality-of-life issues is critical within medical education.

There are several ways organizations, educators, and individuals can prevent and address burnout. Interventions must be at the level of the organization (to enhance organizational resilience), as well as the level of the individual (to enhance personal resilience). Typically, interventions within medicine have focussed on personal resilience, at the expense of the critical role of organizations. Interventions across organizational and individual levels to address burnout and promote resilience include:

- organizational leadership in building a positive well-being culture, and promoting help-seeking behaviours
- organizational leadership in making changes and advocating for system-level improvements to the healthcare system including on issues pertaining to fair treatment of staff, and fair pay
- promoting academic support services
- support to develop stress management strategies
- recognizing threats to self-care and appreciating the need to maintain self-care
- encouraging a safe and supportive learning environment, where students are valued and respected, and
- addressing curriculum issues, such as overassessment

In the fifth challenge, Epstein explores the problems of assessing expertise especially when more than one answer can satisfy the question, suggesting that assessment of process may become more important than assessment of content. One clear issue relates to the assessment of clinical reasoning especially when there are high variability items (creating a lack of consensus between examiners), suggesting a more programmatic approach to assessment would be preferable. The assessment of clinical reasoning becomes more complex and blurred when considering the startling prevalence of medically unexplained symptoms and the difficulties in which this term is being addressed.

Epstein's last challenge raises the issue of assessments that predict future performance in the clinical environment. This is likely to be the Holy Grail of medical assessment but, like the Holy Grail, very difficult, if not impossible, to reach. As Epstein states,[27] ' ... robust measures of outcome that can be directly attributed to the effects of training have not been defined'.

➲ See Chapter 6: Assessment principles, and 7: Assessment techniques.

Educational environment

The term educational environment encapsulates some of the ideas presented above, and within the medical education context could be considered as the physical, educational, and social spaces in which learning occurs. Goodyear[23] perceives the educational setting as 'a way of representing the coming together of tasks, activities, environment and people'. Though the educational environment includes elements of the curriculum, it also transcends it, and can be seen more broadly as the ways in which physical and social settings (which may be part of a hospital, university, community, or small group teaching session) interact.

In medical education, the key goal is the optimization of the transfer of knowledge, skills, and attitudes to ensure quality patient care. From a systems approach, the educational setting therefore, needs to be of a manageable scale to ensure all components are working in a comprehensive, balanced, and fluid manner creating exemplary learning opportunities. The system needs to be designed and managed in a practical, authentic, and long-sighted manner. At times the setting may be artificial and constructed but in medicine there are unique opportunities to draw from and develop learning experiences from the clinical workplace. For example, moving to developing concordant strategies that aim to negotiate agreement between the healthcare professional and patient regarding their care and adherence to following a particular medication regimen; this empowers the patient rather than focusses on compliance, which is a more doctor-centric approach to patient care.

One of the major challenges when creating a learning space or environment is not to proffer mixed or confusing messages, such as teaching the importance of the community and health promotion when the hidden curriculum of an institution (e.g. through student timetabling, institutional leader comments and actions) suggests that student priority should be hospital practice, curative medicine, and research.

A further issue is deciding the best way to collect data about the clinical learning environment, so that student experiences can be explored and necessary improvements made. This is crucial given that medical students need to gain first-hand clinical knowledge and skills through working alongside expert clinicians and interacting with patients. There are two ways in which data on clinical learning environments may be collected.

1. Clinical learning environments can be explored using quantitative educational measures. Several measures are mentioned in the literature, for example:

   The Dundee Ready Education Environment Measure (DREEM), has been used in many contexts and adapted to different disciplines. In many cases, it is considered useful for finding out about students' experiences whilst on clinical rotations.

   The Johns Hopkins Learning Environment Scale has been developed and provides useful measures of students' perceptions of their community of peers, faculty relationships, academic climate, meaningful engagement, mentoring, inclusion and safety, and physical space.

   These measures are useful for developing a sense of the medical students' experiences whilst learning in the clinical environment, although more work is required to develop more culturally responsive instruments that can tap into students' experience in diverse clinical environments.

2. There is also a role for qualitative research in exploring the lived experience of medical students within clinical learning environments. Qualitative approaches (such as interviews and focus groups) can provide rich data about diversity in experiences, and the multidimensional influence of culture on the ways in which students interact with, and experience, healthcare environments.

Conclusions: Identifying and synthesizing the challenges

The ultimate aim of medical education is graduating competent health professionals who are ready to take their place in the profession. In accomplishing this goal, medical educators need to continue to address the major challenges in medical education, such as recruitment issues, pedagogical issues, and so forth. In this chapter, we have presented a structured approach to identifying and discussing many of these challenges. Clearly there are challenges in every element of the educational and clinical landscape. The key educational elements that need to be addressed include those related to:

- Providing pragmatic guidelines to signpost how professional development could be enacted within medical education, such as utilizing the UK GMC professional capabilities document
- Developing sophisticated and equitable recruitment and admission processes so that medical schools acquire the best students and teachers that are representative of the communities they serve
- Developing learning technology and integrating advancements in technology with the facilitation of learning
- Synthesizing patients, students, clinician teachers, and healthcare professionals in the learning process
- Exploring what is communicated through different types of curricula, such as the taught and hidden curricula
- Integrating, developing, and evaluating formal and informal learning strategies
- Developing a wide array of assessment procedures to assure the 'true' competency levels of students at all levels of the lifelong learning cycle
- Ensuring good research measures and a wide range of research methodologies are used to assess the quality of the learning environments
- Optimizing the transfer of knowledge, skills, and attitudes and being aware of cognitive load issues
- Addressing the overarching themes of medical education associated with societal, political, technological, and professional issues

References

1. Hafferty FW, Franks R. The hidden curriculum, ethics teaching, and the structure of medical education. *Acad Med* 1994;69(11):861–871.
2. Brice J, Corrigan O. The changing landscape of medical education in the UK. *Med Teach* 2010;32(9):727–732.
3. Pastorino R, De Vito C, Migliara G, Glocker K, Binenbaum I, Ricciardi W, Boccia S. Benefits and challenges of Big Data in healthcare: an overview of the European initiatives. *Eur J Public Health* 2019;29(Supplement_3):23–27.
4. Cohen JJ. Our compact with tomorrow's doctors. *Acad Med* 2002;77(6):475–480.
5. General Medical Council. Generic professional capabilities framework. 2017. https://www.gmc-uk.org/-/media/documents/generic-professional-capabilities-framework--0817_pdf-70417127.pdf.
6. Brown JVE, Crampton PES, Finn GM, et al. From the sticky floor to the glass ceiling and everything in between: a systematic review and qualitative study focusing on gender inequalities in clinical academic careers. Final report. Comm by: *NIHR Acad, Acad Med Sci, Cancer Res UK, Health Educ Eng, Med Res Coun, Wellcome Trust.* 2020. https://www.hyms.ac.uk/research/research-centres-and-groups/hpeu/gender-inequalities-in-clinical-academic-careers. https://doi.org/10.13140/RG.2.2.35907.32809.

7. Razack S, Hodges B, Steinert Y, Maguire M. Seeking inclusion in an exclusive process: discourses of medical school student selection. *Med Educ* 2015;49(1):36–47.
8. Rodríguez JE, Campbell KM, Mouratidis RW. Where are the rest of us? Improving representation of minority faculty in academic medicine. *South Med J* 2014;107(12):739–744.
9. Nguyen BM, Guh J, Freeman B. Black Lives Matter: moving from passion to action in academic medical institutions. *J Natl Med Assoc* 2022;114(2):193–198.
10. Mbaki Y, Todorova E, Hagan P. Diversifying the medical curriculum as part of the wider decolonising effort: A proposed framework and self-assessment resource toolbox. *Clin Teach* 2021;18(5):459–466.
11. Irby DM. What clinical teachers in medicine need to know. *Acad Med* 1994;69(5):333–342.
12. Dodds AE, Reid KJ, Conn JJ, Elliott SL, McColl GJ. Comparing the academic performance of graduate and undergraduate entry medical students. *Med Educ* 2010;44(2):197–204.
13. Feeley AM, Biggerstaff DL. Exam success at undergraduate and graduate-entry medical schools: is learning style or learning approach more important? A critical review exploring links between academic success, learning styles, and learning approaches among school-leaver entry ('traditional') and graduate-entry ('nontraditional') medical students. *Teach Learn Med* 2015;27(3):237–244.
14. Dahlstrom J, Dorai-Raj A, McGill D, Owen C, Tymms K, Watson DAR. What motivates senior clinicians to teach medical students? *BMC Med Educ* 2005;5(1):27.
15. Steinert Y, Mann K, Centeno A, et al. A systematic review of faculty development initiatives designed to improve teaching effectiveness in medical education: BEME Guide No. 8. *Med Teach* 2006;28(6):497–526.
16. Eraut M. Non-formal learning and tacit knowledge in professional work. *Br J Educ Psychol* 2000;70(1):113–136.
17. Hussey T, Smith P. The trouble with learning outcomes. *Act Learn High Educ* 2002;3(3):220–233.
18. Barman L, Bolander-Laksov K, Silén C. Policy enacted–teachers' approaches to an outcome-based framework for course design. *Teach High Educ* 2014;19(7):735–746.
19. Norman GR, Shannon SI, Marrin ML. The need for needs assessment in continuing medical education. *BMJ* 2004;328(7446):999–1001.
20. Young JQ, Van Merrienboer J, Durning S, Ten Cate O. Cognitive load theory: implications for medical education: AMEE Guide No. 86. *Med Teach* 2014;36(5):371–384.
21. Swanwick T. Understanding medical education. In: Swanwick T, Forrest K (Eds.), *Understanding medical education: evidence, theory, and practice* (pp. 1–6). Oxford: Wiley, 2018.
22. Peña A. The Dreyfus model of clinical problem-solving skills acquisition: a critical perspective. *Med Educ Online* 2010;15(1):4846.
23. Goodyear P. Educational design and networked learning: patterns, pattern languages and design practice. *Aust J Educ Technol* 2005;21(1):82–101.
24. Lazda-Cazers R. A course wiki: challenges in facilitating and assessing student-generated learning content for the humanities classroom. *J Gen Educ* 2010;59(4):193–222.
25. Lockyer J, Carraccio C, Chan M-K, et al. Core principles of assessment in competency-based medical education. *Med Teach* 2017;39(6):609–616.
26. van der Vleuten CPM, Schuwirth LWT, Driessen EW, et al. A model for programmatic assessment fit for purpose. *Med Teach* 2012;34(3):205–214.
27. Epstein RM. Assessment in medical education. *N Engl J Med* 2007;356(4):387–396.
28. Hosseini M, Heydari A, Reihani H, Kareshki H. Elements of teamwork in resuscitation: an integrative review. *Bull Emerg Trauma* 2022;10(3):95–102.

The future
of medical education

*Matthew H.V. Byrne, Megan E.L. Brown,
Helen R. Church, and Gabrielle M. Finn*

The future of medical education

Healthcare is evolving rapidly and necessitates changes in medical education. Medical education involves all health professionals for the entirety of their careers. As such the future of medical education involves everyone. Traditions can be firmly rooted, and change can be challenging, but as Abraham Lincoln said, 'the most reliable way to predict the future is to create it'.

Changing populations

As medical educators, we must be responsive to the needs of our partners in medical education. By this, we mean the requirements and the flourishing of healthcare students and patients.

Medical education is in the process of shifting practices to better meet the needs of students from a variety of backgrounds. Traditionally, medical education has been exclusive—reserved largely for a privileged few. Now, and moving forwards, widening access, participation, and success initiatives across medical schools are opening doors to those from minoritized backgrounds to study medicine and become doctors. These initiatives are important, as diversity within the healthcare workforce across many demographics and experiences improves the quality of care that patients receive.[1] Though the work done so far in this area is impressive and important, we are sure that most working within medical education would agree that further progress is required to enhance the inclusivity of medical education, and so graduate a workforce that is representative of the population it serves. Research and actions within medical education that challenge the systemic barriers that people who are minoritized (e.g. racialized people, disabled people, LGBTQIA+ people) face are critical to the advancement of equity within the field. ▶▶ Further, there needs to be a continued drive to educate all healthcare professionals on social inequality and its relationship to socio-political environments, and steps taken to empower healthcare professionals to draw on their privilege to advocate more actively for their colleagues and patients when they do witness inequality.

The patient population that healthcare professionals serve is also changing, which will have an impact on the format and delivery of medical education in the future. An ageing population with high levels of chronic disease and multimorbidity means that working in multi-professional teams to deliver coordinated, integrated care is essential. We anticipate that this will lead to an amplified need for interprofessional education that prepares medical students to work in diverse clinical teams and deliver complex, person-centred care. ▶ To date, interprofessional education is still not a widespread or integrated practice within many medical curricula[2]—a renewed emphasis on the criticality of this approach to evolving patient demographics globally is crucial in advancing the quality of medical education and patient care.

As the advent and progression of the COVID-19 and Mpox pandemics have demonstrated, medical education must be 'future proofed' for disaster or emergency situations within healthcare to prevent disruptions to healthcare training and service provision. We are likely to see an enhanced focus on novel diseases and pandemic preparedness in the future of medical education.[3] Alongside pandemic responses, personalized medicine is another emerging field that medical education will likely expand to encompass. Medical schools will need to adapt their curricula to incorporate the principles of personalized medicine such as genetic testing, genomic analysis, and precision medicine.[4] As will be described below, these principles will require medical students (and, by extension, educators) to become comfortable with the use of new technologies such as artificial intelligence and machine learning, and new skills such as data analysis and the interpretation of genetic information.

Curriculum

Modern medical education, and indeed societal expectations of such, present a number of major challenges when future proofing curricula. Firstly, the time available for medical education remains static, yet the content augments as the practice of medicine evolves. The coverage of the basic sciences, in particular anatomy, has been significantly reduced, often cited as a reason for subsequent surgical error within clinical practice.[5] Future medical education will face increased pressure to reform curricula, negotiating the tension between foundational sciences and the need to keep pace with technological and pharmacological advancements, as well as emerging diseases.

While presented with the challenge of ensuring a contemporaneous curriculum, the historical wrongs of colonialism much also be addressed. Future medical education must be decolonized, and inclusive. Inclusive curricula are those which are designed to improve the experience and attainment of all students including those in protected characteristic groups. Within the sphere of medical education, inclusivity can be all encompassing in that it can be inclusive of diverse learners and their needs, but also the diversity of the future patients that they will serve. Within increases in global migration, and the resulting healthcare issues that this presents, the need for curricula to evolve will be magnified. The changing needs of the global population have outpaced the lexicon of medical education. For example, sex, sexuality, and gender are given little space for exploration within the curriculum.[6] ▶ Medical education of the future needs to be more considered with respect to diversity of imagery, resources, and language. Examples of this include the spectrum of gender, or racial diversity.[7]

Societal expectations are not limited to the cognitive knowledge acquired during medical education, but also extend to holding medical educators to account with global initiatives such as sustainability and green curricula. This encompasses what we teach, how we teach, and what we use to teach. Many institutions are making marvellous strides forwards in their reduction of the use of disposable plastics, for example, within their laboratory teaching sessions by instead utilizing glass and ensuring recycling efforts are maximized. One can imagine that there will be more enforced metrics to manage performance and reward institutions with respect to green initiatives in the not-too-distant future.

The content of an evolving curriculum is not the only consideration, how we teach is of equal importance. Medical education is going back to its roots, with increasing use of apprenticeship-based models of curriculum delivery. This is either through literal apprenticeship-based programmes, such as those being implemented within the UK, or longitudinal clerkships.

Curricula structural changes should be underpinned by further evolution in pedagogy, for example a focus on individual learning, medical humanities, educating for empathy, holistic approaches to reflection, interprofessional education, or technological pedagogy such as simulation and virtual reality. Integrating meaningful pedagogy within curricular, while simultaneously balancing preparedness for practice, and for new assessments such as the impending medical licencing assessment (MLA) in the UK,[8] are at the forefront of educators' minds as they navigate the changing landscape of medical education. It is important to consider critically whether, prior to/during/following implementation, models of curriculum delivery are faithful to the educational theory and principles supporting their benefit. Divorcing curriculum delivery models from their evidence-base is inefficient, ineffective, and unsustainable.

Healthcare systems

While our research colleagues in health sciences and pharmaceuticals are developing the latest cutting-edge advancements in medical science, these are redundant unless there are adequate numbers of highly skilled healthcare professionals to deliver this care. Similarly, these advances aim to prolong and/or improve quality of life; thus, also contributing to the increasing, and ageing, population. While efforts have been made to expand medical school places to train more doctors, these long-term plans are no quick fix. The development of new allied health professional roles, such as the Physician Associate, which has been utilized to good effect in many other countries, have become increasingly popular in the UK in the past 10 years. These initiatives have not escaped scrutiny. Blurring of roles, confusing acronyms, and diluting learning opportunities for resident doctors have all been criticisms of the development of new professions ●

The number of locally employed doctors has increased dramatically over the past five years, choosing alternative career pathways to the traditional Completion of Training route to become a Consultant, or simply taking time out of training.[10] Currently, however, this is not an option for those who wish to work as General Practitioners (GP) where doctors who have not completed, or are currently enrolled in, a formal GP training programme cannot work as GPs.[11] It seems inevitable that the restrictions on non-GP specialists to work in general practice will be lifted and could represent a turning point in restoring the GP workforce to better serve patients in the community.

On the horizon too is the implementation of medical student 'apprenticeship' programmes in the UK. Reportedly to build on efforts in widening participation, and a key component of the Long Term Workforce Plan, students will enter their undergraduate training as apprentices—simultaneously studying and working throughout their degree. There are still lots of unanswered questions about the initiative, and the medical education community awaits its implementation and progression with bated breath. ● Will the clinically situated learning experiences afforded within the 'service provision' aspect of the apprenticeship enhance students' professional development, or will this erode the more traditional 'academic' side of a medical degree.

Much has been made of physician mental health in recent years, in no small effect due to the fallout of the COVID-19 pandemic. Increased rates of intention to leave the profession, as well more serious consequences of burnout, including self-harm and even suicide have been attributed not only to relentless working patterns but also to the toxic working environment in which bullying, sexism, and racism still exist.[12] ▶▶ The retention of the workforce relies upon initiatives to prioritize readiness for practice at undergraduate level, and initiatives to promote well-being throughout the career of the health professional. Awareness of this during undergraduate training is slowly but surely being integrated into the curriculum, and these sentiments are being echoed in the post-graduate training schemes through use of resident doctor forums and home-grown initiatives. Nationally, working patterns being reduced to 4 days a week (80% of full time) is being piloted in areas across the UK for foundation doctors, and the option to train less-than-full-time became available to doctors purely for personal choice (rather than due to a prescribed list of limited options which mainly included carer/childcare duties) was introduced in 2021.

While there are changes afoot in the workforce of the NHS, no one can predict the potential future of the NHS within the UK. Chronic underfunding and the additional strain of COVID-19 have left devastating effects on waiting times for referrals, surgical delays, and difficulty with accessing doctors in both primary and secondary care. While many hope that the NHS will continue to recover and thrive, equally there is a question over its longevity—in which case, the training and practice of our future workforce is likely to change unrecognizably ●

New technologies

New technologies are exciting and offer the prospect of transforming learning. In particular, new technologies can make learning more efficient—something that is becoming increasingly important as the volume of knowledge increases. However, new technologies are seldom a 'quick fix' and often require a large amount of work to implement successfully and to subsequently assess their effectiveness.

Simulation and virtual reality will become more common as it continues to become more realistic and provide more detailed feedback. This will allow learners to practice within a safe environment, reduce risk to patients, encounter rare conditions, and reduce the cost of consumables.[13] Instead of the outdated adage: see one, do one, teach one; we will simulate many first.

New technologies also influence the delivery of healthcare. For example, within the span of a surgeon's career, open surgery has evolved to laparoscopic surgery, and subsequently to robot-assisted surgery. The education delivered to learners needs to reflect changes in clinical practice. Healthcare systems will become increasingly digitalized and now we are seeing the advent of genomic medicine, big data, and artificial intelligence.[13] Sequencing of the first human genome in 2003 was a pivotal moment in medicine. Since then, we have seen increasing consideration given to precision medicine. While genetic sequencing was initially prohibitively expensive, its price has now decreased to the point where its use in clinical practice is feasible. Soon we may see widespread adoption of genetic testing to inform personalized risk stratification and management plans for many conditions. Similarly, big data has become increasingly common within healthcare, as hundreds of thousands of data points can be collected during a patient's interactions with a healthcare provider. This data can be used to help identify conditions, interpret investigations, and inform decision-making. However, the advent of these technologies brings their own sets of challenges. This data is often complex and heterogeneous between patients, and as a consequence it is difficult to interpret. Currently, we do not know yet whether all clinicians will need to learn these skills, or if the skills will be siloed among highly specialized clinicians that require unique training pathways. Artificial intelligence may assist practitioners in interpreting increasingly large volumes of data. These technologies could develop to the point where minimal understanding of the systems is needed, and users simply ask the programme to generate recommendations.

Artificial intelligence in education also presents its own issues. ChatGPT is an artificial intelligence chatbot that has passed a wide range of university and postgraduate level examinations. These programmes can be used to personalize learning and improve critical thinking. ▶ However, there are concerns that these programmes may generate incorrect information and be used to cheat in examinations. As such, there have been subsequent bans on their use from some institutions, and debates whether this constitutes cheating or plagiarism.[14]

COVID-19 transformed the delivery of education. Pandemic lockdowns mandated a transition to online remote learning facilitated by videoconferencing technologies. Similarly, in place of face-to-face clinical appointments, healthcare providers pivoted to telephone and video consultations—with many of these clinical changes remaining after COVID-19. While students value face-to-face interactions and practical hands-on experiences, this change has challenged us to reflect on prior teaching styles and re-invent educational techniques. Much of the curriculum has already been translated into an online format, and as a consequence we may see increased use of hybrid curricula going forward. This could result in increased flexibility in learning and more efficient knowledge acquisition,[15] and could better prepare learners for remote practice in the future.

Social media is used by nearly all students and health professionals. It can be a tool that can improve communication between students and educators and improve short-term retention of information. However, its influence on long term knowledge remains unclear. As the use of social media in education is likely going to continue to increase, more robust guidance and research methodologies are needed to understand its impact.[16]

Collaboration

While knowledge and clinical reasoning may be supplemented by artificial intelligence programmes, the humanistic elements of patient care will remain.[13] Greater collaboration with patients may arise as less time is required for administrative tasks, this could lead to deeper relationships with patients. Consequently, we may see a shift towards increased communications and empathy training.[13]

As previously discussed, we will also see increased interdisciplinary team learning. Increased collaboration with multi-disciplinary colleagues will provide a better understanding of role awareness, challenges different professions face, and understand of how multi-disciplinary approaches can lead to better holistic patient care.[13]

As well as collaboration with colleagues we will see greater collaboration across institutions. Globalization of medical education will mean that these collaborations can occur at institutions in geographically separate locations, thus increasing the scope of opportunities available and revealing exciting new partnerships. Funding opportunities are decreasing, and increased collaboration will mean that institutions can deliver high-impact activities on a larger scale.[17]

As the use of online educational platforms and social media expand, we will see further growth of free open-access medicine. This will help to increase the number of learning opportunities available and reduce the monetary burden on students who are graduating with increasing debts.

Within educational research, we will see increased collaboration with fields outside of medical education. For example, collaborations with philosophers, or the use of theories from other fields. These interdisciplinary collaborations will provide novel insights, greater depth of understanding, and faster evolution of the field.[18]

References

1. Jackson CS, Gracia JN. Addressing health and health-care disparities: the role of a diverse workforce and the social determinants of health. *Public Health Rep* 2014;129(Suppl 2):57–61.
2. Herath C, Zhou Y, Gan Y, Nakandawire N, Gong Y, Lu Z. A comparative study of interprofessional education in global health care: a systematic review. *Medicine (Baltimore)* 2017;96(38):e7336.
3. Ashcroft J, Byrne MHV, Brennan PA, Davies RJ, Davies RJ. Preparing medical students for a pandemic: a systematic review of student disaster training programmes. *Postgrad Med J* 2020;0:1–12.
4. Matuchansky C. The promise of personalised medicine. *Lancet* 2015;386(9995):742.
5. Kumar R, Singh R. Model pedagogy of human anatomy in medical education. *Surg Radiol Anat* 2020;42(3):355–365.
6. Finn GM, Ballard W, Politis M, Brown ME. It's not alphabet soup—supporting the inclusion of inclusive queer curricula in medical education. *Br Stud Dr J* 2021;5(2):27.
7. Finn GM, Danquah A, Matthan J. Colonization, cadavers, and color: considering decolonization of anatomy curricula. *Anat Rec* 2022;305(4):938–951.
8. Hateley P. A new national exam for medical students. *BMJ* 2015;351:h4208.
9. Roberts S, Howarth S, Millott H, Stroud L. Experience of the impact of physician associates on postgraduate medical training: a mixed methods exploratory study. *Clin Med (Lond)* 2019;19(1):4–10.
10. Church HR, Agius SJ. The F3 phenomenon: early-career training breaks in medical training. A scoping review. *Med Educ* 2021;55(9):1033–1046.
11. Waters A. Let SAS doctors work in general practice, says GMC. *BMJ* 2022;379:o2505.
12. Oliver D. David Oliver: No wonder training grade doctors are unhappy. *BMJ* 2022;378:o2245.
13. Han ER, Yeo S, Kim MJ, Lee YH, Park KH, Roh H. Medical education trends for future physicians in the era of advanced technology and artificial intelligence: an integrative review. *BMC Med Educ* 2019;19:460.
14. Sallam M. ChatGPT utility in healthcare education, research, and practice: systematic review on the promising perspectives and valid concerns. *Healthcare (Basel)* 2023;11(6):887.
15. Khamees D, Peterson W, Patricio M, et al. Remote learning developments in postgraduate medical education in response to the COVID-19 pandemic—a BEME systematic review: BEME Guide No. 71. *Med Teach* 2022;44(5):466–485.
16. Guckian J, Utukuri M, Asif A, et al. Social media in undergraduate medical education: a systematic review. *Med Educ* 2021;55(11):1227–1241.
17. Lundy K, Ladd H. Why collaboration is key to the future of higher education. 2020. https://www.ey.com/en_gl/strategy/strategies-for-collaborating-in-a-new-era-for-higher-education
18. Albert M, Rowland P, Friesen F, Laberge S. Interdisciplinarity in medical education research: myth and reality. *Adv Health Sci Educ Theory Pract* 2020;25(5):1243–1253.

Index

For the benefit of digital users, indexed terms that span two pages (e.g., 52–53) may, on occasion, appear on only one of those pages.

Tables, figures, and boxes are indicated by an italic *t* , *f* , and *b* following the page/paragraph number.